Thoracic Ultrasound and Integrated Imaging

Francesco Feletti
Bruna Malta • Andrea Aliverti
Editors

Thoracic Ultrasound and Integrated Imaging

EXTREMESPORTMED
SOCIETY OF OUTDOOR SPORTS & PERFORMANCE MEDICINE

Springer

Editors
Francesco Feletti
Dipartimento di Diagnostica per Immagini
Ausl della Romagna, Ospedale S. Maria delle Croci
Ravenna
Italy

Dipartimento di Elettronica
Informazione e Bioingegneria
Politecnico di Milano
Milan
Italy

Andrea Aliverti
Dipartimento di Elettronica
Informazione e Bioingegneria
Politecnico di Milano
Milan
Italy

Bruna Malta
Dipartimento di Diagnostica per Immagini
Ausl di Ferrara
Ospedale Universitario di Ferrara
Ferrara
Italy

This project has benefited from the support of the international association **EXTREME**SPORT**MED**

ISBN 978-3-319-93054-1 ISBN 978-3-319-93055-8 (eBook)
https://doi.org/10.1007/978-3-319-93055-8

This Springer imprint is published by the registered company Springer Nature Switzerland AG
The registered company address is: Gewerbestrasse 11, 6330 Cham, Switzerland

Preface

Thoracic ultrasound provides critical diagnostic information in many conditions and situations, which can contribute to a correct diagnosis or therapeutic approach.

Thanks to portable and handheld ultrasound systems, thoracic ultrasound is now available not only at the patient's bedside but also outside healthcare facilities and even in wild and remote locations.

Today the method is part of any physician's primary diagnostic resources and doctors must be aware of its role, possibilities and limitations.

This volume collects the contributions of some of the most distingushed experts in this imaging technique, inevitably presenting different points of view due to the different kinds of training and experience of the authors.

Specific attention is paid to the principles governing the formation of images and the role of artefacts which are particularly important aspects in chest sonography because of the abundance of reflective and eco-impermeable elements like air and bone in this area.

Specific chapters are dedicated to thoracic ultrasound applications in neonatology, pediatrics, and emergency medicine as well as guided procedures and diaphragm function studies.

In many cases, the imaging findings are presented together with relevant clinical information and images provided by other imaging methods in order to highlight the role of thoracic ultrasound.

This integrated approach provides medical practitioners with essential know-how for using thoracic ultrasound as an extension of their physical examinations.

Ravenna, Italy — Francesco Feletti
Ferrara, Italy — Bruna Malta
Milan, Italy — Andrea Aliverti

Contents

Part I

Technique

Physical Principles and Image Creation

1

Francesco Feletti, Bruna Malta, and Andrea Aliverti

1.1 Introduction

Ultrasound images derive from the interaction between ultrasounds and anatomical structures. Ultrasounds are sound waves with frequencies superior to 20 kHz, i.e. higher than the frequency audible by the human ear.

In order to correctly read an ultrasonic image, it is necessary to understand how the ultrasounds interact with biological tissues and how the ultrasound constructs the image. In particular, when studying the thorax, due to pulmonary air and the bones of the ribcage which both alter the propagation of ultrasounds, a perfect reading of both real and artefactual images is indispensable.

In thoracic ultrasound (TUS), the highest frequencies, i.e. those between 5 and 15 MHz, are reserved for the structures of the chest wall, while lower frequencies, i.e. those between 3.5 and 5 MHz, are generally used for exploring the pleura, lungs and mediastinal structures.

1.2 B-Mode

1.2.1 Transducer Frequencies in Thoracic Ultrasound

Ultrasounds are longitudinal mechanical waves; that is to say, they consist of periodic compressions and rarefactions of the medium.

The wavelength (λ) is inversely related to the frequency (η), i.e.

$$\lambda = V / \eta$$

Ultrasounds propagate (Fig. 1.1) with slightly different velocities in biological tissues; however, the ultrasound scanner assumes a standard value of 1540 m/s in all the intervals of the frequencies used in order to render the anatomic image.

In order to improve sonographic signals originating from structures of a small dimension, it is necessary to reduce the dimensions of the wavelength and therefore increase the insonation frequency.

However, in crossing tissues, the ultrasonic beam is gradually attenuated as a consequence of

F. Feletti (✉)
Dipartimento di Diagnostica per Immagini, Ausl della Romagna, Ospedale S. Maria delle Croci, Ravenna, Italy

Dipartimento di Elettronica, Informazione e Bioingegneria, Politecnico di Milano, Milan, Italy
e-mail: francesco.feletti@auslromagna.it

B. Malta
Dipartimento di Diagnostica per Immagini, Ausl di Ferrara, Ospedale Universitario di Ferrara, Ferrara, Italy
e-mail: mltbrn@unife.it

A. Aliverti
Dipartimento di Elettronica, Informazione e Bioingegneria, Politecnico di Milano, Milan, Italy
e-mail: andrea.aliverti@polimi.it

F. Feletti et al. (eds.), *Thoracic Ultrasound and Integrated Imaging*,
https://doi.org/10.1007/978-3-319-93055-8_1

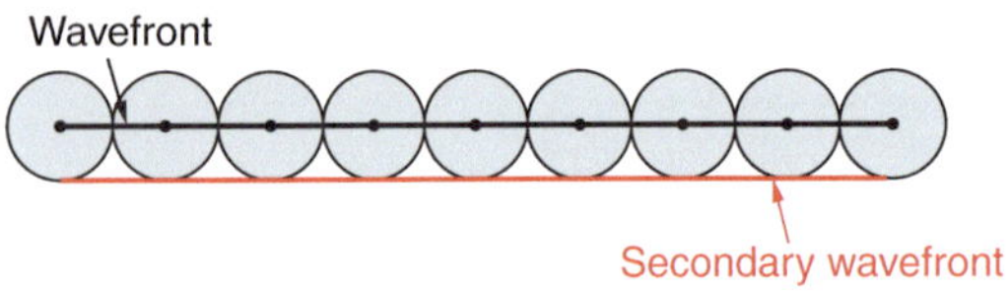

Fig. 1.1 The propagation of ultrasounds. According to the Huygens principle, a wavefront can be broken down into point sources of spherical waves in phase with one another. The wavefront in subsequent moments is given by the superimposition of secondary spherical waves and is represented by their tangents

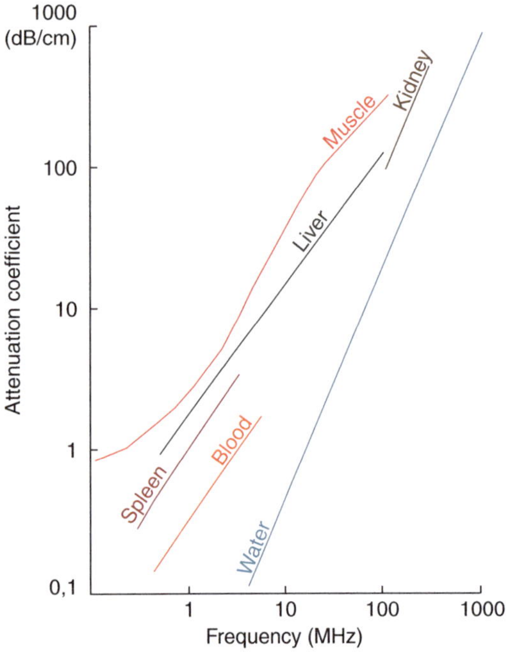

Fig. 1.2 The relation between attenuation coefficient and frequency. In all tissues, attenuation increases very rapidly when increasing the frequency, and this limits the resolution in the sonographic representation of deeper structures. (Figure adapted from Valli and Coppini [1])

the transformation of acoustic energy into thermic energy, and the attenuation depends on the frequency. In particular, the attenuation is quantified in 1–2 dB/cm/MHz; therefore, the higher the frequency of the ultrasound, the lesser the capacity that they have to penetrate (Fig. 1.2).

The dependence of attenuation on frequency limits the resolution of deep structures in sonography.

In TUS, the use of frequencies in the range between 1 and 20 MHz allows for an anatomic detail to the millimetre.

In fact, for $\eta = 1$ MHz, we have $\lambda = 1.5$ mm; for $\eta = 20$ MHz, we have $\lambda = 0.077$ mm.

In TUS, higher frequency bands, i.e. bands between 5 and 15 MHz, are used for the structures of the chest wall or are reserved for small children [2], while lower frequencies, between 3.5 and 5 MHz, are generally used to explore the pleura, lungs, and mediastinal structures.

1.2.2 Image Creation

In TUS, the transducer emits ultrasounds through the piezoelectric effect as a result of electrical pulse agitation and, alternatively, acts as an ultrasonic generator and receiver [3].

The emission of ultrasounds comes in the form of brief sets and is repeated with a periodic cadence according to the pulse repetition frequency (PRF) spaced out by rest periods when the sonogram receives the tissue signals and elaborates them (Fig. 1.3) [4].

Generally, the emission phase lasts about one-hundredth of the listening phase.

Ultrasounds are emitted by the sonogram in the form of opportunely focused beams and are propagated in tissues and interact with them in a way similar to a ray of light, i.e. they are reflected, refracted, diffused, and partially attenuated [4, 5].

In particular, most of the sonographic image is formed by the echoes produced through being reflected by the contacting surfaces between tissues with different acoustic impedance, which are represented on the sonographic monitor as light signals.

When ultrasound beams meet an anatomical surface, part of them are reflected. They cease to be part of the original beam and constitute a new one that travels in different directions [6].

If the insonated surface is perpendicular to the incident beam, the reflected beam returns to the transducer to be represented, while the part of the beam that is not reflected continues to move deeper, interacting with other anatomical structures.

The successive reflections progressively attenuate the beam while, in the reception phase, the

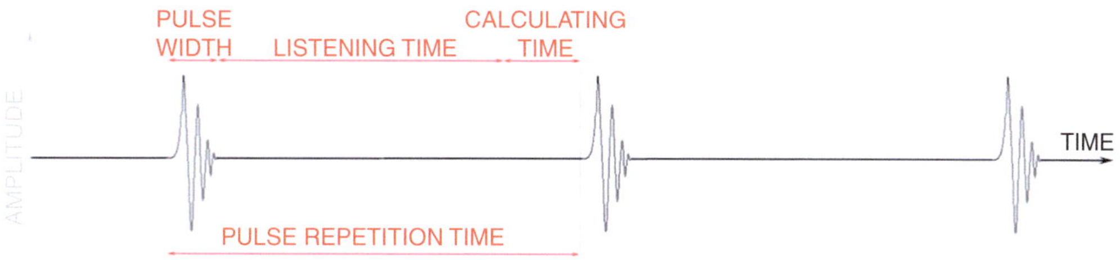

Fig. 1.3 This graphic demonstrates and simplifies the electrical signals that the central processing unit sends to the transducer in order to generate ultrasound beams. The pulse repetition time, listening time, and calculating time are represented

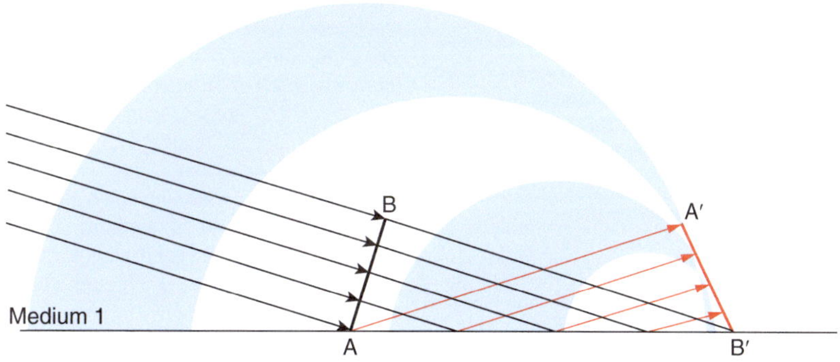

Fig. 1.4 Huygens principle applied to reflection explains why the angle of incidence and the angle of reflection are equal. Since the wavefront is perpendicular to the radius, triangles *ABB* and *AAB′* are right-angled; moreover, they are congruent, having a common hypotenuse and having the same velocity of wave propagation as medium 1. Thus, the angle of incidence of *BAB* is equal to the angle of reflection *ABA*. (Figure adapted from Violino and Robutti [7])

transducer is struck by a succession of echoes produced by the interfaces found at further distances from the transducer.

The vibration created in the transducer by the echoes generates successive electrical signals that are represented on the monitor as points of light with an intensity proportional to the entity of the echo received.

The depth of the image is estimated taking into account the time passed between the emission of the ultrasounds and the reception of the signals (time of flight).

1.2.3 Reflection

Reflection is the physical phenomenon that presides over the creation of sonographic signals.

Reflection depends both on the difference of the acoustic impedance at the interface and on the angle of insonation.

Acoustic impedance is a measure of the resistance that every medium opposes to the passage of ultrasounds.

The higher the difference of acoustic impedance between the two mediums, the higher the intensity of the sonographic signals while the lesser the difference, the further the penetration of the beam in depth.

For every surface of separation between the two mediums, the reflection is highest if the beam strikes perpendicularly. However, if the incidence arrives obliquely, the beam is partially reflected and partially refracted.

The angle of reflection is equal to the angle of incidence (Fig. 1.4); refraction will be described later.

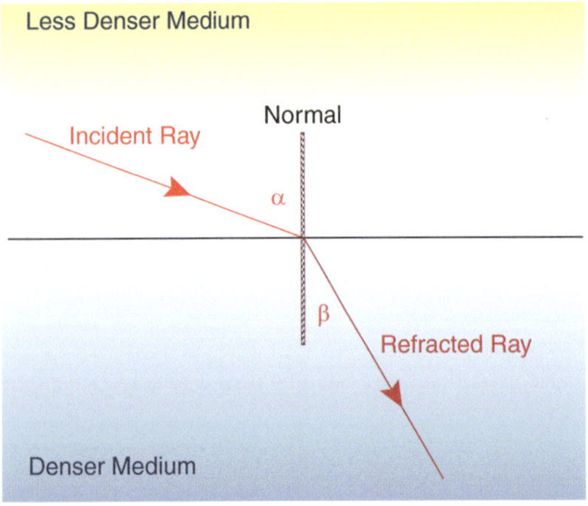

Fig. 1.5 According to Snell's law, the relation between the sine of the angle of refraction (β) and the sine of the angle of incidence (α) is equal to the relation between the propagation velocity of the wave in the two mediums: $\sin\beta/\sin\alpha = V2/V1$. The angle of incidence and refraction are the angles included between the wavefront and the interface before and after the refraction

1.2.4 Refraction

When ultrasounds enter into a medium with different acoustic impedance, not only does the velocity change but so do the direction, the ray, and the wavefront: that is to say the refraction of the wave that takes place (Figs. 1.5 and 1.6).

For every interface, a critical angle of insonation beyond which the refracted sound runs along with the interface and is not transmitted: this phenomenon is involved in the generation of lateral acoustic shadows, described in Chap. 2.

1.2.5 Angle of Insonation

Anatomical surfaces are almost all curved; thus, the ultrasound beam obliquely strikes most of them. Consequently, the echoes produced by reflection are of moderate-intensity, while posterior attenuation is contained. Furthermore, only a fraction of the ultrasounds reflected by inclined or curved surfaces is intercepted by the transducer during the reception, while a large part of the beam reflected ends up outside of the transducer, and energy is lost (Fig. 1.7a–c).

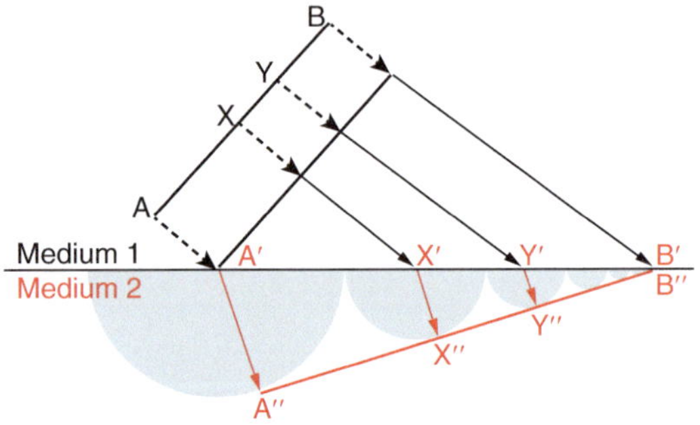

Fig. 1.6 Description of refraction according to Huygens principle. *AB* is the initial wavefront, while *x* and *y* are two of the points located along with it; every point of the wavefront can be considered as a centre wave point. The wave reaches the interface in point A' at time $t = 1$ and strikes the interface in points x', y', and B' in successive moments. Each of these points later generates new spherical waves that propagate in medium 2 with a velocity that's different with respect to medium 1. In particular, at time $t = 2$, the spherical wave generated in A' has already reached point A'', while the wave generated in B' has just started to propagate in medium 2. Consequently, the wavefront $A''B''$ is deviated with respect to the direction of the wave in medium 1. (Figure adapted from Violino and Robutti [7])

The angle of insonation plays a role in the reduction of intensity and sensibility.

Therefore, when the incidence of the beam is oblique, increasing distance reduces the detail and definition of the image.

At the same time, however, the visualization of the posterior structures can be improved by obliquely insinuating a specular surface because reflection is reduced. Anyhow, inclination results in refraction phenomena and can determine artefacts, as described in Chap. 2.

1.2.6 Scattering

Scattering happens when the beam encounters particles with dimensions that are comparable to the wavelength of ultrasounds and consists in a series of physical interactions that provoke the interspersion of ultrasounds in all directions.

Scattering contributes significantly to the attenuation of the beam and is generally more notable in tissues with abundant connective or cellular components [8].

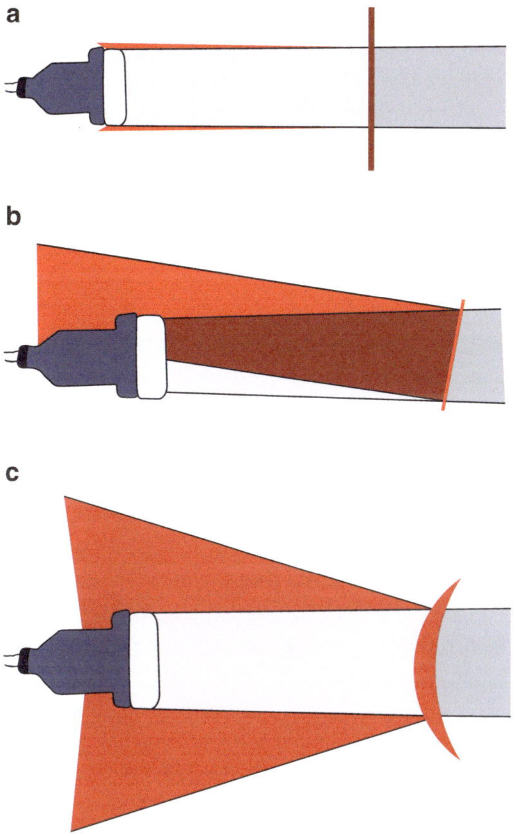

Fig. 1.7 (**a**–**c**) Reflected signals have maximum intensity when a hyper-reflective surface is insonated perpendicularly (**a**). If the explored structure has an inclined (**b**) or convex (**c**) surface, reflected ultrasounds are only partially intercepted by the transducer, and the sonographic signals have a reduced intensity

1.2.7 Diffuse Reflection

Diffuse reflection is a phenomenon of interspersion in which the diffusers are aligned along a surface.

The small irregularities with dimensions that are comparable to the wavelength of the beam reflect ultrasounds in different directions and send reflected signals back to the transducer at significantly wide angles of incidence (Fig. 1.8).

Since the surfaces of anatomical separation are prevalently curved and are rarely reached by the beam perpendicularly, diffuse reflection brings a fundamental contribution to the creation of sonographic images, which otherwise would be limited to a few reflections coming from specular surfaces that are perpendicularly insonated.

In conclusion, the angle of insonation changes the images produced by specular reflection but does not significantly influence signals produced by diffuse reflection.

It follows that, in order to visualize a specular reflection, for example, a smooth septum inside a cystic mass, it must be insonated perpendicularly, while the angle of incidence of the beam does not influence the visualization of small vegetations with irregular profiles that act as diffusers.

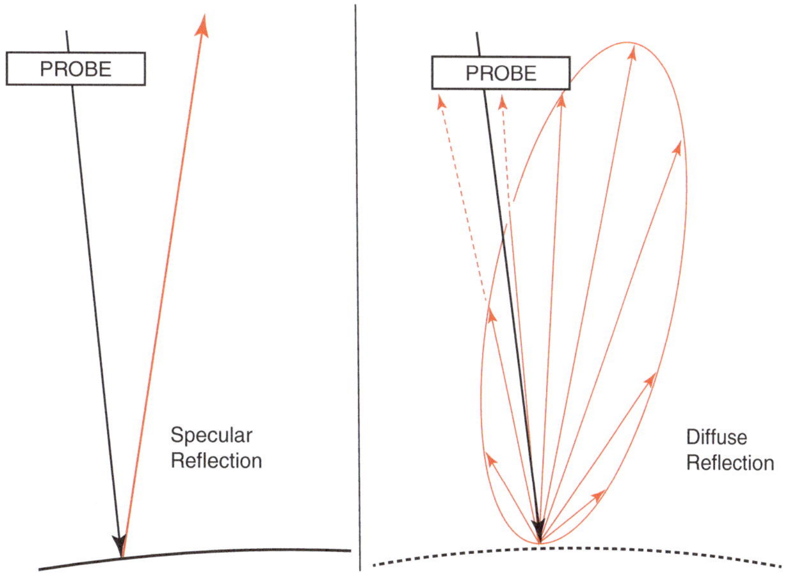

Fig. 1.8 Unlike specular reflection, diffuse reflection allows the probe to receive signals reflected by a much wider angle of incidences

1.3 Doppler Applications

1.3.1 The Doppler effect

The Doppler effect, used in sonography to study blood flow and similar, consists in the frequency variation of a wave perceived by an observer when they are moving toward or away from the source.

The frequency varies in a way that is directly proportional way to the velocity and increases if the movement is approaching, while it is reduced when moving away.

The Doppler effect is double in sonography, in that the Doppler effect is the sum of the transducer and red blood cells during the insonation phase and the red blood cells and the transducer during the reception.

The Doppler signal is the frequency difference between the signal emitted and received by the ultrasound probe.

$$D = 2 \times f \times v \times \cos\alpha$$

- *D*—Doppler signal
- *f*—insonation signal
- *v*—absolute value of the blood/velocity of the ultrasound
- *α*—the angle of insonation between the axis of the beam and the direction of the blood

Given the order of magnitude of the blood velocity (m/s) and the frequencies used in ultrasound (MHz), the values of Doppler signals fall into the range of audible sound (kHz), and they can, therefore, be heard.

The sound evokes the sense of speed since the sound is low if the velocity is low and acute if the velocity is high.

The operator must know how to correctly position and manoeuvre the probe.

If the vessel is perpendicularly insonated (angle $\alpha = 90°$; $\cos \alpha = 0$), the Doppler effect is null, and no flow signal is represented in the spectrum or colour box.

The Doppler effect's dependency on the cosine of the angle of insonation makes it necessary to insonate the vessel with angles as close to 0° as possible; however, for anatomical reasons, this is often impossible, and, for quantitative evaluations, angles under 60° are considered acceptable.

Furthermore, since under 30° the movement of the vessel walls can interfere with measurements, leading to an underestimated signal, the optimal angle for the study is between 30° and 60°.

1.3.2 Continuous Wave Doppler

In continuous-wave Doppler, two distinct transducers are used, one that emits ultrasounds and another that receives the signal. The Doppler signals represent the average of all the flows encountered in the exploring beam along its path, and the spatial data is missing.

Information regarding the angle of insonation is also lacking, so this approach only allows for a qualitative study.

1.3.3 Pulse Wave Doppler

In pulse wave Doppler, the same probe used for creating grayscale B-mode images is used, generating and receiving ultrasound groups dedicated to studying Doppler signals.

The time that passes between the emission of ultrasounds and the reception of Doppler signals allows for depth to be established.

Thus, pulse wave Doppler can overlap, on the grayscale image, a sample volume where measurements (i.e. Doppler spectrum, flow velocity, and the resistance of the vessels) can be sampled or a *colour box* representing Doppler colour or power analysis.

1.3.4 Spectral Analysis

Since blood flow does not have a uniform velocity, in order to know how many red blood cells are travelling at a specific velocity, the different frequencies that compose the signal must be distinguished. For this purpose, a fast Fourier transform is used.

The Fourier spectral analysis of Doppler signals shows the time on the abscissa and the frequency that corresponds to the speed of the blood cells on the ordinate.

The approaching and receding signals are represented, above and below the baseline, respectively.

The light points that make up the path indicate the number of red blood cells that have a determined velocity; the amplitude and the width of the path indicate the dispersion of the velocity in the sampled volume.

In particular, the upper profile of the path indicates the highest velocities and the window, i.e. the area between the lower margin of the path. The baseline represents an index of the homogeneity of the flow.

Since modern sonography must rapidly elaborate large quantities of data, it sometimes uses alternative methods to estimate velocity instead of the fast Fourier transform.

For example, the so-called autocorrelation method consists of multiplying and summing the signal with a series of versions of itself staggered over time.

Instead, *colour velocity imaging* successively recognizes the echoes reflected by red blood cells and, detecting their movement over time, measures the velocity. This system, unlike the classic Doppler method, does not include aliasing, but the angle of insonation must, in any case, be taken into consideration when measuring velocity.

1.3.5 Colour Doppler

The colour Doppler can overlap, on the grayscale image, a map of the direction and velocity of flows on a colour scale.

Red and blue are used to indicate the direction of the flow, approaching or moving away from the probe; a higher saturation of the colour corresponds to slow flows, while signals with less intense colouring correspond to higher velocities.

The sample of the flows can be extended to the whole scan or can be conveniently limited to a frame, the so-called colour box [9].

In particular, the area examined is subdivided into many small sample volumes along the probe's parallel sight lines (multi-gating) and is therefore fractionated into pixels that are assigned a colour.

In most sonography, the information of the grayscale image and the Doppler information are acquired either asynchronously or alternated along the line of sight.

The ultrasound groups dedicated to the grayscale are brief, in order to optimize spatial resolution; in Doppler analysis, they are long for improving the sensibility for slow flows.

In order to reconcile the small angles of insonation necessary for optimizing the grayscale image with the angles required for obtaining Doppler signals, it is possible to selectively tilt the ultrasonic beam dedicated to the Doppler by activating the steering.

The steering tilts the beam, electronically regulating the activation sequence of the piezoelectric crystals that are ordered in series which make up the transducer [9].

1.3.6 Aliasing

According to Shannon's theorem, the highest measurable frequency, both in pulse wave Doppler and in colour Doppler, is limited to a value equal to ½ of the PRF, a value that is also called the Nyquist limit.

As a result, if the velocity of the blood is too high with respect to the PRF, a phenomenon called aliasing occurs, where an overturning of the Doppler signals that exceed the Nyquist limit takes place.

In spectral analysis, this translates into a flattened systolic peak, and the missing apex is represented below the baseline [9].

Aliasing can simulate an inversion of the vessel flow and cause interpretive problems.

Sometimes, however, it can also help diagnose stenosis, since its appearance can demonstrate acceleration in the flow.

A gradual increase in PRF eliminates aliasing; however, if the examined vessel runs deep, the PRF cannot be increased indefinitely.

An alternative for avoiding aliasing in these cases can be reducing the frequency of insonation, possibly changing the transducer.

Alternatively, the angle of insonation can be increased, even if this correction can produce ambiguity in the attribution of the direction of the flow and negatively influence the quantitative analysis of the velocity.

Lowering the baseline is often the easiest way to eliminate aliasing, although the analysis is limited to a unidirectional study, thus renouncing the identification of a possible associated retrograde flow.

In the case of extremely high flows and cardiac applications, specifically to avoid aliasing, it may be preferable to use equipment with continuous emission probes.

1.3.7 Clutter and Wall Filters

"Clutter" means the undesired component of the signal produced by the movement of anatomical structures (vessel walls, cardiac pulsation, respiratory excursions) other than blood flow. Clutter has low frequencies since these movements are slower than those of red blood cells in vessels and much higher amplitudes because the tissue masses in the movement are much higher than those of blood.

These characteristics allow the undesired signals to be easily cut out with the so-called wall filter; this is a mathematical elaboration filter that allows for the elimination of frequencies below a determined level, defined as "cutoff," suitably chosen by the operator [10].

In regulating the wall filter, an elevated value setting eliminates clutter but, on the other hand, it reduces sensitivity in as much as it establishes that the sample starts from higher velocity values and information relative to slow flows is lost.

1.4 Contrast-Enhanced Ultrasound (CEUS)

1.4.1 Contrast Medium

Sonography contrast mediums currently in use are those of the second generation, formed by gaseous microbubbles that have a nonlinear echogenic behaviour when they are insonated with their resonance frequency [11].

In these conditions, the contrast medium itself becomes a source of ultrasounds and generates an ample spectrum of frequencies with a clear predominance of the second harmonic.

The factors on which resonance is based are the dimensions of the microbubbles and the frequency of insonation. Since the harmonic signal produced by the contrast medium is decidedly more intense than that generated by the surrounding tissues, the signals relative to the microcirculation can be differentiated from the echo signals generated by adjacent tissues.

Previously, this was not possible with Doppler due to various limitations, including the "clutter" effect in particular.

With harmonic images used in CEUS, it is possible to eliminate clutter from the adjacent tissues without affecting the flow signal, unlike what happens with the use of wall filters.

Therefore, CEUS allows the study of microcirculation from the angle of insonation to be freed from the movement of adjacent organs (i.e. the heart or great vessels).

This method is particularly helpful for slow intralesional flows, which would be eliminated by the filters used in traditional Doppler imaging; with CEUS, therefore, the vascular map of lesions becomes more precise [12].

To work around the problem of the fragility of microbubbles, nowadays a low mechanical index (MI) is used.

MI is a measure of the elastic deformation imposed upon the material by applied ultrasounds. MI = Pressure of maximum depletion/square root of the insonated frequency.

Currently, the values MI < 1 kPa are used in CEUS, together with the use of selective filters for the second harmonic, offering the advantage of significantly reducing the interference of tissue signals.

The focus influences MI and should be kept outside of the region of study, in the 2/3 distal of the field of view, in order to limit the breakage of microbubbles [13].

However, even in CEUS, the focus should be shifted depending on the structures to be examined.

Another technique adopted in order to preserve the most microbubbles possible is the use of specific software that employs lower framerate values than those used for standard B-Mode imaging.

1.4.2 Optimizing and Interpreting CEUS Images

While structures are much more visible as they are superficial in B-Mode, CEUS provides the best results at around the middle of the field of view: it is therefore advisable to look for the acoustic window and the angle of insonation that allow the placement of the region of interest at more or less half the depth of insonation.

The gain compensation, in general, must be balanced, and the setting levers should all be arranged approximately in the middle range; in some ultrasound scanners, with abdominal probes, the most superficial levers should be reset and therefore, from a practical point of view, a few preliminary tests may prove useful.

The overall gain should be set to medium-low levels; before the administration of the contrast medium, this should allow for the estimation of the most evident specular interfaces, namely rib cage surfaces, vessel walls, the pleural line and the diaphragm.

1.5 Conclusions

In this chapter, we have discussed the physical phenomena that preside over the creation of sonographic images, i.e. reflection, refraction and the diffusion of ultrasounds.

Although these phenomena are no different with respect to the sonographic study of other areas, in TUS being aware of them is of practical interest for interpreting images, both real and artificial, correctly, due to the abundant presence of pulmonary air and the bones of the rib cage that condition and change the propagation of ultrasounds.

Doppler applications allow for the study of vascular flows, and, in particular, spectral analysis can describe blood flow velocity over time. Colour Doppler permits the overlapping a map in colour scale of the direction and average velocity of flows over grayscale images. Finally, CEUS is useful for studying microcirculation and slow intralesional flows and requires a few specific adjustments to ultrasound settings.

References

1. Valli G, Coppini G. Bioimaging. Bologna: Pàtron Editore; 2002. p. 185–93.
2. Feletti F, Gardelli G, Mughetti M. Thoracic ultrasonography in paediatrics: a tecnique often neglected. Quaderni acp 2009;16(3):97–8.
3. Rizzatto G. Ultrasound transducers. Eur J Radiol. 1998;27(Suppl 2):S188–95.
4. Kremkau FW. Sonography principles and instruments. 8th ed. Amsterdam: Elsevier Saunders; 2011. p. 292.
5. Jensen JA. Medical ultrasound imaging. Prog Biophys Mol Biol. 2007;93:153–65. https://doi.org/10.1016/j.pbiomolbio.2006.07.025.
6. Case TD. Ultrasound physics and instrumentation. Surg Clin North Am. 1998;78(2):197–217.
7. Violino P, Robutti O. La fisica e i suoi modelli. Zanichelli, Bologna 1995. 3, 1; 36-37.
8. Fetzer DT, Rafailidis V, Peterson C, Grant EG, Sidhu P, Barr RG. Artifacts in contrast-enhanced ultrasound: a pictorial essay. Abdom Radiol (NY). 2018;43(4):977–97. https://doi.org/10.1007/s00261-017-1417-8.
9. Derchi LE, Martinoli C, Solbiati L, Rizzatto G. Power Doppler: physical and constructive principles and comparison with Doppler color. Radiol Med. 1997;93(4):329–35.
10. Bjaerum S, Torp H, Kristoffersen K. Clutter filter design for ultrasound color flow imaging. IEEE Trans Ultrason Ferroelectr Freq Control. 2002;49(2):204–16.
11. Gummadi S, Eisenbrey JR, Lyshchik A. Contrast-enhanced ultrasonography in interventional oncology. Abdom Radiol (NY). 2018;43(11):3166–75. https://doi.org/10.1007/s00261-018-1581-5.
12. Piscaglia F, Nolsøe C, Dietrich CF. The EFSUMB guidelines and recommendations on the clinical practice of contrast enhanced ultrasound (CEUS). Update 2011 on non-hepatic applications. Ultraschall Med. 2011;32:1–27.
13. Dietrich CF, Ignee A, Hocke M, Schreiber-Dietrich D, Greis C. Pitfalls and artefacts using contrast enhanced ultrasound. Z Gastroenterol. 2011;49(3):350–6. https://doi.org/10.1055/s-0029-1245851.

2 Artefacts in Thoracic Ultrasound

Francesco Feletti, Bruna Malta, and Andrea Aliverti

2.1 Introduction

Today, technological evolution increasingly improves the quality of ultrasound images, making artefacts less visible; the sonographer thus risks not paying enough attention to them.

In general terms, artefacts in medical imaging often hamper the diagnostic process since, by definition, they are altered representations of anatomical reality.

In ultrasound, however, this is not always true because by understanding artefacts we are provided with information on the type of interaction that ultrasounds have with anatomical structures and this can help us to interpret images correctly [1].

In particular, in thoracic ultrasound (TUS) some artefacts are responsible for fundamental semiological signs (e.g. B-lines).

2.2 Artefacts in B-Mode

2.2.1 Classification of Artefacts

From a practical point of view, we can consider three main groups of ultrasound artefacts (Table 2.1). Some depend to varying degrees on the operator and the parameters of the ultrasound system; others can be modified with appropriate insonation angles or postural expedients, while still others depend solely on the intrinsic characteristics of the ultrasound machine.

2.3 Ultrasound/Tissue Interaction Artefacts

2.3.1 Reflection Artefacts

2.3.1.1 Reverberation Artefacts

Reverberation artefacts depend on reflection and are therefore more evident in the case of orthogonal insonation and a considerable difference in acoustic impedance.

Electronic Supplementary Material The online version of this chapter (https://doi.org/10.1007/978-3-319-93055-8_2) contains supplementary material, which is available to authorized users.

F. Feletti (✉)
Dipartimento di Diagnostica per Immagini, Ausl della Romagna, Ospedale S. Maria delle Croci, Ravenna, Italy

Dipartimento di Elettronica, Informazione e Bioingegneria, Politecnico di Milano, Milan, Italy
e-mail: francesco.feletti@auslromagna.it

B. Malta
Dipartimento di Diagnostica per Immagini, Ausl di Ferrara, Ospedale Universitario di Ferrara, Ferrara, Italy
e-mail: mltbrn@unife.it

A. Aliverti
Dipartimento di Elettronica, Informazione e Bioingegneria, Politecnico di Milano, Milan, Italy
e-mail: andrea.aliverti@polimi.it

F. Feletti et al. (eds.), *Thoracic Ultrasound and Integrated Imaging*,
https://doi.org/10.1007/978-3-319-93055-8_2

Table 2.1 Classification of ultrasound artefacts in B-Mode [1, 2]

Mechanisms involved	Artefact classification	
1. Ultrasound/tissue interaction artefacts	I. Reflection artefacts	• Reverberation artefacts • Mirror image artefacts • Comet-tail artefacts • "Rain" artefacts
	II. Refraction artefacts	• Lateral shadow cones • Lateral displacement • Image doubling
	III. Beam attenuation artefacts	• Posterior reinforcement • Acoustic shadows
	IV. Ultrasound beam speed artefacts	
	V. Ring down artefact	
	VI. Ultrasound beam characteristic artefacts	• Side-lobe artefacts • Partial volume artefacts
2. Incorrect device use artefacts	I. Range ambiguity artefacts	
	II. Fish echo	
3. Interference or malfunction artefacts	I. Antenna artefacts	

In these conditions, the insonated structure reflects most ultrasounds toward the transducer.

In turn, the transducer behaves like a specular reflector and returns most of the ultrasounds it receives, even without the ultrasound producing a new impulse.

The ultrasound beam, therefore, rebounds between the insonated anatomic surface and the transducer, generating ultrasound signals repeated at regular intervals. The insonated surface is reproduced several times in the ultrasound image at multiple depths with respect to the real image. The depths depend on the time between the emission of the beam and each successive echo (Fig. 2.1).

The reverberation artefact therefore consists of multiple parallel and equidistant hyperechoic lines that are repeated, with gradually less intensity due to the beam's progressive loss of energy.

The so-called A-lines (Fig. 2.2a, b) are reverberation artefacts and are very important in TUS because they indicate that the pleura behaves like a specular reflector because the lung has regular air content [3]. A-lines are absent in cases where the lung's ultrasound permeability is increased due to interstitial pathologies or the loss of normal alveolar content.

Reverberation artefacts are attenuated by harmonic tissue imaging and when the gain is set to low values [1].

In TUS, reverberation effects devoid of diagnostic utility can be generated between the transducer and the ambient air if the transducer does not perfectly adhere to the skin, as can sometimes happen due to the convexity of the chest wall.

2.3.1.2 Comet Tail Artefacts

When the ultrasonic beam encounters small reflective structures located in successive short distances, the ultrasounds, as a result of reflection, bounce between them several times, before returning to the transducer (internal reverberation; see Fig. 2.1).

The ultrasound system therefore registers multiple reflections of the beam and represents a series of small hyperechoic bands arranged perpendicularly to the ultrasound beam and parallel to each other, forming the comet-tail artefact.

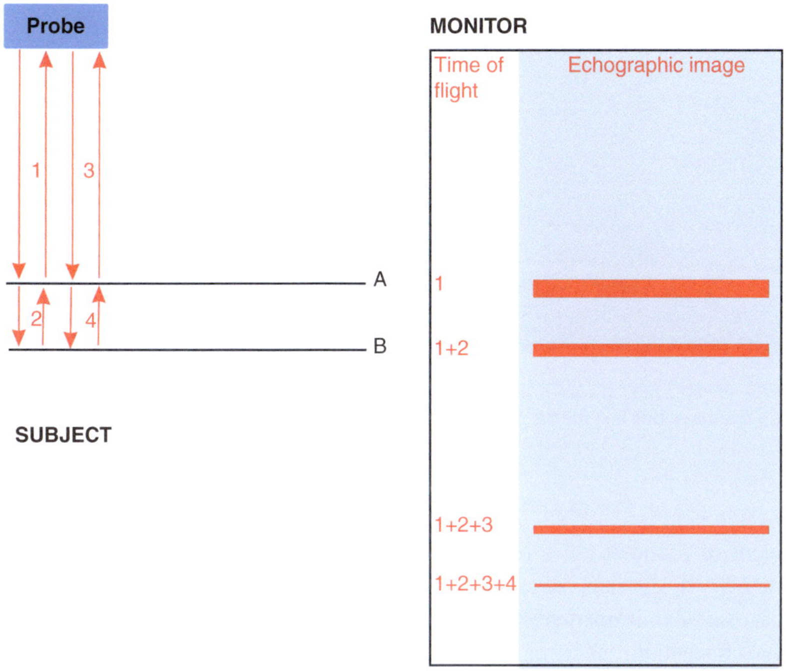

Fig. 2.1 Generation of reverberation artefacts. The ultrasonic beam generated by the transducer reaches the specular surface A. The reflected beam in A gives rise to the echo placed at depth 1. The energy refracted by A reaches interface B where it is reflected and makes the transducer register a second echo that is placed on the monitor at the depth that corresponds to the time of flight 1 + 2. A fraction of the energy received by the transducer is reflected. Therefore, without any new ultrasound emission from the transducer, a second reflection is generated both on A (image 1 + 2 + 3) and on B (1 + 2 + 3 + 4). Also, a part of the energy reflected by B on its return path to the transducer can be reflected by A. The beam can be reflected several times between A and B, thus giving rise to so-called internal reverberation

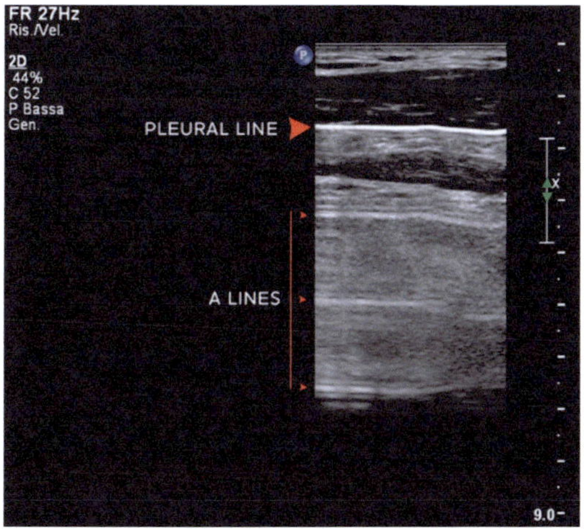

Fig. 2.2 A-lines; the artefact is more evident if the incidence of the ultrasound beam is perpendicular to the pleural line

The *chimney phenomenon* [4] is a comet-tail artefact that occurs between bone fragments in the rib fractures (Fig. 2.3).

Irregularities of diaphragm muscle fibers also generate comet-tail artefacts.

Other structures that can produce comet tail artefacts are scleral calcification of vessels or viscera walls, crystal deposits, foreign bodies in soft tissues (e.g., projectiles, fragments of glass or wood [5]), bone cortical fragments, clips, plastic or metal probes and catheters [6, 7].

Spatial compound imaging can make these artefacts less noticeable, while tissue harmonic imaging can make them more evident and define them [1].

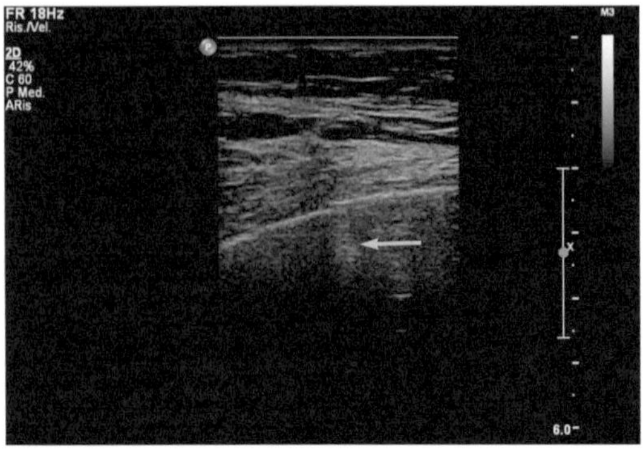

Fig. 2.3 Chimney phenomenon (arrow). In the case of non-displaced rib fractures, this may be the only sign visible by TUS

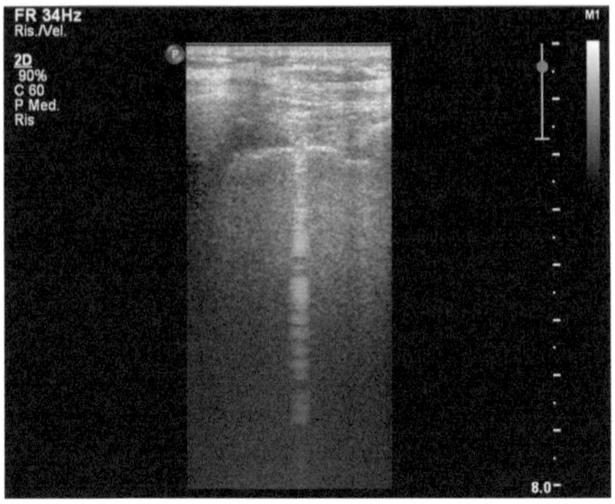

Fig. 2.4 Single B-line artefact

An equivalent of a comet-tail artefact is the twinkling artefact. It consists of scintillating colour-Doppler signals, immediately below a hyper-reflective formation, and, in TUS, can favour the identification of small calcified foci on vessel walls, anatomical structures, surgical clips, and foreign bodies [8].

2.3.1.3 B-Line Artefacts

For their importance in TUS and the complexity of the topic, these artefacts deserve a specific treatment.

Recent international recommendations based on evidence defined B-line artefacts as discrete laser-like vertical hyperechoic bands (Figs. 2.4 and 2.5) which, starting from the pleural line, extend toward the bottom of the field of view without fading and shift concomitantly to lung sliding [9, 10] (Fig. 2.6) (Video 2.1).

Based on animal experiments, B-line artefacts have been attributed to misleading interpretation by machines of complex acoustic phenomena (reflections in closed spaces, induction of stationary waves, resonance) that wave energy undergoes in the presence of alterations in the geometry of the peripheral aerial spaces related to different situations: folded alveolar spaces, interstitial lung diseases, free intra-alveolar bubbles, and oedema [11, 12].

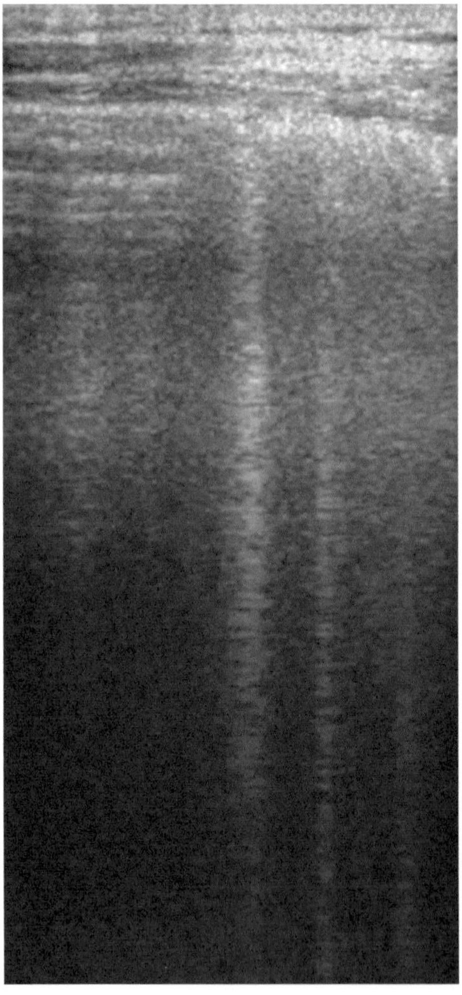

Fig. 2.5 B-lines

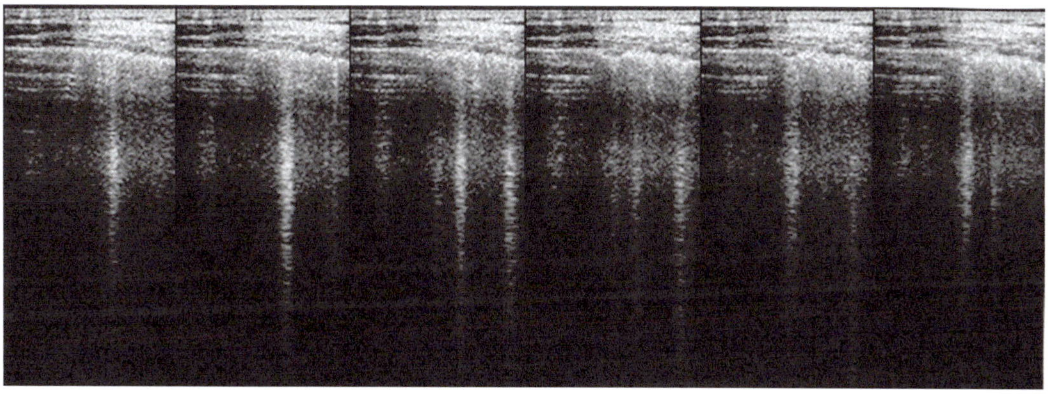

Fig. 2.6 B-lines. Intercostal scanning with high-frequency probe (7–12 MHz): B-lines change depending on location and appearance with respiratory acts

Fig. 2.7 (**a**) Mirror image produced by axial reflection. (**b**) Mirror image produced by non-axial reflection. *S* reflective surface, *R* real image, *F* false image

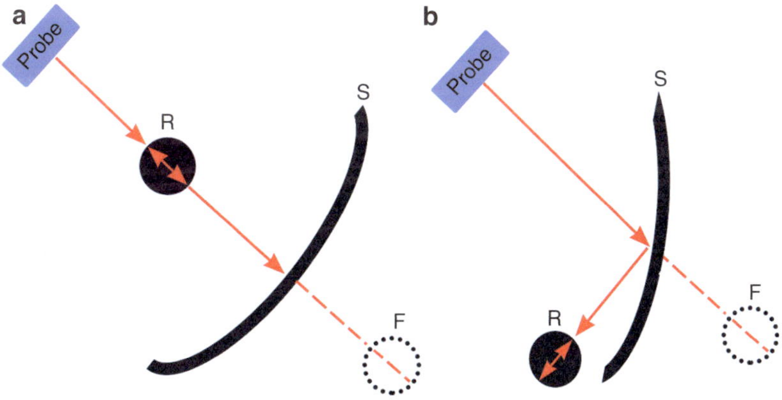

They correspond to CT findings of abnormalities of the secondary pulmonary lobule such as thickening of the interlobular septa and diffuse, alveolar opacities, areas of ground-glass opacity [13–15].

B-line artefacts correspond to three types of anatomopathological substrates, namely, increased interstitial fluid, infiltrative processes of the interstitium and interstitial inflammation, or fibrosis related to infections [9, 13]. Hence, B-line artefacts can be found in a variety of diffuse pulmonary conditions characterised by the aforementioned anatomopathological patterns.

These artefacts are made less evident by compound and harmonic imaging and made more evident by the high gain settings [13, 16].

2.3.1.4 Mirror Image Artefacts

The mirror image artefact duplicates an image and depends on reflection.

It occurs in different ways according to the mutual position of the specular reflector and the structure under examination (Fig. 2.7a, b).

A first circumstance is when ultrasounds meet an anatomical formation and subsequently perpendicularly affect a specular reflector.

In this case, it produces a second artefact image of the anatomical structure, which is represented distally from the reflective surface and in the direction of the ultrasound beam propagation.

In fact, after the first interaction with the object, the beam is reflected from the more profound surface and encounters the object for the second time.

A second echo of the object is generated that, retracing the route in reverse, is again reflected and, returning to the transducer, forms the second image of the object.

A different situation occurs when the beam obliquely hits the specular surface before reaching the object.

In this case, the reflected beam reaches the anatomical formation under examination from a direction that is different from the emission, while the ultrasound machine, insensitive to this deviation, places the false image beyond the interface, in the direction of the original beam.

In both cases, the ultrasound system establishes the false image placement based on the time elapsed between the emission of the impulse and the arrival of the echoes (time of flight).

These artefacts are typically generated by the diaphragmatic pleura surface which behaves like an extended specular curved surface (Figs. 2.8a, b, 2.9, and 2.10).

The diaphragm, due to mirror image artefacts, frequently appears as an ultrasound image composed of three parallel hyper-echogenic lines (Fig. 2.11a, b).

The bottom line depends on the real interface between the liver and the diaphragm. The middle line is created from the interface between soft tissues and pulmonary air. These two lines are always visible and are separated by a hypoechoic layer that corresponds to the muscular thickness of the diaphragm whereas, the third line is inconstant and represents the mirror image artefact of the first line.

Recognizing mirror image artefacts is crucial because they can simulate pathological conditions (Fig. 2.12), including pulmonary consolidation [1].

Another common mirror image artefact in TUS involves the subclavian artery, the image of which can be mirrored by the pleural line [17].

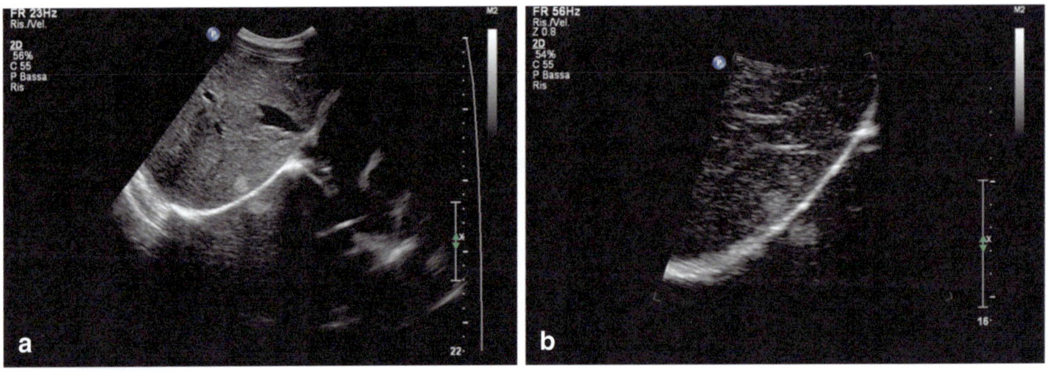

Fig. 2.8 Mirror image artefact (**a**, **b**) of a focal liver lesion (angioma) on the diaphragm. Since the diaphragm dome does not have a constant radius, the artefact only appears if the specific insonation angles occur

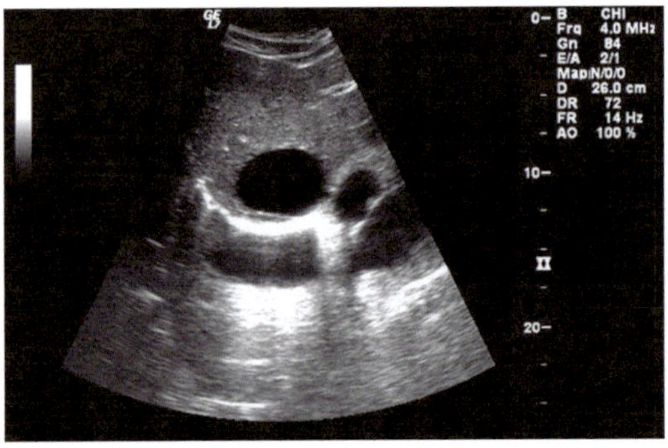

Fig. 2.9 Mirror image artefact of a focal liver lesion (cyst) on the diaphragm. Such an image should not be mistaken for a small pleural effusion

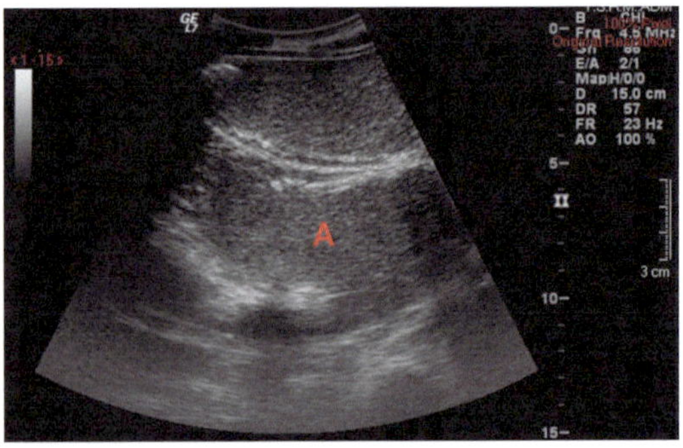

Fig. 2.10 Mirror artefact of the left hepatic lobe. If not recognized as such, this artefact (A) could be mistaken for pulmonary consolidation, since the consolidated lung looks similar to the liver parenchyma

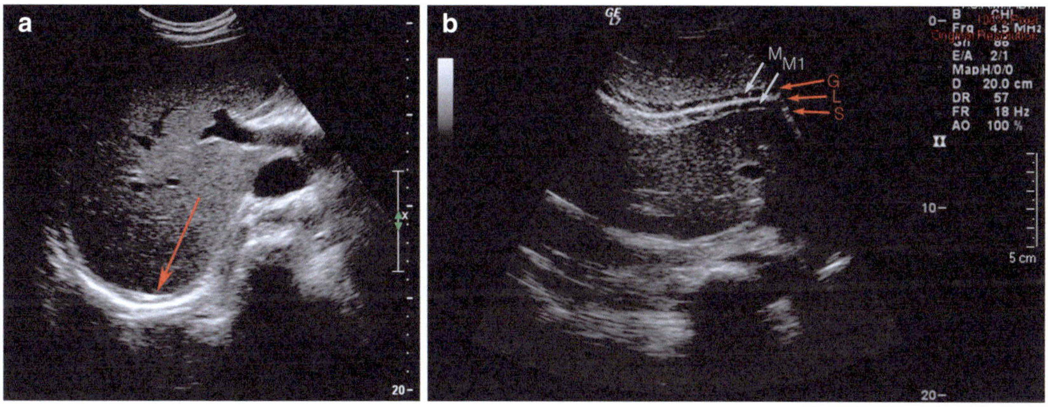

Fig. 2.11 Mirror effect and ultrasound representation of the diaphragm. (**a**) The diaphragm appears to consist of three parallel hyperechogenic linear images. (**b**) The glissonian hyperechogenic interface (G), the pleural line (L), and the mirror effect (S) that more deeply replicates the glissonian image are indicated. The muscle layer of the diaphragm (M) is also reproduced by a mirror effect (M1)

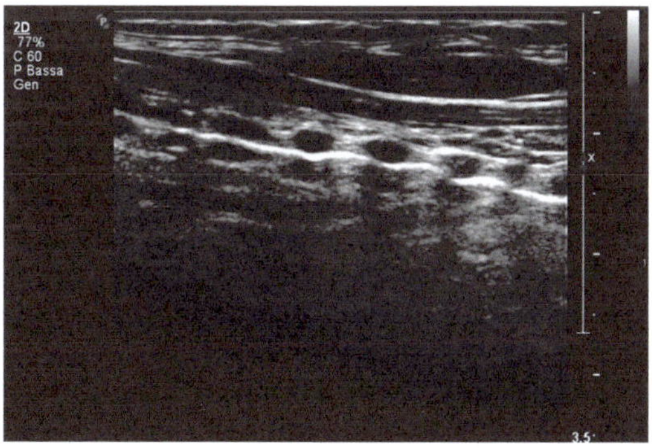

Fig. 2.12 The mirror effect of the trachea. The cartilaginous rings of the trachea are mirrored at the interface between the tissues and the tracheal air

2.3.1.5 Rain Artefacts

Rain artefacts depend on the low-intensity echoes generated by the micro-discontinuity of soft tissues, which reverberate within an underlying anechoic liquid deposit.

These are diffuse echoes below the upper wall of the liquid structures, which progressively decrease in intensity with depth until they disappear altogether.

The intensity is directly proportional to the echogenicity and inversely proportional to the thickness of the diffuser tissues interposed between the transducer and the liquid deposit.

The particular arrangement and the variation according to gain allow the rain artefact to be differentiated from the actual presence of corpuscular material in the liquid being examined.

In TUS, rain artefacts can occur in pleural effusion or in cystic lesions.

This artefact, together with internal reverberations and posterior reinforcement, is an essential semiological sign, useful for differentiating the cystic or solid nature of examined structures.

2.3.2 Refraction Artefacts

Reflection and refraction are two phenomena that always coexist, although in different proportions depending on the ultrasound's angle of incidence and the interface characteristics.

2.3.2.1 Lateral Shadow Cones

Lateral shadow cones are typically generated in liquid structures with a rounded section and thick walls, such as large vessels or cysts with a thick wall.

Upon encountering a formation with these characteristics, ultrasounds are refracted and then deviated both to the upper and lower walls, while on both sides the refraction gradually increases as the ultrasounds strike evermore obliquely until becoming tangents. Refraction diverts ultrasounds, and forms a thin conical shadow behind each side of a round liquid form.

These artefacts are called lateral shadow cones, and they are much more intense, the more the acoustic impedance of the two mediums is different.

At the point of origin of the lateral shadows, the wall of the formation that determines them does not appear and thus is interrupted; this aspect must be taken into account when, for example, studying an aneurysm. Similarly, diaphragmatic gaps consist in apparent diaphragm discontinuities where ultrasound beams reach it obliquely [18].

2.3.2.2 Tendon Anisotropy

When the beam does not strike tendons perpendicularly, they may appear hypoechoic, due to phenomena of reflection and refraction, simulating echo-structural alterations.

This artefact makes the study of superficial tendons that are anatomically curved or obliquely placed at the cutaneous level particularly delicate and makes linear probes more suitable for the study of musculoskeletal pathology.

2.3.2.3 Artefacts from Lateral Displacement and Image Doubling

If the ultrasound beam is refracted and deviated before meeting a structure, the echo generated by the structure retraces the path in reverse back to the transducer.

Since the ultrasound scanner ignores the refraction, the image is represented along the beam's original trajectory and at the distance corresponding to the time of flight.

Lateral displacement artefacts may occur when using intercostal acoustic windows due to the refraction against costal cartilage, muscle aponeurosis, and fibrotic bands.

A particular case of artefacts from an altered image position linked to multiple refraction phenomena is the image doubling artefact. Generally, objects of about 1 cm are doubled, including bioptic needles and the aorta when in axial section [19] (Figs. 2.13a, b and 2.14), while larger objects appear enlarged or deformed or with discontinuous contours. The incorrect calculation of distances or the wrong location of structures may result, which is particularly dangerous during an ultrasound-guided procedure.

Like all refractive artefacts, lateral displacement is related to the angle of insonation, the size and shape of the transducer, the width of the refracting surface.

2.3.3 Beam Attenuation Artefacts

2.3.3.1 Posterior Reinforcement

Posterior reinforcement is the enhancement of the ultrasound signals successive to liquid formations and is generated through the interaction of several factors.

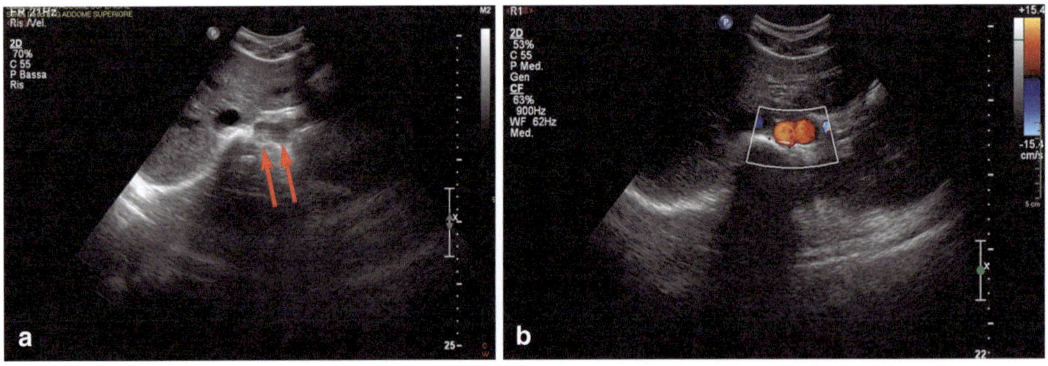

Fig. 2.13 Artefact by splitting the aorta image into axial scan (**a**, **b**) with convex probe (3–5 MHz). The geometry of the bands of muscles, in this case, the rectus muscles of the abdomen, can determine refraction phenomena responsible for the splitting of the ultrasound images

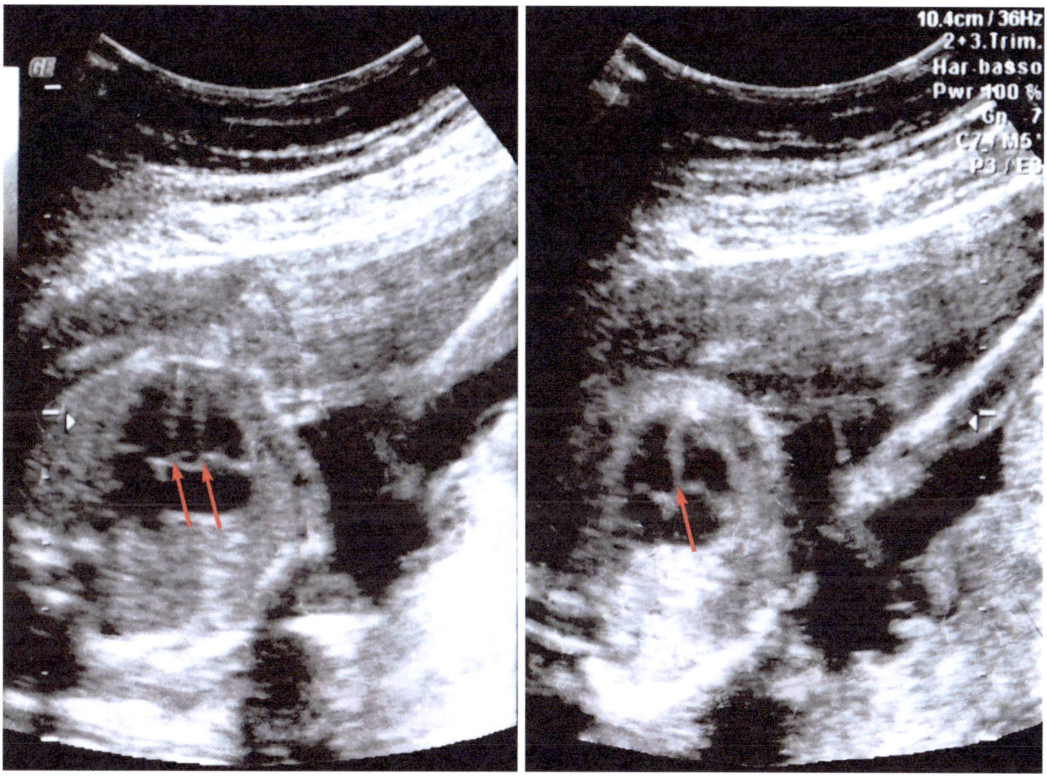

Fig. 2.14 Image doubling of the cardiac septum

Firstly, when crossing liquids, the intensity reduction of the ultrasound beam is lower than when crossing the surrounding tissues. This effect is amplified by the fact that ultrasounds amplify the deeper signals more than the superficial ones to compensate for the progressive attenuation of the beam with the depth.

Furthermore, the velocity of ultrasonic propagation in liquids is lower than in the surrounding soft tissues and liquid pockets since refraction behaves like converging lenses; thus, the posterior structures appear enlarged and more evident.

Due to posterior reinforcement, when the diaphragm is visualized below pleural effusion, it may appear focally thickened, blurred and distorted, sometimes creating the diagnostic suspicion of pleural or diaphragmatic lesions [20] (Fig. 2.15).

Particularly echo-permeable solid materials like lymphomatous tissue, adipose tissue, and angiomas can sometimes produce posterior reinforcements.

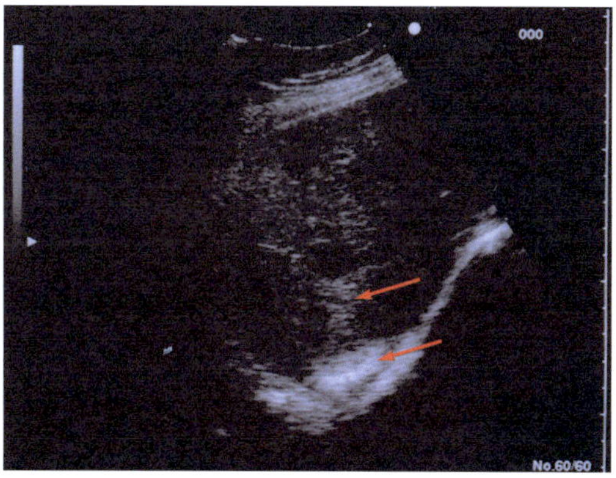

Fig. 2.15 Rear reinforcement and slow effect in a hepatic cyst. Because of the posterior reinforcement, the diaphragm below the cyst appears thicker and more distorted, simulating a possible pleural or diaphragmatic lesion

This artefact may however be lacking in the case of small liquid pockets that are far from the focus or only partially included in the explorative beam.

The use of tissue harmonic imaging can accentuate posterior reinforcement.

2.3.3.2 Acoustic Shadows

Both reflection and absorption prevent the deeper propagation of ultrasounds and, consequently, block ultrasound signals.

Both phenomena, therefore, give rise to acoustic shadows.

In particular, the ribs and calcifications produce *clean* acoustic shadows which are very evident and with sharp margins; in fact, ultrasounds are both reflected by the surface and, in the case of the ribs, intensely absorbed by bone tissue.

On the other hand, the acoustic shadows generated by gaseous bubbles are subtler, have less defined contours, and are defined as *dirty* because posterior attenuation is accompanied by reverberation phenomena, amorphous reflections, and refractions that disperse the ultrasounds [21].

In TUS, acoustic shadows can indicate various pathological conditions, including subcutaneous emphysema (Fig. 2.16) and calcified pleural plaques from asbestosis (Fig. 2.17).

The reduction or interruption of the costal shadow cone may however be a sign of an osteolytic lesion or a costal fracture.

Yet small formations, far from the focal zone of the beam, may not present the shadow cone.

The use of a digital compound significantly reduces the width of the back shadows, changing their shape. Acoustic shadows are also attenuated by excessive beam widths and by incorrect focus positioning.

Acoustic shadows are however strengthened by increasing insonation frequency and by using tissue harmonics [1].

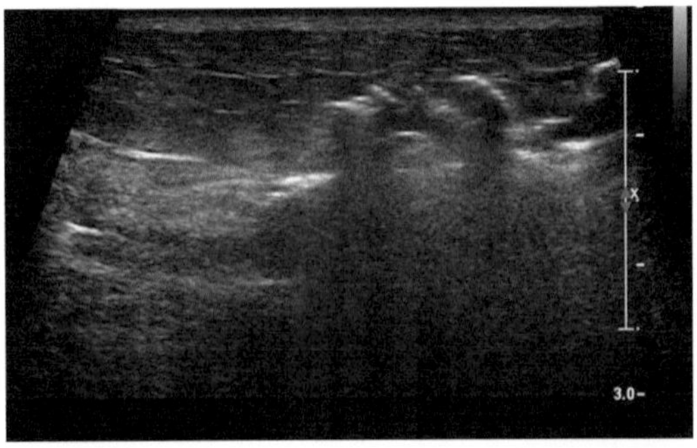

Fig. 2.16 Dirty acoustic shadows caused by subcutaneous emphysema

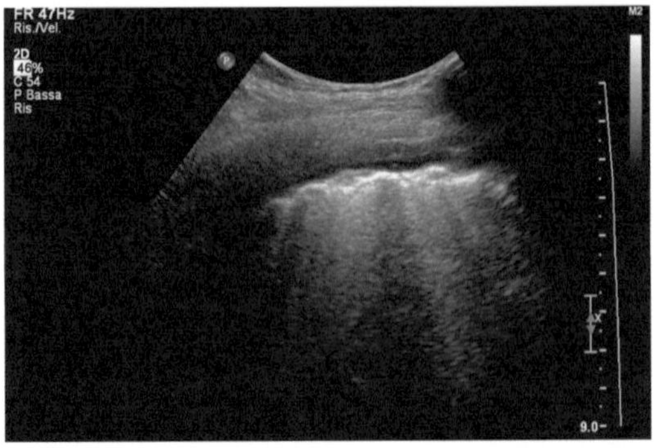

Fig. 2.17 Acoustic shadows in calcified pleural plaques from asbestosis

2.3.4 Ultrasound Beam Speed Artefacts

This artefact depends on the fact that the ultrasound system assigns depth to anatomical structures based on the time of flight calculated on a standard ultrasound speed of 1540 m/s, while in reality ultrasound speed varies in different tissues.

Consequently, if ultrasound speed in a structure is sufficiently higher than the surrounding tissue, the size of the formation will be reduced along the ultrasound's axis of propagation and vice versa [22] (Fig. 2.18).

2.3.5 Ring Down Artefact

This particular artefact is produced when ultrasounds strike thin liquid flaps situated between microbubbles, which, as a result, begin to vibrate, generating a continuous and fluctuating signal with decreasing intensity [23]. The artefact consists of a hyperechoic strip that goes down in the direction of the beam; it is made up of thin parallel bands that are closely juxtaposed with each other.

The periodicity and the thickness of the bands are two typical aspects of this artefact [1]; both are constant for each but *ring down* change concomitantly from one *ring down* to the next.

Another feature of this artefact is its dynamic nature; in fact, it varies in location and appearance over short periods.

The periodic and dynamic nature of this artefact distinguishes it from the comet tail artefact [23].

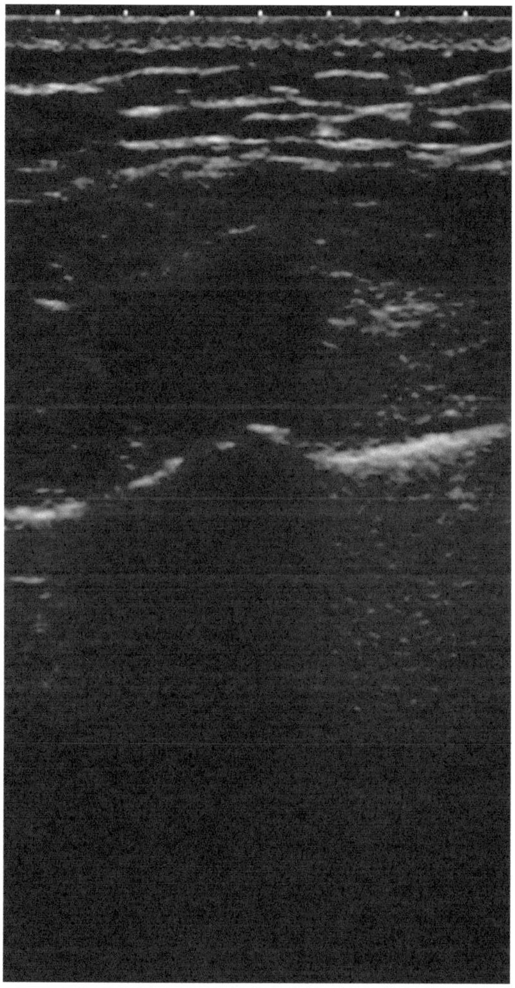

Fig. 2.18 Costal cartilage transmits ultrasounds more rapidly than the soft tissues of the chest wall. Its image is therefore deformed, and the underlying pleural line appears convex, simulating the presence of an expansive pulmonary lesion with compressive effects on the pleura

2.3.6 Ultrasound Beam Characteristic Artefacts

2.3.6.1 Partial Volume Artefact

This artefact is produced when a structure with liquid content has a diameter smaller than the thickness of the insonated layer or when it is only partially included within it.

In these circumstances, echoes formed in the beam width but outside the liquid component are represented as superimposed over it.

Due to this artefact, in ultrasound-guided procedures involving ducts or vessels, it is necessary to orient the transducer so as to visualize these anatomical structures transversely.

If a duct or a vessel is displayed longitudinally, the needle could be represented as if the tip were inside the duct even though it is merely adjacent to it.

2.3.6.2 Side-Lobe Artefacts

Side lobes are lateral and divergent components of the beam of lower intensity than the main beam.

In the presence of a concave specular surface, the reflection of the main beam produces the actual image, while the side lobes generate artefact reflections and diffusions that the ultrasound scanner cannot distinguish from the signals of the main beam.

Side-lobe artefacts are diffused or arched echoes with a shape and appearance that depends on the design and the constructive characteristics of the transducer [17].

In TUS, side lobes reflected on the pleura can confer to a non-echogenic pleural effusion, a falsely corpuscular or septate appearance.

Side-lobe artefacts occupy slopes but are recognizable as veritable sediments because they have a concave upper edge; the area occupied by the artefact extends, increasing the gain, and the artefact can disappear by changing the orientation of the probe or the point of insonation.

Finally, these artefacts can be reduced with the use of tissue harmonic or with the use of advanced transducers designed to reduce the amplitude and amplification of the signals coming from the most external elements of the transducer [1, 24].

2.4 Incorrect Device-Use Artefacts

2.4.1 Range Ambiguity Artefacts

The pulse repetition frequency (PRF) is the sum of the ultrasonic emission time and the pulse reception period (PRP) (see Chap. 1).

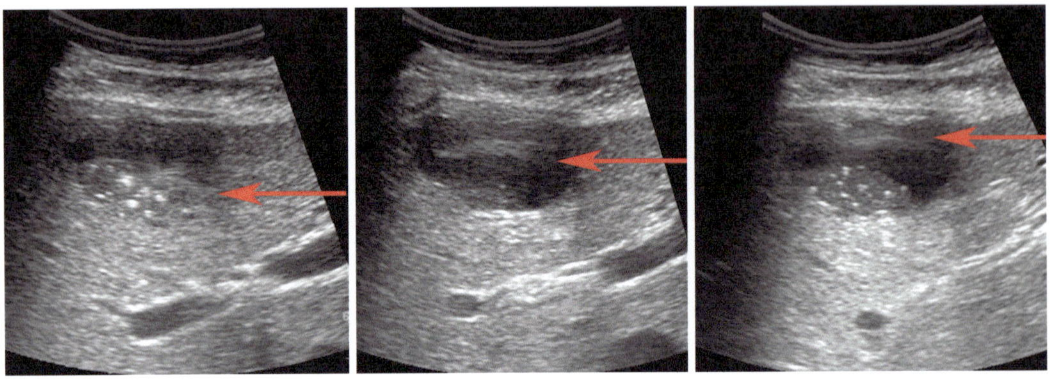

Fig. 2.19 Range ambiguity artefacts in a juxtadiaphragmatic hepatic cyst; a linear mobile hyperechogenic image was visible within the anechogenic formation, simulating a floating membrane. The image moved synchronously with the respiratory acts and moved out of the way when the PRF was modified, allowing the artefactual nature of the artefact to be clarified

In general, the transducer uses less than 1% of the PRF to generate the pulse and operates as a receiver for most of the time.

Usually, the PRP is abundantly sufficient for the ultrasound to travel the entire distance, both to and from, that separates the probe from the examined structure.

However, if the object of study is profound, considering that the ultrasounds always travel more or less at the same speed (about 1540 m/s), if the PRF is set to high values (short PRF), the echoes may fail to reenter the transducer during the corresponding PRF.

The ultrasound signals are thus received and interpreted only after the subsequent ultrasounds are sent. They are therefore attributed to the last ultrasound emission and positioned at an incorrect depth.

These artefacts are generated when deep reflecting surfaces are reached from the most distal part of the beam, producing linear images of weak intensity that overlap with non-echogenic structures included in the closest part of the beam.

Cardiac walls typically produce ambiguity range artefacts that fluctuate in synchronicity with the cardiac cycle and are therefore easily recognizable.

The depth of the artefact is modified by changing the values of the PRF. In particular, the lower the PRF, the more the echoes become superficial and vice versa (Fig. 2.19). The elimination of this artefact, can be achieved by lowering the PRF. Modern ultrasounds use higher PRF than in the past, and this makes this artefact more frequent; in order to solve this problem, specific systems have recently been introduced to reduce the PRF.

2.4.2 Fish Echo

Fish echoes occur as a result of the contamination of the gel or spacing systems, for example, in the presence of gaseous or oily bubbles. They consist of superficial bright spots and are easily recognizable.

2.5 Interference or Malfunction Artefacts

2.5.1 Antenna Artefacts

Interferences due to high-frequency (shortwave) radio signals and other electrical equipment in the vicinity of the ultrasound machine determine artefact images in the form of waves, lines or bands that overlap the real anatomical structures. In order to eliminate the antenna effect, the ultrasound should be properly shielded with a grounded Faraday cage, and a voltage stabilizer should be installed on the power supply network. However, similar artefacts can still commonly occur.

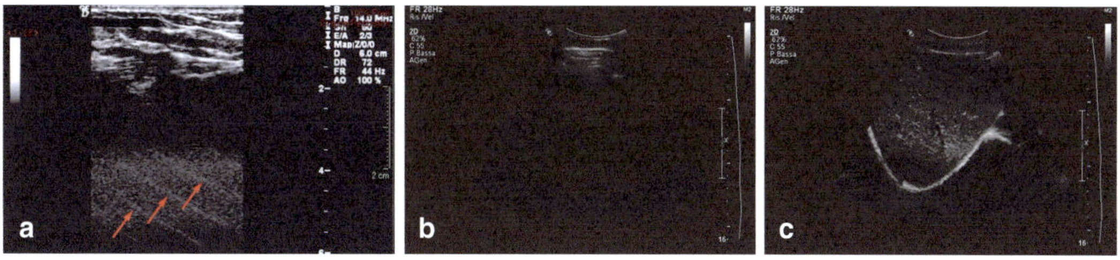

Fig. 2.20 Antenna effect. These images (**a**–**c**) should not be confused with A-lines

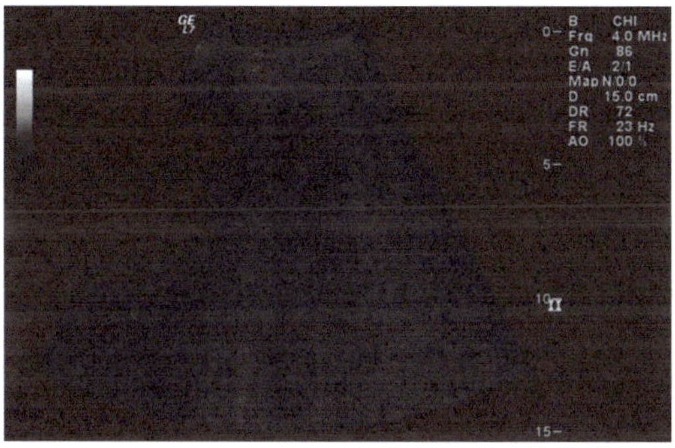

Fig. 2.21 Antenna effect. These images should not be misinterpreted as B-lines

In TUS, it is imperative to distinguish these artefacts from others with diagnostic significance, like A- (Fig. 2.20a–c) or B-lines (Fig. 2.21).

2.6 Artefacts in CEUS Images

2.6.1 Nonlinear Artefacts

When microbubbles in the contrast medium are hit, they manifest nonlinear behaviour, i.e., they contract and expand, spending much more time near their maximum size than near their minimum size.

This response generates valuable harmonic frequencies that make it possible to distinguish the signals of the microbubbles from most of the tissues that instead manifest linear behaviour, that is, they respond to ultrasounds with symmetric contractions and rarefactions [25].

However, specific structures such as organ capsules, vessel walls, and the diaphragm, in addition to determining hyper-reflective interfaces, generate phase aberrations indistinguishable from microbubble signals.

In dubious situations, in order to confirm the nature of the structures mentioned above and distinguish them from contrast signals, a high-power flash pulse can be used to eliminate the microbubbles [25].

2.6.2 Pseudoenhancement

Pseudoenhancement depends on spontaneously hyperechoic structures that, when contrast enhancement is reduced, tend to reappear from the background, becoming more evident and giving the impression of being vascularized (late hyperperfusion simulation) [25, 26]. To avoid interpretative errors, it is therefore indispensable to carry out a careful ultrasound or B-mode study before moving on the examination with the contrast medium.

2.6.3 Near-Field Signal Loss

Near the transducer, acoustic pressure is stronger than in the rest of the insonation sector, and this often leads to a progressive reduction of signal in the near field. Near-field signal loss happens in particular if high values of the mechanical index (MI), high scanning frequencies, or high framerates are used [27].

2.6.4 Image Plane Signal Loss

A prolonged insonation of the same structure, keeping the transducer in the same position, leads to accelerated destruction of bubbles along the direction of the beam. The result is a wide broad band of low signal when the transducer is moved to another plane that is orthogonal to the previous one.

In order to reduce this phenomenon, it is essential to maintain low MI levels, limit framerates, and perform intermittent and sweeping scans rather than keeping the probe fixed at one point.

2.6.5 Pseudowashout

Lesions with slowed blood flow are subject to greater persistence of the contrast medium under the acoustic pressure of the beam. The consequently increased destruction of bubbles can simulate a quick washout.

In addition to the preventive measures already described about image plane signal loss, it is essential to position the focus well below the lesion, since the acoustic pressure is higher in focus.

2.6.6 Signal Saturation

If quantitative evaluations are carried out, it is crucial to consider that in angiographic exams or highly vascularized lesions, depending on the probe's output power, the contrast dose and the gain setting, the received signals can exceed the display range. Signals that reach this level are represented at the maximum brightness level of the reference scale, while any further increment exceeding this level is not shown.

2.6.7 Shadowing

In exceptional cases, an excessive amount of contrast medium in superficial tissues can impede the study of deeper structures, producing the formation of posterior acoustic shadows. In TUS, this artefact can be generated in the presence of voluminous hyper vascularized angiomas of the chest wall. This artefact can be limited or eliminated by delaying the administration of the contrast agent through a series of successive infusions, increasing the destruction of the bubbles by moving the focus up or increasing the MI.

2.6.8 Doppler Applications

Although the measurements of peak speed, average speed, resistance indices, and spectral analysis do not appear to be altered after the administration of a contrast agent with modern systems, it is conservatively advisable to carry out the evaluations of the Doppler duplex parameters before administering the contrast medium [28–30]. The spectrum is altered because contrast mediums cause an increase in Doppler bandwidth, while the cavitation of microbubbles generates sharp spikes that are superimposed on the Doppler waveform (Fig. 2.22) [25].

Contrast mediums may instead be employed to amplify colour Doppler signals, although a few possible artefacts should be taken into account.

The colour signal amplified by contrast mediums via bolus injection may exceed the limits of the colour-write priority filters that allow the pixel to be assigned a colour or shade of grey. The result is the emergence of so-called blooming, which consists of artefact Doppler signals outside the vessels (Fig. 2.23). Increasing the PRF and reducing the Doppler gain can reduce but not eliminate these artefacts [31].

In addition, decorrelation errors result when a portion of the microbubbles is destroyed within the time that elapses between the first and the second Doppler pulse; this can result in a mosaic of red and blue pixels.

Many interpretation problems generated by these artefacts can be prevented with a colour Doppler study before the administration of a contrast medium.

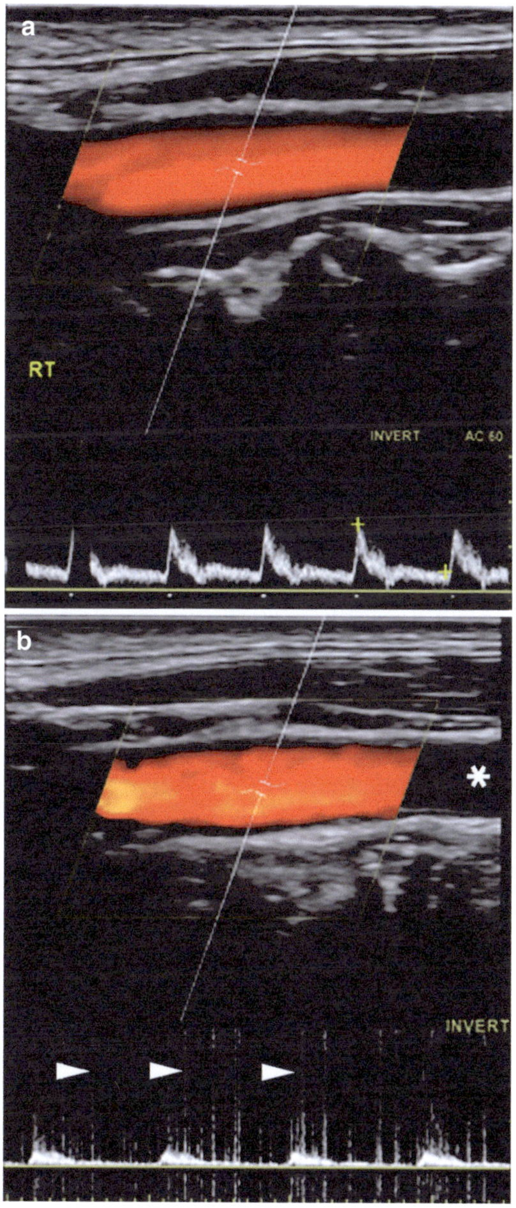

Fig. 2.22 Colour Doppler image of the common carotid artery (**a**) showing a typical common carotid artery waveform. Colour Doppler image after contrast administration (**b**) shows the presence of short high-intensity spikes (arrowheads) projecting over Doppler waveform. Note the presence of microbubbles being visualized as moving echogenic focus on the B-mode image (asterisk). (Reprinted with permission from Fetzer et al. [25])

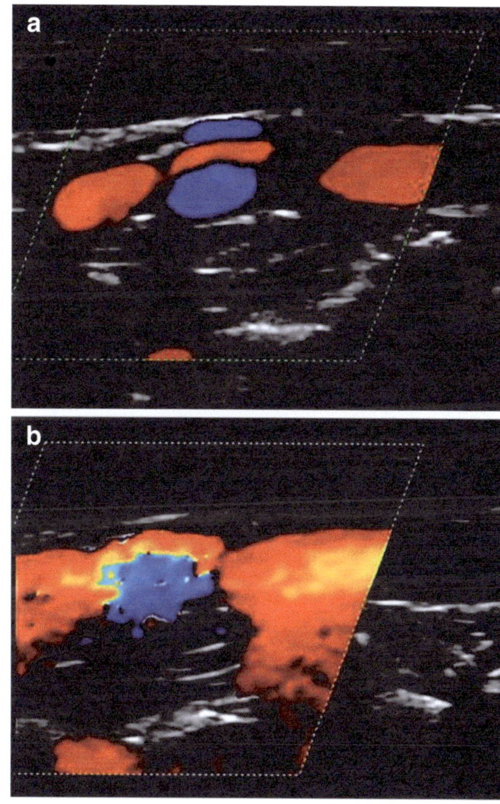

Fig. 2.23 Colour Doppler image of the proximal internal carotid artery before (**a**) and after contrast administration (**b**). Microbubbles significantly increase the colour Doppler signal, causing blooming artefact with colour outside the vascular lumen. This artefact can be decreased by reducing colour gain or setting a higher pulse repetition frequency. Aliasing (as seen in **b**) could be misinterpreted as turbulent flow associated with vessel stenosis. (Reprinted with permission from Fetzer et al. [25])

2.7 Artefacts Related to the Use of Doppler and Colour Doppler

The primary artefacts in the study of vascular flows regard limits in determining their presence or absence in a vessel, the direction and speed of the flow, and the spatial localization of the vessels.

2.7.1 Signal Presence Where No Flow Is Present

The overlap of false colour-Doppler signals in anechoic structures can be misinterpreted as signs of vascular dilatation.

By only over-amplifying signals, electronic noise can be represented inside hypo-anechoic structures and simulate flow signals. Moreover, the movements of organs, like the heartbeat or respiratory cycles, can produce false flow signals when not adequately removed with wall filters.

Nevertheless, vibrations are not always eliminated and can be so numerous and intense (typically near arteriovenous fistulas) as to spread throughout all perivascular tissues, even to the point of making it impossible to display the vessel.

2.7.2 Failure to Represent Real Flows

A too slow flow present in a vessel may not be observed.

Firstly, generally speaking, flows with speeds of less than 3 cm/s are eliminated by wall filters.

Furthermore, the PRF must be set to appropriate values, proportional to the flow velocity, and excessively high values do not allow for the examination of low-speed flows.

Finally, the Doppler signal depends on the angle of insonation, and, for nearly perpendicular angles, Doppler signals may be null.

2.7.3 Determining Flow Direction

Sometimes in tortuous course vessels, both coming and going flows can be sampled; much experience is needed to interpret Doppler signals in these particular anatomical conditions correctly. In other circumstances, an excessive amplification of the signal can lead to the saturation of the receiving system, resulting in specular spectra both above and below the baseline, making it impossible to discern the actual flow direction. In these cases, it is still possible to reduce the artefact spectrum by lowering the gain.

Finally, if the angle of insonation is too large (>60°), the colour signal can appear ambiguous, while the spectral curve may be partly above and partly below the baseline, making the interpretation of flow direction difficult.

2.7.4 Measurement of the Flow Velocity

Sometimes following the course of smaller vessels is complicated, so the angle between the incident beam and direction and flow are difficult to evaluate: in this case, reliable flow speed analyses are not possible. Without the proper attribution of the insonation angle, the examination must be limited to qualitative analysis (presence, direction, arterial or venous flow) or semiquantitative analysis (waveform, systolic-diastolic ratio).

Wall filter settings should be kept at the lowest possible levels, since elevated levels can lead to measurement errors of the slower speeds in the diastolic phase, simulating an increase in vascular resistance. However, in TUS it is often necessary to set wall filters somewhat higher than the 50 and 100 Hz levels generally used in most other anatomical areas. Indeed, the signals of motion transmitted by the respiratory muscles, the heart and great vessels must be eliminated when studying the chest.

2.7.5 Spatial Localization of Vessels

The Doppler signals of the subclavian artery can be duplicated by the mirror effect on the clavicle bone surface.

Similarly, the so-called *ghost carotid* is a reverberation artefact resulting from the vessel walls themselves, which behave as specular reflectors, leading to duplication of the vessel and the respective Doppler spectrum in the tissues below.

When using the hepatic acoustic window, the mirror effect can also duplicate the image of the suprahepatic veins above the pleural line (Fig. 2.24).

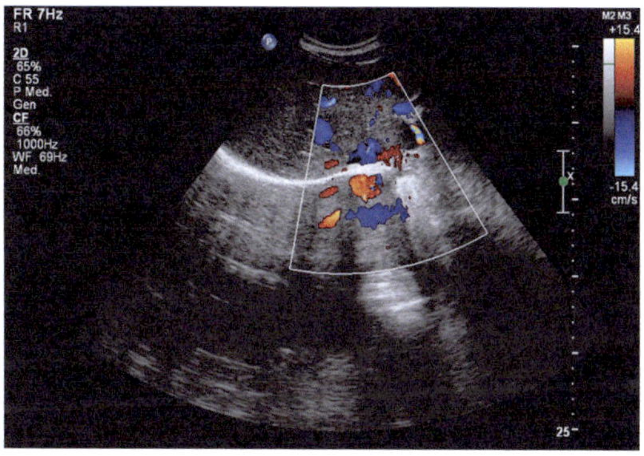

Fig. 2.24 Mirror artefact of the colour suprahepatic veins on the diaphragm with colour Doppler

2.8 Conclusions

Ultrasound artefacts are very common, and, although many of them are undesirable, others provide essential information for interpreting ultrasound images. Some artefacts, such as the A- and B-lines, are even preeminent semiological signs in TUS.

For these reasons, physicians studying TUS must have a thorough understanding of how these artefacts are formed, their meaning, and how to make them more or less visible. Training with simulators allows standardized ultrasound learning and teaching, and even virtual reality could facilitate students to learn how to read the images [32–34].

References

1. Baad M, Feng Lu Z, Reiser I, Paushter D. Clinical significance of US artifacts. Radiographics. 2017;37:1408–23. https://doi.org/10.1148/rg.2017160175.
2. Oliva L. Gli Artefatti in Ecotomografia. Milano; Masson S.p.A. 1989;2.3:5.
3. Wongwaisaywan S, Suwannanon R, Sawatmongkorngul S, Kaewlai R. Emergency thoracic US: the essentials. Radiographics. 2016;36(3):640–59.
4. Dubs-Kunz B. Sonographische Diagnostik von Rippenfrakturen. In: Anderegg A, Despland P, Henner H, editors. Ultraschalldiagnostik, vol. 91. Berlin: Springer; 1992. p. 268–73.
5. Desai A, Parihar R, Mathews J, Akduman L. Occult wooden posterior segment intraocular foreign body. Ophthalmic Surg Lasers Imaging Retina. 2014;45(1):58–61. https://doi.org/10.3928/23258160-20131220-09.
6. Reißig A, Kroegel C. Transthoracic sonography of diffuse parenchymal lung disease: the role of comet tail artifacts. J Ultrasound Med. 2003;22:173–80.
7. Bönhof JA. Ultrasound artifacts—part 1. Ultraschall Med. 2016;37:140–56.
8. Kim HC, Yang DM, Jin W, Ryu JK, Shin HC. Color Doppler twinkling artifacts in various conditions during abdominal and pelvic sonography. J Ultrasound Med. 2010;29(4):621–32.
9. Volpicelli G, Elbarbary M, Blaivas M, et al. International evidence-based recommendations for point-of-care lung ultrasound. Intensive Care Med. 2012;38:577–91. https://doi.org/10.1007/s00134-012-2513-4.
10. Dietrich CF, Mathis G, Blaivas M, et al. Lung B-line artifacts and their use. J Thorac Dis. 2016;8(6):1356–65. https://doi.org/10.21037/jtd.2016.04.55.
11. Soldati G, Smargiassi A, Inchingolo R, Sher S, Neanna R, Valente S, Inchingolo CD, Corbo GM. Lung ultrasonography and vertical artifacts: the shape of air. Respiration. 2015;90:86. https://doi.org/10.1159/000430483.
12. Soldati G, Smargiassi A, Inchingolo R, Sher S, Neanna R, Valente S, Inchingolo CD, Corbo GM. Lung ultrasonography may provide an indirect estimation of lung porosity and airspace geometry. Respiration. 2014;88:458–68.
13. Dietrich CF, Mathis G, Blaivas M, Volpicelli G, Seibel A, Atkinson NS, Cui XW, Mei F, Schreiber-Dietrich D, Yi D. Lung artifacts and their use. Med Ultrason. 2016;18(4):488–99. https://doi.org/10.11152/mu-878.
14. Chiesa AM, Ciccarese F, Gardelli G, Regina UM, Feletti F, Bacchi Reggiani ML, Zompatori M. Sonography of the normal lung: Comparison between young and elderly subjects. J Clin Ultrasound. 2015;43(4):230–34. https://doi.org/10.1002/jcu.22225. Epub 2014 Sep 15.
15. Ciccarese F, Chiesa AM, Feletti F, Vizioli L, Pasquali M, Forti P, Zoli M, Zompatori M. The Senile Lung as a Possible Source of Pitfalls on Chest Ultrasonography and Computed Tomography. Respiration. 2015;90(1):56–62. https://doi.org/10.1159/000430994. Epub 2015 Jun 4.
16. Heng HG, Widmer WR. Appearance of common ultrasound artifacts in conventional vs. spatial compound imaging. Vet Radiol Ultrasound. 2010;51(6):621–7.
17. Schuler A. Image artifacts and pitfalls. In: Mathis G, editor. Chest sonography. Switzerland: Springer; 2017. p. 166.
18. Schuler A. Image artifacts and pittfalls. In: Mathis G, editor. Chest sonography. Switzerland: Springer; 2017. p. 165.
19. Hadzik R, Bombiński P, Brzewski M. Double aorta artifact in sonography - a diagnostic challenge. J Ultrason. 2017;17(68):36–40. https://doi.org/10.15557/JoU.2017.0005. Epub 2017 Mar 31.
20. Schuler A. Image artifacts and pittfalls. In: Mathis G, editor. Chest sonography. Switzerland: Springer; 2017. p. 168.
21. Filipczynkski L, Kujawska T, WÚjcik J. Grey scale imaging of ultrasonic shadow behind rigid, elastic and gaseous spheres in a tissue-like attenuating medium.

In: Tortoli P, Masotti M, editors. Acoustical imaging, vol. 22. New York: Plenum Press; 1996. p. 215–20.
22. Bönhof JA, Linhart P. A pseudolesion of the liver caused by rib cartilage in B-mode ultrasonography. J Ultrasound Med. 1985;4:135–7.
23. Avruch L, Cooperberg PL. The ring-down artifact. J Ultrasound Med. 1985;4(1):21–8.
24. Gill R. The physics and technology of diagnostic ultrasound: a practitioner's guide. Sydney: High Frequency Publishing; 2012.
25. Fetzer DT, Rafailidis V, Peterson C, Grant EG, Sidhu P, Barr RG. Artifacts in contrast—enhanced ultrasound: a pictorial essay. Abdom Radiol (NY). 2018;43(4):977–97. https://doi.org/10.1007/s00261-017-1417-8.
26. Jo PC, et al. Integration of contrast-enhanced US into a multimodality approach to imaging of nodules in a cirrhotic liver: how I do it. Radiology. 2017;282(2):317–31.
27. Dietrich CF, et al. Artifacts and pitfalls in contrast-enhanced ultrasound of the liver. Ultraschall Med. 2014;35(2):108–25.
28. Gutberlet M, et al. Do ultrasonic contrast agents artificially increase maximum Doppler shift? In vivo study of human common carotid arteries. J Ultrasound Med. 1998;17(2):97–102.
29. Terslev L, et al. Doppler ultrasound findings in healthy wrists and finger joints before and after use of two different contrast agents. Ann Rheum Dis. 2005;64(6):824–7.
30. Kono Y, et al. Carotid arteries: contrast-enhanced US angiography–preliminary clinical experience. Radiology. 2004;230(2):561–8.
31. Forsberg F, et al. Artifacts in ultrasonic contrast agent studies. J Ultrasound Med. 1994;13(5):357–65.
32. Heer IM, Middendorf K, Müller-Egloff S, et al. Ultrasound training: the virtual patient. Ultrasound Obstet Gynecol. 2004;24(4):440–4.
33. Jelacic A, Bowdle K, Togashi K, Vonhomeyer P. The use of TEE simulation in teaching basic echocardiography skills to senior anesthesiology residents. J Cardiothorac Vasc Anesth. 2013;27(4):670–5.
34. Feletti F, Mucci V, Aliverti A. Chest ultrasonography in modern day extreme settings: from military setting and natural disasters to space flights and extreme sports. Can Respir J. 2018:9p. https://doi.org/10.1155/2018/8739704.

Technical Execution

3

Francesco Feletti, Bruna Malta,
and Andrea Aliverti

3.1 Introduction

One of the advantages of Thoracic Ultrasound (TUS) is that it can be done with the same equipment commonly used in abdominal or musculoskeletal echography; however, a specific methodological approach that takes into consideration the particular methodical challenges and objectives is advantageous.

After having discussed some indispensable methodological considerations, we will then consider the study of the chest wall and the structures contained in the thorax.

Finally, we will present a few aspects relative to conducting exams in critical patients and newborns.

3.2 General Considerations

The execution of TUS meets two significant physical barriers: alveolar air and the bone structures of the rib cage.

The air almost entirely reflects the ultrasounds, resulting in reverberation objects and posterior "dirty" shadows; bone absorbs nearly all ultrasounds, generating considerable shadows with well-defined outlines (see Tables 3.1 and 3.2).

Both the air and bone prevent the visualization of the deeper-lying structures.

For these reasons, in TUS, the search for more adequate acoustic windows each time for visualizing the examined structures is fundamental.

Furthermore, the selection of the transducer must take into account the fact that the structures examined in TUS can be found at widely varying depths (see Table 3.3).

In choosing the adequate acoustic windows (Fig. 3.1), it must also be considered that the study can be limited by stitches, medication, and scabs resulting from trauma or surgery.

In practical terms, when conducting TUS, it is useful to consider the study of the chest wall and

Table 3.1 Reflection coefficient of critical medium in TUS [1]

Interface	Reflection coefficient (%)
Intercostal muscle/fat	0.69
Intercostal muscle/bone	43
Intercostal muscle/lung	52

F. Feletti (✉)
Dipartimento di Diagnostica per Immagini, Ausl della Romagna, Ospedale S. Maria delle Croci, Ravenna, Italy

Dipartimento di Elettronica, Informazione e Bioingegneria, Politecnico di Milano, Milan, Italy
e-mail: francesco.feletti@auslromagna.it

B. Malta
Dipartimento di Diagnostica per Immagini, Ausl di Ferrara, Ospedale Universitario di Ferrara, Ferrara, Italy
e-mail: mltbrn@unife.it

A. Aliverti
Dipartimento di Elettronica, Informazione e Bioingegneria, Politecnico di Milano, Milan, Italy
e-mail: andrea.aliverti@polimi.it

F. Feletti et al. (eds.), *Thoracic Ultrasound and Integrated Imaging*,
https://doi.org/10.1007/978-3-319-93055-8_3

Table 3.2 Acoustic absorption coefficient of critical medium in TUS [2]

Tissue	Absorption coefficient (dB/cm) at 1 MHz
Muscle	2
Fat	0.6
Bone	20
Air	35

Table 3.3 Frequency/depth relation of ultrasound spread

Examined structure	Depth (cm)	Frequency (MHz)
Skin, subcutaneous tissue, breast	1–2	<10
Thickness of the chest wall	2–4	7–10
Pleura and lung	6–8	5–7
Mediastinum (adults)	10–20	<5

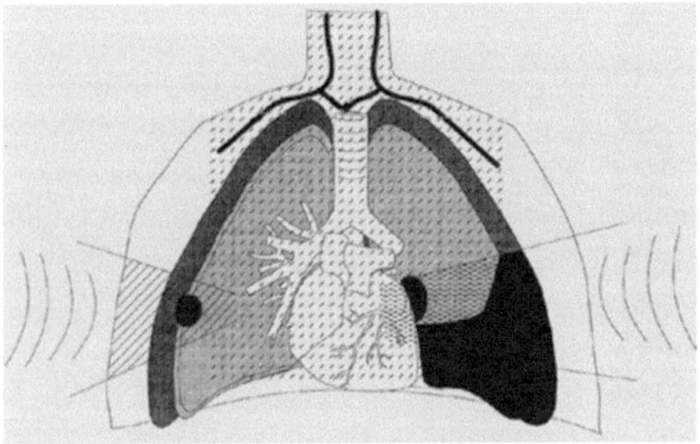

Fig. 3.1 Structures and pathological changes accessible to sonography

the structures contained within the rib cage separately and to distinguish the following regions topographically: apical, anterolateral, dorsal, and basal.

3.3 Study of the Chest Wall

Linear probes at high frequency (5–15 MHz) are generally preferred when the chest wall is examined.

It is above all necessary to recognize anatomical landmarks: ribs, costal cartilages, pleura, subcutaneous tissue, and muscle planes.

The study makes use of longitudinal and transversal scans aimed at clinical landmarks.

Dynamic evaluations can also be useful, for example, in studying traumatic muscular lesions; scans in phases of relaxation and contraction can be useful.

In practical terms, it is useful to outline schematically the structures of interest in the various topographical regions considered.

3.3.1 Apical Region

This region extends back to the clavicle and is dorsally circumscribed by the first rib; it is crossed by the brachial plexus and is covered by various muscles including the scalene, trapezius, and levator scapulae.

The best resolution for studying the brachial plexus is found through linear probes at high frequency (12–15 MHz) [3].

Colour and power Doppler help distinguish vascular structures.

The probe should be moved laterally starting from the base of the neck, and the principal landmarks are represented by the trapezius muscle and the middle and anterior scalene muscles.

It is precisely in the space between these muscles that the branches of the brachial plexus start and are identifiable with a hypoechoic appearance on the sides of the neck through supraclavicular scans (Fig. 3.2a–c).

Nerves can be followed along the way, parallel to the axillary artery (Fig. 3.3a, b), before reaching the axilla (Fig. 3.4a, b), through subclavian scans between the clavicle and the first rib.

Studying the branches of the brachial plexus is useful for patients with trauma (including childbirth trauma), for ultrasound-guided anaesthesia during upper limb interventions [4], for surgical procedures with supraclavicular access or for detecting possible infiltration in Pancoast tumours [5].

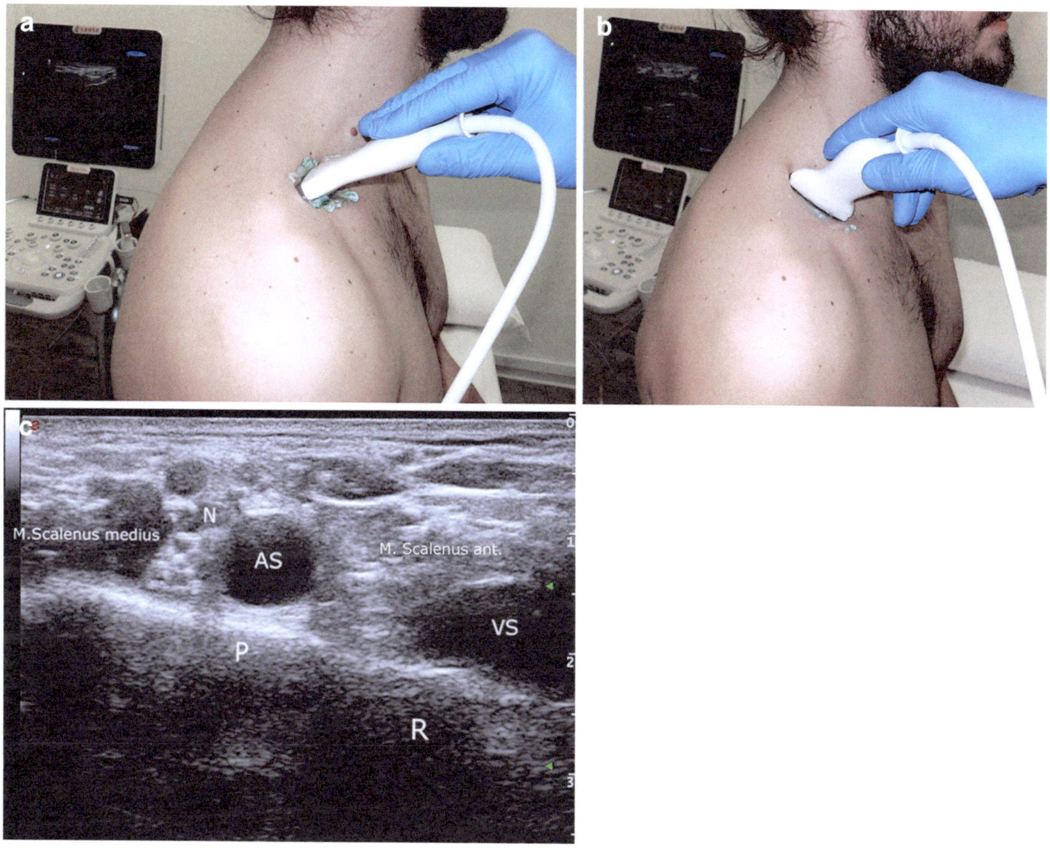

Fig. 3.2 Study of the supraclavicular region. (**a**) Horizontal scan with a linear probe placed at the base of the neck, sideways. (**b**) Sagittal scan with the linear probe placed at the base of the neck, sideways. (**c**) Sagittal scan with the linear probe, sonographic image: *AS* a. subclavia, *VS* v. subclavia, *R* rib, *P* pleura, *N* branches of brachial plexus

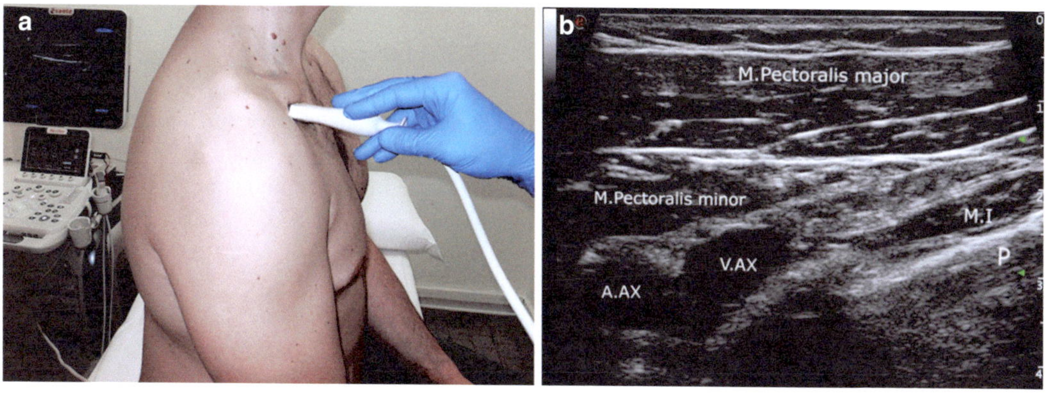

Fig. 3.3 (**a**) Subclavian transverse scan with a linear probe placed along the midclavicular line. (**b**) Corresponding sonographic image: *A. AX a. axillaris*, *V. AX* v. axillaris, *MI* m. intercostalis, *P* pleura

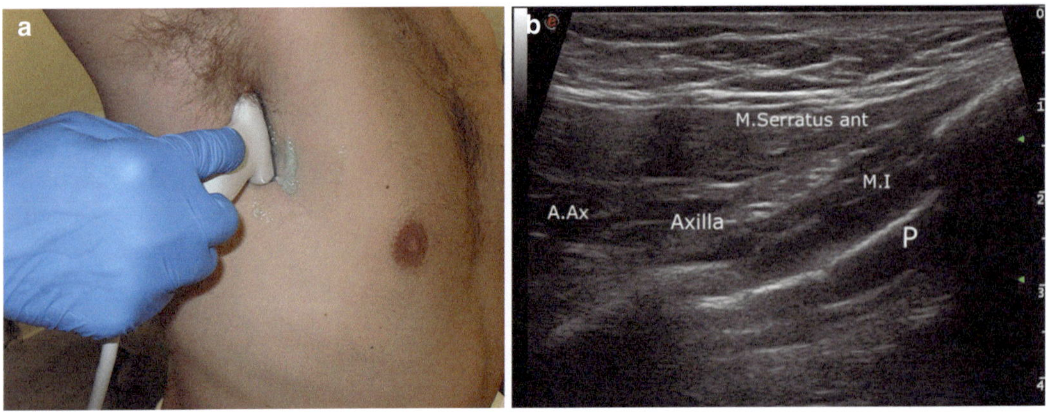

Fig. 3.4 (**a**) Longitudinal scan with a linear probe in the armpit. (**b**) Corresponding sonographic image: *A. AX a. axillaris*, *M.I* m. intercostalis; *P* pleura

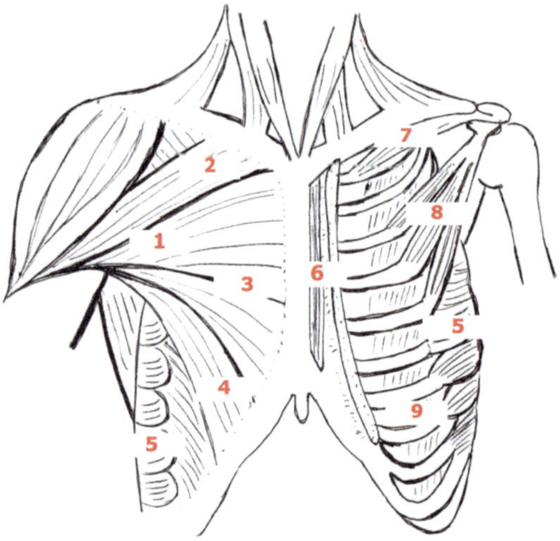

Fig. 3.5 Anatomical relations of the anterolateral chest wall muscles: (1) Pectoralis major and corresponding parts (2–4); (2) Pars clavicularis; (3) Pars sternocostalis; (4) Pars abdominalis; (5) Serratus anterior; (6) Sternalis muscle; (7) Subclavius; (8) Pectoralis minor; (9) Intercostales externi muscles. Figure adapted from [6]

3.3.2 Anterolateral Region

The pectoralis major muscle presents an ample medical insertion that extends from the medial of the front edge of the clavicle to the front surface of the sternum and from the first seven costal cartilages to the aponeurosis of the rectus muscles of the abdomen and external oblique muscle (Fig. 3.5).

It is laterally inserted with a single tendon on the crest of the greater tubercle of the humerus [7].

The pectoralis minor muscle starts from the external surfaces of the third to the fifth rib and is inserted in the coracoid process of the scapula.

The subclavian muscle runs from the bottom side of the clavicle to the first rib.

The serratus muscle extends from the outer surfaces of the first to the tenth rib up to the front surface of the vertebral edge of the scapula.

Intercostal muscles are arranged diagonally from the lower profile to the upper profile of the ribs.

The transverse thoracic muscle fits from the fourth to the sixth costal cartilage up to the posterior surface of the xiphoid process [8].

3.3.3 Dorsal Region

The shoulder blades cover the intercostal muscles and are stabilized by rhomboid muscles, which are inserted on the spinous processes of the thoracic vertebrae (Fig. 3.6).

3.3.4 Basal Region

The diaphragmatic dome separates the chest cavity from the abdominal cavity; it is inserted posteriorly through the pillars on the front surface of the soma of L1 and L2 and at the front of the inner surface of the last six ribs and the xiphoid process of the sternum (Fig. 3.7).

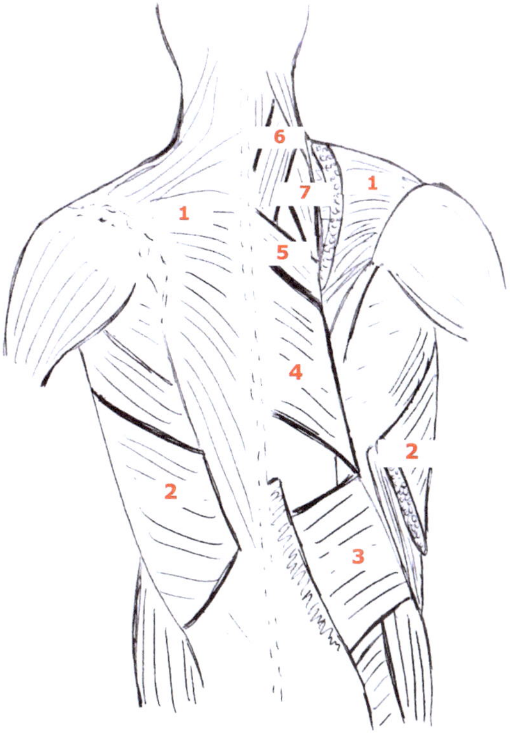

Fig. 3.6 Anatomy of the dorsal region of the chest wall: (1) Trapezius; (2) Latissimus dorsi; (3) Serratus posterior inferior; (4) Rhomboid major; (5) Rhomboideus minor; (6) Splenius capitis; (7) Levator scapulae. Figure adapted from [9]

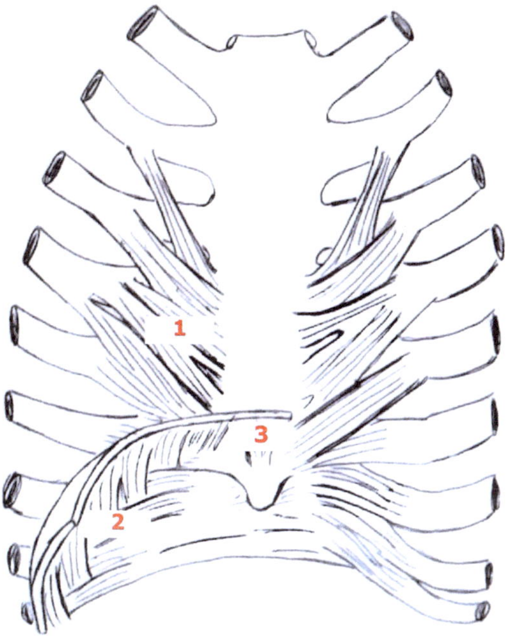

Fig. 3.7 Anatomy of the basal region of the chest wall: (1) Transversus thoracis muscle; (2) Pars costalis diaphragm; (3) Pars sternalis diaphragm. Figure adapted from [10]

In TUS, it is always necessary to interpret the presence of elements in the wall thickness that limit the penetration of the beam.

These may include calcifications that can indicate myositis ossificans or are neoplastic and must not be confused with calcifications of the costal cartilages.

Air in the wall thickness can be a sign of subcutaneous emphysema or abscesses.

Objects determined by subcutaneous emphysema (Line E, consult the next chapter) determine an acoustic barrier that masks the view of the ribs.

TUS is often used to answer specific diagnostic questions [11, 12], and often a targeted approach is sufficient, in particular, when the chest wall is studied.

However, when the study concerns the pleura or the lung, a more systematic approach may be useful.

3.4 Studying the Structures Contained in the Thorax

To optimize penetration depth in order to study the pleura and the lungs, generally, a convex transducer with frequencies 3.5–5 MHz is used.

Sometimes however it is useful to turn to aimed scans with linear probes at higher frequencies, above all if it is necessary to evaluate lung sliding in order to exclude a pneumothorax to examine in greater detail the mantle zone of the lung.

Integrating studies and scans using a linear probe can show small echogenic differences in peripheral portions of a pathological process, for example, small cystic components or fluid bronchogram in the context of pulmonary condensation.

A systematic study generally requires starting from the top, moving toward the bottom and in a ventral-dorsal direction: first parasternal and along the midclavicular line, then along the axillary and finally interscapular lines.

Having to overcome the ribs and having to scan at least two orthogonal planes, generally, the intercostal planes, perpendicular to the rib axis, are used.

Generally, patient cooperation is asked; patients should inhale and exhale deeply, holding their breath or coughing when required, for example, to assess lung sliding [13].

In order to identify the best acoustic windows and the adequate positioning of the patient, it can be useful to turn again to the topographic distinctions already noted.

3.4.1 Apical Region

This study can begin in the supine position.

Subsequently, with the patient seated, supraclavicular scans (Fig. 3.8a) allow for the exploration of the pulmonary apexes, while suprasternal access (Fig. 3.8b) allows for the exploration of the anterior mediastinum.

3.4.2 Anterolateral Region

This region can be evaluated in the supine position, but the study of the structures along the axillary line (Figs. 3.9a–c and 3.10a, b) can be aided

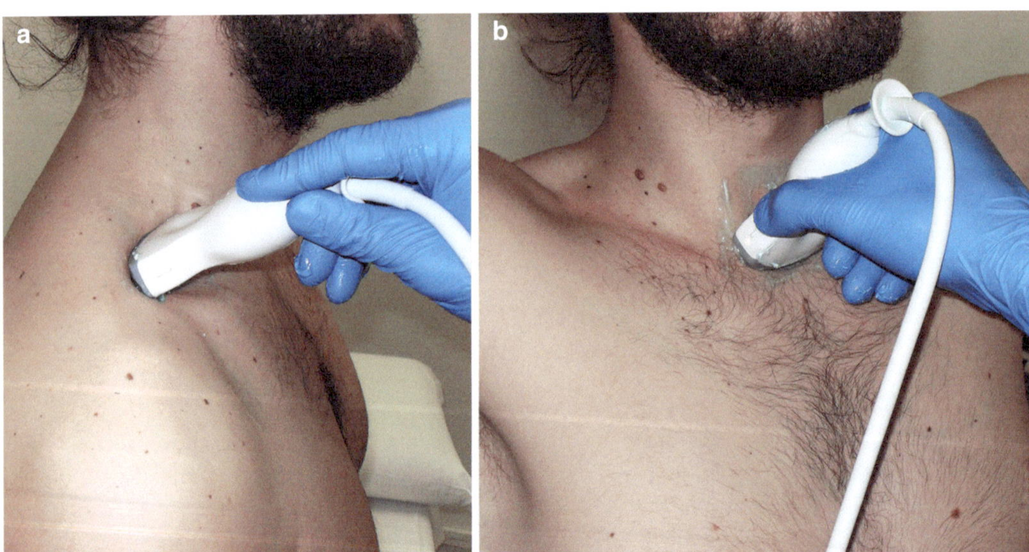

Fig. 3.8 (**a**) Supraclavicular scan for the study of lung apices. (**b**) Parasternal scan for the study of the anterior mediastinum

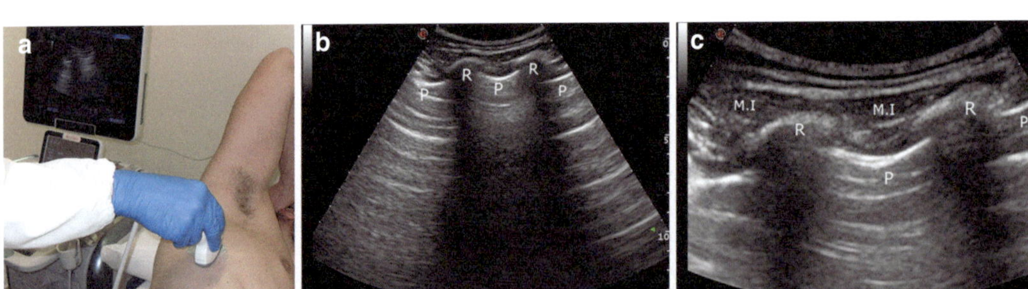

Fig. 3.9 (**a**) Longitudinal scan, along with the axillary line (**a**) and corresponding sonographic images (**b**, **c**). (**b**) The setting for the study of the chest wall. (**c**) Setting for the study of the lung

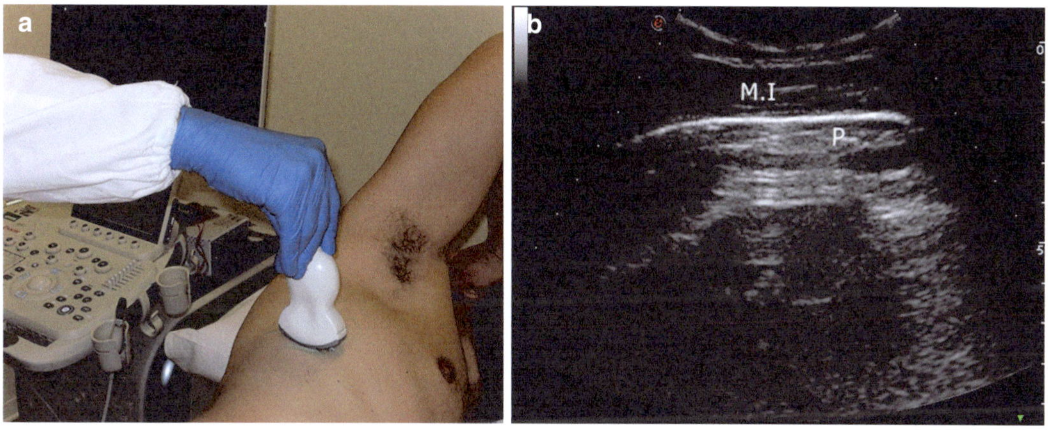

Fig. 3.10 (**a**) Transverse scan along the axillary line. (**b**) Corresponding sonographic image

by placing the patient in the lateral decubitus position.

The patient may also be asked to sit, with their arms raised and hands resting on the neck, to maximize intercostal spaces.

3.4.3 Dorsal Region

This region is studied in lateral and prone positions.

In the evaluation of subscapular structures, the patient is usually asked to extend the arm and to embrace the contralateral shoulder.

In asking the patient to assume a hyperkyphosis posture, it is possible to expand the intercostal acoustic windows (Fig. 3.11).

3.4.4 Basal Region

The diaphragmatic surface can be evaluated in the supine position with a variable degree of inclination to one side.

The transhepatic or trans-splenic subcostal approach allows for the viewing of the diaphragmatic surface of the lung (Fig. 3.12a, b).

In addition, a sitting position can be adopted, especially useful in searching for pleural effusion, particularly if in small quantities, usually found in the posterior costophrenic recess.

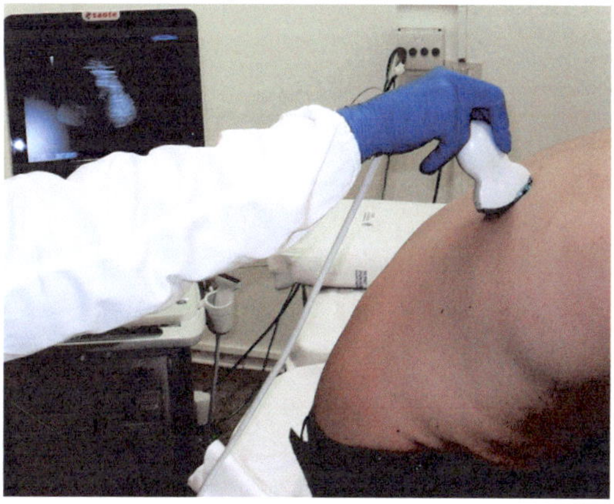

Fig. 3.11 Subscapularis scan while the patient is sitting in kyphosis position

Cranially tilting the probe around the subxiphoid (Figs. 3.13a, b and 3.14a, b), the pericardium can be evaluated in order to identify any possible spilling; and this scan should always be conducted in traumatized patients.

3.5 Studying Critical Patients

Sometimes it is impossible or ill-advisable to move the patient, for example, in polytraumatic cases, and scans must be limited to those possible with the patient in the supine position. It must be considered that, since air tends to come about in

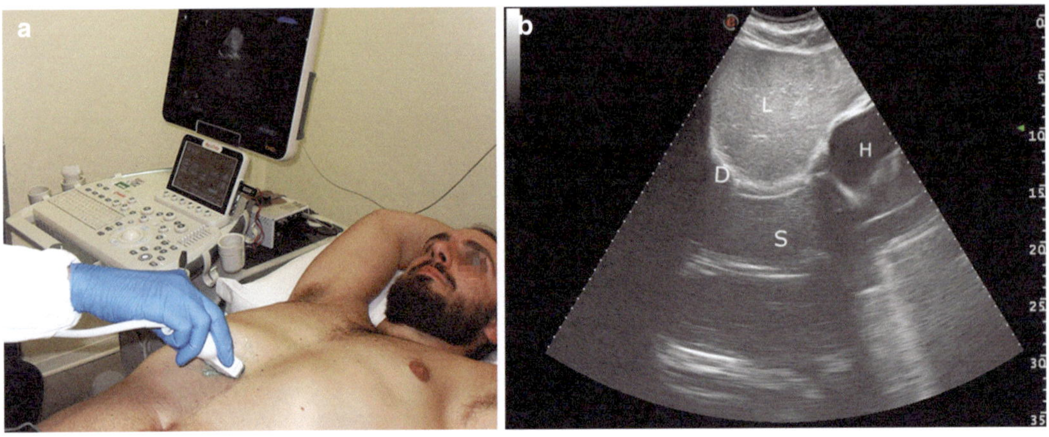

Fig. 3.12 (**a**) Subcostal transhepatic scan to visualize the base of the lung. Corresponding sonographic image: *L* liver, *D* diaphragm, *S* reflection of the liver above the diaphragm, *H* heart

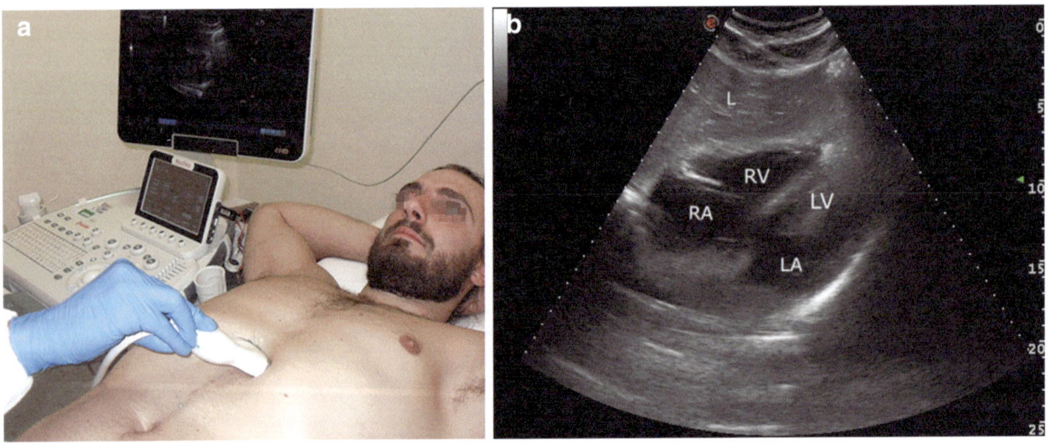

Fig. 3.13 (**a**) Subxiphoid scan to identify possible pericardial effusions. Corresponding sonographic image: *RA* right atrium, *RV* right ventricle, *LA* left atrium, *LV* left ventricle, *L* liver

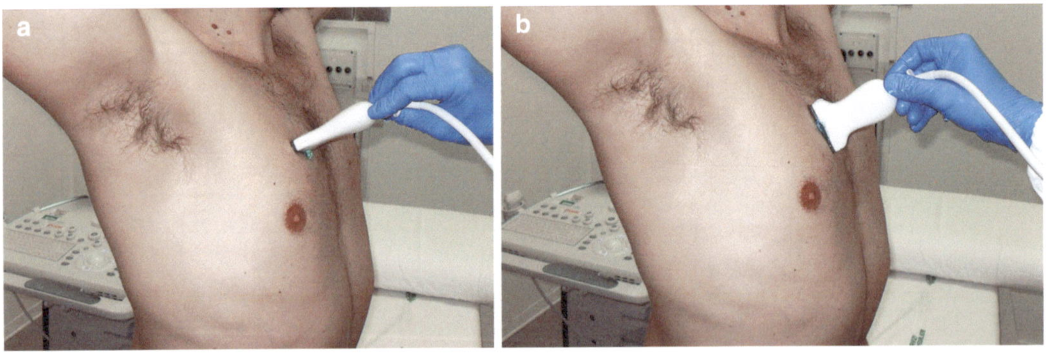

Fig. 3.14 Transverse (**a**) and longitudinal (**b**) parasternal scan

Trendelenburg positions when patients are in the supine position, small pneumothoraxes can come about in parasternal and juxta-cardiac locations, which are easily evaluated with TUS without moving the patient.

In studying inpatients in intensive care units, if clinical conditions allow, it may be useful to enlist the help of qualified personnel to perform mobilization manoeuvres that consent for TUS scans in lateral or oblique decubitus, to reach the posterior zones of the lungs and pleura.

3.6 Studying the Lungs in Newborns

In newborn and premature patients, when a dedicated pediatric probe at high frequencies (5–8 MHz) is not available, a linear probe at high frequencies (5–10 MHz) similar to that used for the thoracic wall and adult peripheral lung regions can be used.

This allows for an optimal examination of the chest cavity, given the reduced volume to explore.

A convex probe can still be used for a quantitative estimation of a massive pleural effusion.

3.7 TUS Training Strategies

In its diverse applications, TUS is a relatively simple method and a low learning curve with respect to ultrasound techniques for other anatomical areas [14, 15].

It should, however, be used only by doctors who have undergone proper theoretical and practical training in ultrasound semiotics for correctly interpreting TUS patterns, including not only real images but also artificial ones like Line A and Line B [14–17].

The use of a simulated environment and animal and artificial or hybrid manikins can be integrated into a didactic course to aid in the learning of both TUS and US-guided invasive procedures [18–21] (Fig. 3.15).

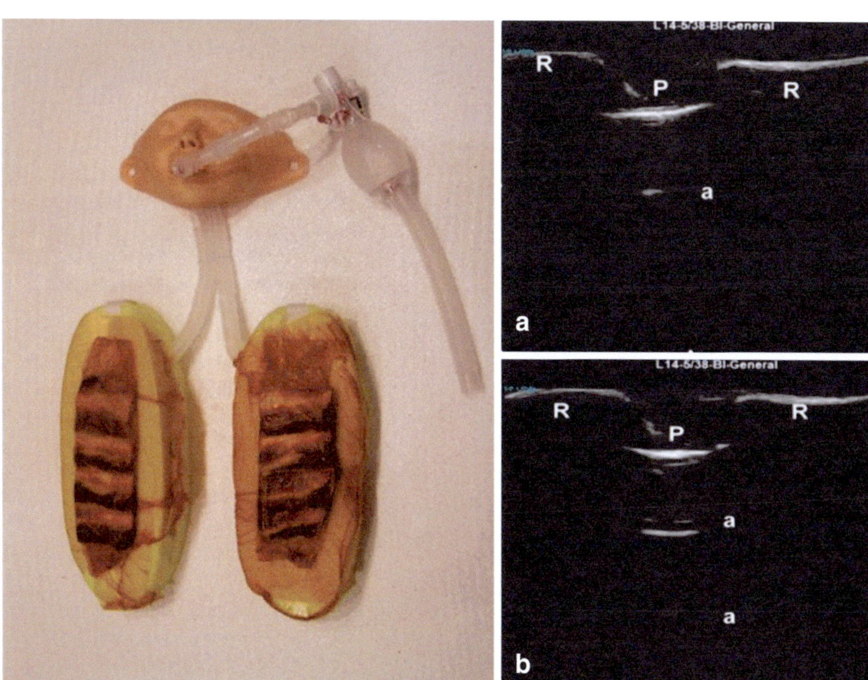

Fig. 3.15 The hybrid simulation model of the lung (foams with the attached pig rib cages wrapped in Ioban™ dressing). (**a**) An intercostal sonogram of the foam. *R:* rib, *P:* pleura, *a:* A line. (**b**): The rib cage elevated above the foam (= pneumothorax). Reprinted with permission from [20]

In fact, with these tools, it is possible to reproduce normal and pathological TUS findings accurately and allows for controlled, supervised learning with immediate feedback.

Training for US-guided manoeuvres, the use of a simulated environment and manikins allows students to acquire hand-eye coordination skills without risk as well as learning to quickly recognize thoracic anatomy and immediately identify complications such as pneumothorax [22].

3.8 Conclusions

The probe, positioning of the patient, and the acoustic window must be chosen each time based on clinical questions.

In practical terms, when performing TUS, it is useful to topographically distinguish the following regions: apical, anterolateral, dorsal, and basal.

Particular considerations can be valid in critical patients and in studying newborns, due to the reduced mobility of the patient and for the reduced dimensions of the thorax, respectively.

References

1. Garagnani M, Lamberti C. Ecografia: Principi fisici e sviluppi tecnologici. Modena: Athena Audiovisuals; 2003.
2. Angiolucci G. Cosa dobbiamo conoscere degli ultrasuoni nella pratica clinica: come si forma l'immagine ecografica e l'artefatto. Ultrasuoni nel Castello di Gargonza, Arezzo, 30 May–3 June 2012.
3. O'Neill J, Dobranowski J. Musculoskeletal ultrasound: anatomy and technique the brachial plexus, vol. 13. Berlin: Springer; 2008. p. 314.
4. Vogel B. Ultrasonographic detection and guided biopsy of thoracic osteolysis. Chest. 1993;104(4):1003–5.
5. Mathis G. Chest sonography. Berlin: Springer; 2008. p. 6.
6. Feneis H. Testo e atlante di anatomia con nomenclatura internazionale. Rome: Verduci; 1989. p. 85. fig.A.
7. Franzi AT. Commento ragionato all'atlante di anatomia umana di Frank H. Netter. Ciba Edizioni; 1995. p. 174–6.
8. Galletti S, Galletti R, Sperandeo M, Trovato G. Patologie della gabbia toracica in ecografia toracica. Edra, Milano: Diagnosi e tecniche interventistiche; 2015. p. 29.
9. Feneis H. Testo e atlante di anatomia con nomenclatura internazionale. Rome: Verduci; 1989. p. 75. fig.A.
10. Feneis H. Testo e atlante di anatomia con nomenclatura internazionale. Berlin: Verduci; 1989. p. 85. fig.C.
11. Lichtenstein D. Lung ultrasound in acute respiratory failure an introduction to the BLUE-protocol. Minerva Anestesiol. 2009;75(5):313–7.
12. Lichtenstein DA. BLUE-protocol and FALLS-protocol: two applications of lung ultrasound in the critically ill. Chest. 2015;147(6):1659–70.
13. Mathis G. Chest sonography. Berlin: Springer; 2008. p. 4.
14. Gargani L, Volpicelli G. How I do it: lung ultrasound. Cardiovasc Ultrasound. 2014;12:25.
15. Gardelli G, Feletti F, Gamberini E, Bonarelli S, Nanni A, Mughetti M. Using sonography to assess lung recruitment in patients with acute respiratory distress syndrome. Emerg Radiol. 2009;16(3):219–21.
16. Gardelli G, Feletti F, Nanni A, Mughetti M, Piraccini A, Zompatori M. Chest ultrasonography in the ICU. Respir Care. 2012;57(5):773–81.
17. Zanforlin A, Giannuzzi R, Nardini S, et al. The role of chest ultrasonography in the management of respiratory diseases: document I. Multidiscip Respir Med. 2013;8(1):54.
18. Rippey J, Gawthrope I. Creating thoracic phantoms for diagnostic and procedural ultrasound training. Aust J Ultrasound Med. 2012;15(2):43–54.
19. Do HH, Lee S. A low-cost training phantom for lung ultrasonography. Chest. 2016;150(6):1417–9.
20. Wojtczak JA. Models to teach lung sonopathology and ultrasound-guided thoracentesis. J Ultrason. 2014;14(59):367–70.
21. Feletti F, Mucci V, Aliverti A. Chest ultrasonography in modern day extreme settings: from military setting and natural disasters to space flights and extreme sports. Can Respir J. 2018: 9p. https://doi.org/10.1155/2018/8739704.
22. Wrightson JM, Fysh E, Maskell NA, Lee YC. Risk reduction in pleural procedures: sonography, simulation and supervision. Curr Opin Pulm Med. 2010;16(4):340–50.

Part II

Semeiotics and Integrated Imaging

4 Lung Consolidation

Gebhard Mathis

4.1 Inflammatory Consolidations in the Lung

4.1.1 Pneumonia

Pneumonia can be verified by US immediately after clinical investigation. The value of chest sonography in pneumonia lies in the assessment of accompanying pleural fluid, timely detection of abscess formation, sonography-guided collection of pathogens, and controls particularly in pregnant women and children.

4.1.2 Sonomorphology of Pneumonia

A number of sonomorphological criteria are characteristic for pneumonic infiltrations. They are of varying intensity in the course of disease.

Echotexture: In the early congestive stage of disease, the echotexture of the pneumonic lung is similar to that of the liver or tissue. Pneumonia shows a bizarre configuration and is rarely segmented in shape like pulmonary infarction or rounded like carcinomas and metastases. Pneumonia is characterized by an irregular, serrated, and somewhat blurred margin.

G. Mathis (✉)
Praxis for Internal Medicine, Rankweil, Austria
e-mail: gebhard.mathis@cable.vol.at

Bronchoaerogram: A marked tree-shaped bronchoaerogram with ramifications was found in 70–87% of the cases [1–6]. A large number of lenticular echo reflections measuring a few millimeters in size are frequently observed up to the pleura (Fig. 4.1). During all stages of this disease, the bronchoaerogram is more pronounced than in cases of pulmonary embolism [7]. In the curative phase of pneumonia, the hyperechoic sections increase, and the depicted lesion becomes smaller on the sonogram (Fig. 4.2, [7]). Viral pneumonias are often less ventilated and/or reveal less pronounced bronchoaerograms. These are smaller and more compact than bacterial pneumonia and

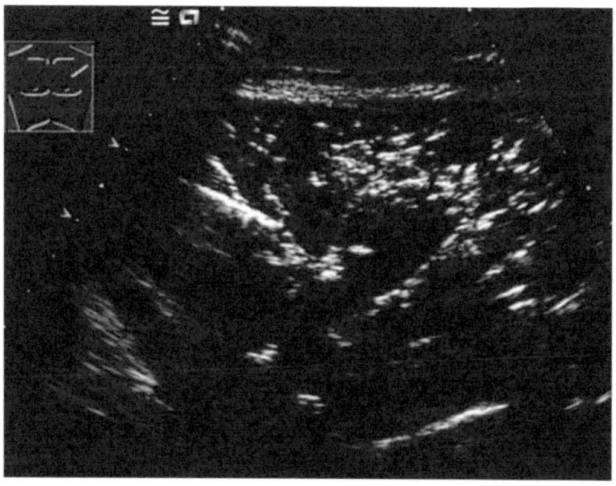

Fig. 4.1 A 68-year-old severely ill man with clinical signs of acute pneumonia. In the upper lobe of the lung on the left side, there is a liver-like consolidation with a bronchoaerogram

F. Feletti et al. (eds.), *Thoracic Ultrasound and Integrated Imaging*,
https://doi.org/10.1007/978-3-319-93055-8_4

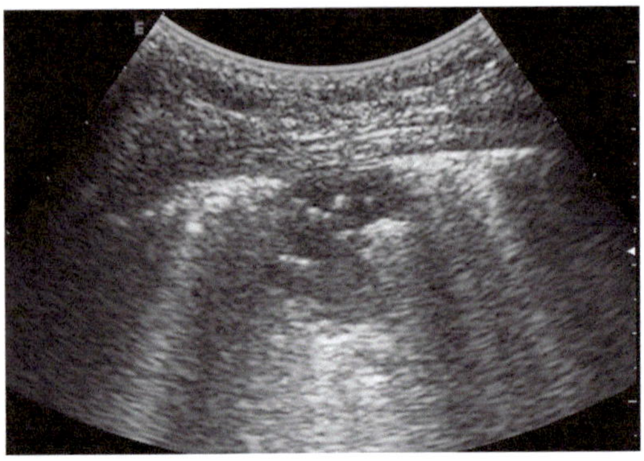

Fig. 4.2 Pneumonia after H1N1 influenza. Small bronchoaerograms up to the pleura. Some B-lines at the margin

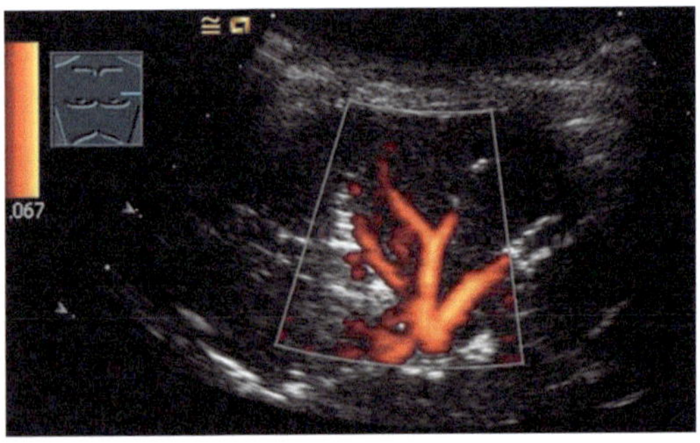

Fig. 4.3 On color-coded duplex sonography, pneumonia is seen as an accentuated, regular pattern of circulation

Table 4.1 Sonomorphology of pneumonia

• Liver- or tissue-like in the early stage
• Bronchoaerogram
• Lentil-shaped air trappings
• Fluid bronchogram (poststenotic?)
• Blurred or serrated margins
• Reverberation echoes at the margin
• Hypoechoic to anechoic in the presence of abscess
• Regular vascularization
• Early and intensive enhancement in CEUS

may resemble large pulmonary infarctions. In contrast to pulmonary infarctions, they are strongly perfused with blood (Fig. 4.3). The air bronchogram moves dynamically in a breath-dependent manner. This is an important difference between an air bronchogram and obstructive atelectasis: the latter is accompanied by a less prominent air bronchogram and is static [8].

Fluid bronchogram: The fluid bronchogram is marked by anechoic tubular structures along the bronchial tree. The bronchial wall is echogenic and the fluid in the segmental bronchi is hypoechoic. The reflexes around the bronchi are wider than those along vessel walls. Given good resolution, the bronchial walls are ribbed, and the vessel walls are smooth; therefore, tubular structures can be easily classified on B-mode image. In the case of doubt, color-coded duplex sonography helps to distinguish between vessels and bronchi. The fluid bronchogram is seen in approximately 8% of patients with pneumonia and develops in the early phase of the disease as a result of bronchial secretion owing to bronchial obstruction. A persistent fluid bronchogram always raises suspicion of poststenotic pneumonia and is an indication for bronchoscopic investigation 3, 7] (Table 4.1).

Vascularization: On color-coded duplex sonography, pneumonia has a typical appearance. Circulation is uniformly increased and ramified, and the vessels run a normal course. In fact, circulation is increased in the entire infiltrate up to beneath the pleura (Figs. 4.3 and 4.4). This can help to differentiate pneumonia from pulmonary infarctions that have poor or no blood flow or even from tumors with an irregular circulation pattern. Carcinomas are strongly vascularized in their margins. Owing to neovascularization, vessels in the margins of carcinomas are characterized by a typical corkscrew pattern [1, 7]. On contrast-enhanced ultrasound (CEUS), pneumonias are rapidly enriched with contrast medium and achieve intensive saturation after just 4–10 s. CEUS can differentiate especially small subpleural consolidations, if they are inflammatory or embolic [9, 10].

On contrast-enhanced ultrasound, pneumonias are rapidly enriched with contrast medium and achieve intensive saturation after just 4–10 s (Fig. 4.5, [9, 10]).

Parapneumonic effusion: Parapneumonic fluid accumulations can be imaged better on ultrasound than on conventional X-rays (55% versus 25%). These must be discovered and their course monitored in order to initiate invasive therapy in terms of puncture or video-assisted thoracoscopy on a timely basis ([1, 3]; Fig. 4.6).

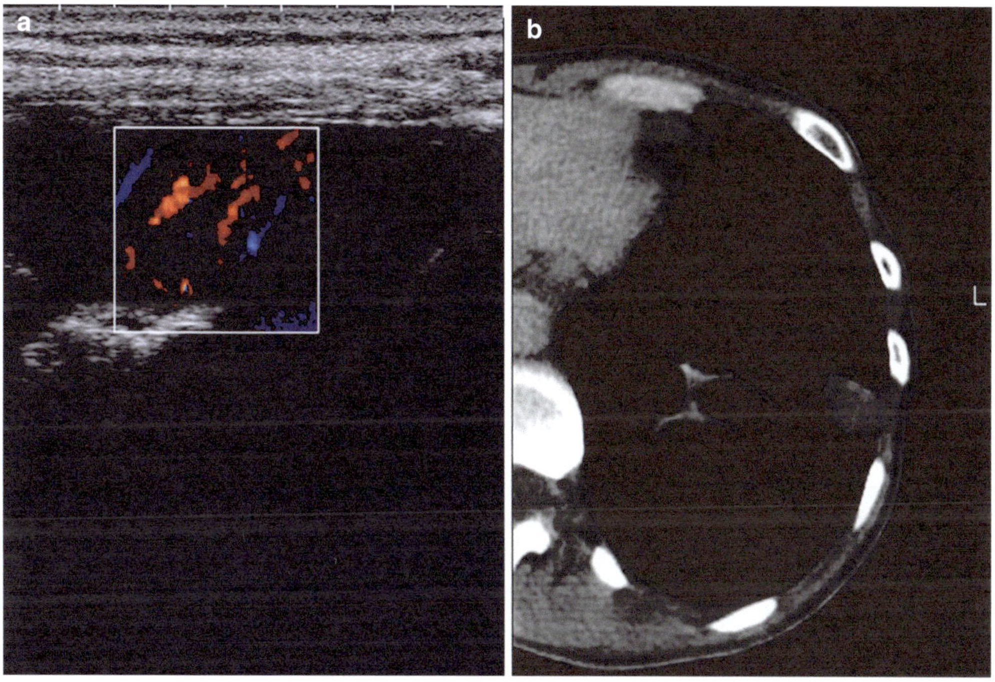

Fig. 4.4 A 52-year-old woman with pain on inspiration, fever, and hemoptysis. (**a**) Sonography reveals a consolidation with less bronchoaerogram but regular vascularization. (**b**) Corresponding CT. Final diagnosis: viral pneumonia

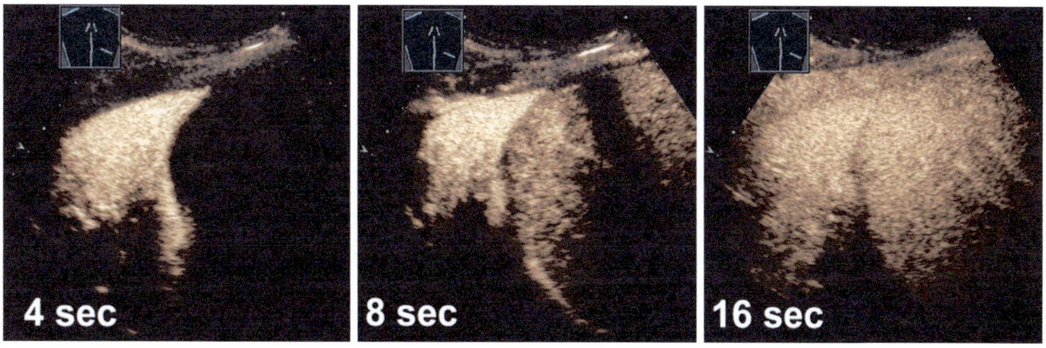

Fig. 4.5 Contrast-enhanced ultrasound (CEUS) of pneumonia. Early and intensive enhancement caused by pulmonary artery supply

Abscess formation: Bacterial pneumonias tend to liquefy and form abscesses. Pulmonary abscesses are depicted as round or oval, mostly echo-free lesions. This is the case in approximately 6% of patients with lobar pneumonia. Sonography more commonly reveals microabscesses (Fig. 4.7, [7, 11, 12]). Considering the scarce quantity of material for bacteriological investigation obtained from the sputum or from bronchial lavage, it is useful to take a specimen for the detection of pathogens by means of sonography-guided aspiration. Lung abscess drainage may be performed under sonographic or computed tomography visual monitoring. The risk of a pneumothorax is minimized when one passes through the chest wall obliquely, in a regular fashion, and enters the lung at the site where the abscess is closest to the pleura. The risk of a dreaded bronchopleural fistula is minimized when the correct approach is used, i.e., when one only traverses the homogeneous infiltrate and avoids ventilated areas [11, 13].

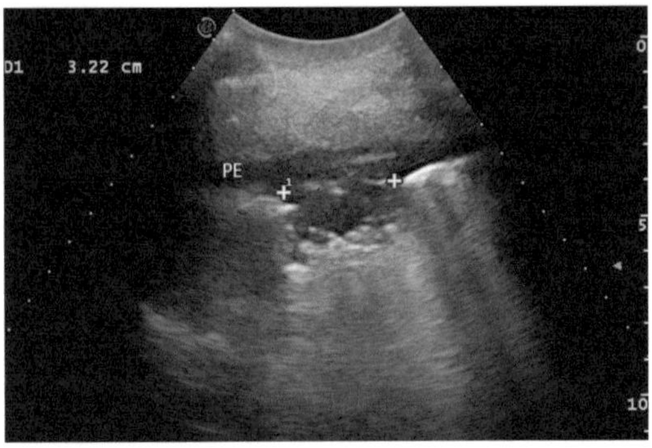

Fig. 4.6 Parapneumonic effusion (PE). Pneumonia (+-+). Remission observed by ultrasound

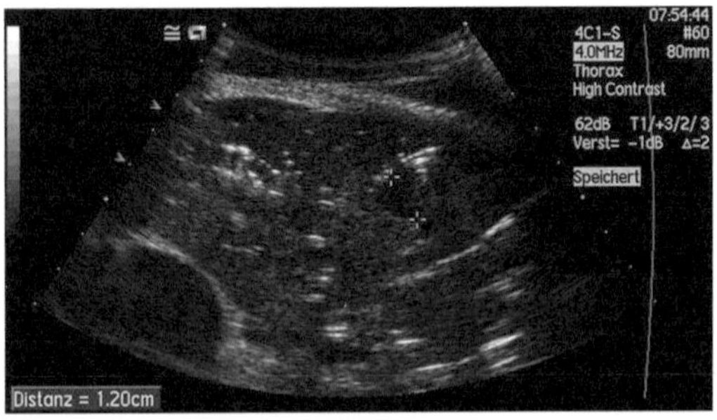

Fig. 4.7 Abscess in a patient with persistent fever (+-+). Sonography-guided aspiration showed a surprisingly large number of tubercle bacilli

4.1.3 Diagnostic Value

In eight meta-analyses of lung ultrasound in community-acquired pneumonia, overall sensitivity (85–97%) and specificity (80–96%) are very high and accuracy is more than 90% [14–16]. Therefore, lung ultrasound is able to rule in pneumonia but not to rule it out.

In cases of persistent clinical suspicion of pneumonia, further radiological investigations will be necessary. However, after the clinical investigation and after obtaining the required laboratory data concerning inflammatory parameters, immediate antibiotic treatment can be initiated almost everywhere: at the medical office, the emergency department, the intensive care unit, and in stroke patients among others [14, 17]. In multimorbid patients admitted to an acute geriatric ward, lung ultrasound (LUS) was more accurate than CXR for the diagnosis of pneumonia, particularly in those with frailty [18]. Bedside chest ultrasound is a reliable tool for the diagnosis of pneumonia in the emergency department, probably being superior to chest X-ray in this setting. It is likely that its wider use will allow a faster diagnosis, conducive to a more appropriate and timely therapy [19].

4.1.4 Tuberculosis

In pulmonary tuberculosis, ultrasonography is helpful in detecting pleural effusions, subpleural consolidations, and pneumonic infiltrates. Ultrasound-guided diagnostic punctures are meaningful in this setting. Chest X-rays and computed tomography are indispensable to obtain an overview of the condition [7, 20, 21]. Tuberculotic lung lesions may be seen on sonography as rounded or irregular structures of relatively homogeneous texture. Depending on the size of the lesion, these infiltrates may also be accompanied by air trappings as in pneumonia. Nodular dissemination, as in miliary tuberculosis, is visualized as multiple subpleural nodes measuring a few millimeters in size. Colliquations can be imaged well, but air in cavities might be a disturbing factor and might limit visualization. Even very small quantities of the specific pleural effusion are seen. Pleural thickening may also be revealed. A patient's response to tuberculostatic therapy can be monitored well with sonography, especially in cases of pleural and subpleural tuberculosis lesions (Fig. 4.8).

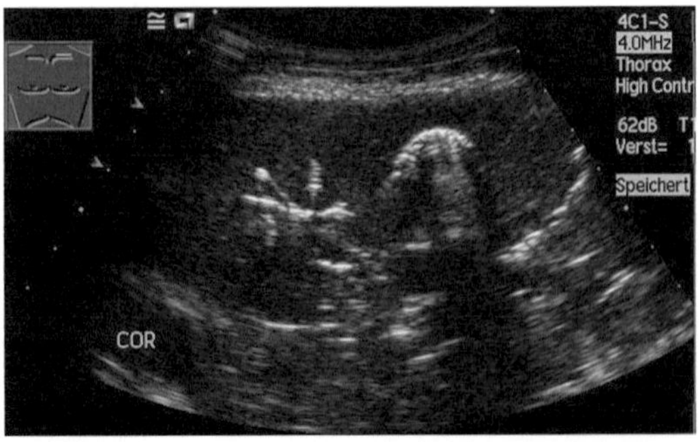

Fig. 4.8 Tuberculosis: pneumonia-like consolidation with an echogen cavern, typical for tuberculosis. Indicated by US-guided biopsy

4.1.5 Interstitial Lung Disease

Technically sonography is entirely unsuitable to diagnose diseases of the lung framework. However, that such diseases are frequently accompanied by pleuritis; the latter being better visualized by sonography than by other imaging procedures, through the following signs:

- minimal pleural effusions
- fragmented pleura with several B-lines
- subpleural consolidations (Fig. 4.9)

The value of the method lies in the detection of a grave condition and in steering the diagnostician's attention toward a specific target. Therapy controls are highly efficient in cases of minimal pleural effusions and subpleural infiltrations; no method is superior to sonography in this regard [22, 23].

4.2 Neoplastic Consolidations in the Lung

In cases of localized chest pain, point-of-care ultrasound (POCUS) immediately can indicate a tumor as the cause of the pain. On the other hand, as a rule, the sonographic investigation is performed when the findings of various radiographic procedures are known. Given specific symptoms, however, a targeted symptom-oriented investigation is meaningful by dynamic investigation.

4.2.1 Sonomorphology of Lung Cancer

Lung cancer and metastases can only be identified with US when they reach the pleura since sound waves will not be reflected by the air-filled lung. In US peripheral lung cancers are usually visualized as relatively well-delineated borders, round or oval, dominantly hypoechoic space-occupying lesions (Fig. 4.10). The echotexture is sometimes inhomogeneous with anechoic necrotic areas (Fig. 4.11) [10]. They reveal an

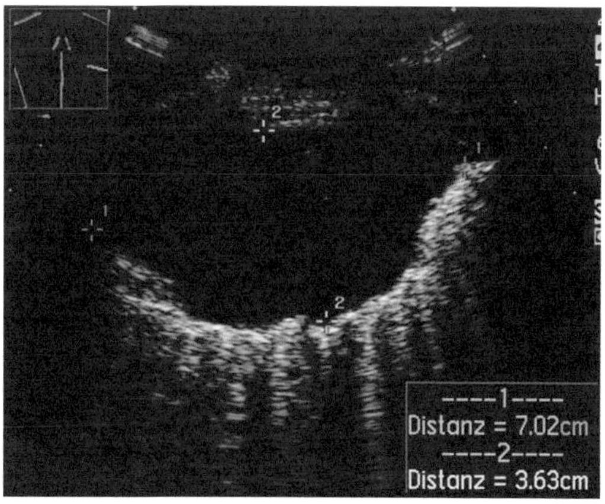

Fig. 4.10 Epidermoid lung cancer infiltrating the chest wall

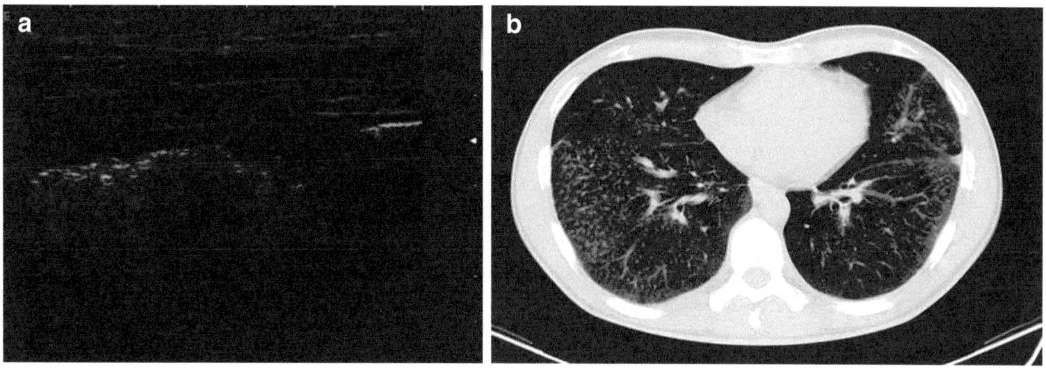

Fig. 4.9 Sarcoidosis. (**a**) Minimal local pleural effusion. Uneven, fragmented visceral pleura with several reverberation echoes. Small subpleural consolidation. (**b**) Corresponding CT

infiltrating growth with ramifications [10]. The margin of the adjacent lung surface characteristically ranges from irregular to knotty (Table 4.2) [7, 24, 25].

Color Doppler sonography identifies vascular displacement and neovascularization along irregular chaotic vascular courses (Figs. 4.12 and 4.13). Since bronchial carcinomas typically have bronchial arterial supply, a delay in contrast agent enhancement occurs in contrast-enhanced ultrasound compared to inflammatory consolidations like pneumonia with pulmonary artery supply (Fig. 4.14) [9, 10].

In the case of central bronchial carcinomas, only atelectasis downstream from the obstruction or poststenotic pneumonia can be delimited in US in many cases. For a long-lasting obstruction, then anechoic, finger-shaped branched tubular structures that correspond to expanded secretion-filled bronchi (known as fluid bronchogram) are often located within the consolidated lung. In some cases the central tumor can be delimited from the atelectasis in B-image sonography and primarily in signal-amplified sonography. In addition, CEUS allows reliable demarcation of necrotic sections within the atelectasis.

In contrast to acute inflammatory infiltrations, the sonomorphology of malignant lesions does not change during a short course of disease. Chronic carnifying pneumonia and peripheral callused cicatricial lesions are problematic in terms of differential diagnosis; it may be difficult to differentiate these entities from malignant disease [7, 24].

4.2.2 Pulmonary Metastases

Pulmonary metastases are documented on sonography when they reach the margin of the lung. Owing to poor visibility in this region, sonogra-

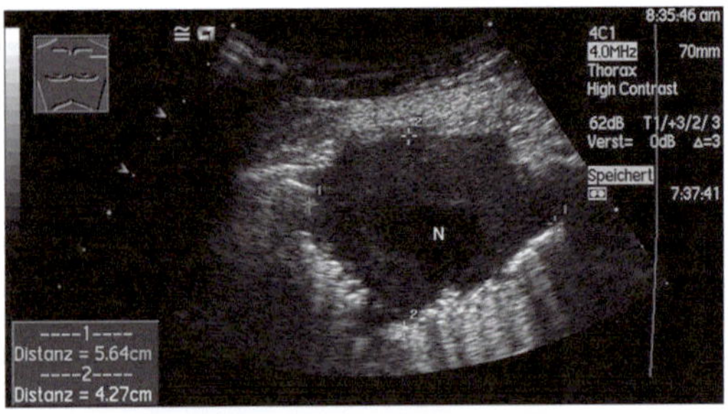

Fig. 4.11 Epidermoid lung cancer with central necrosis (N)

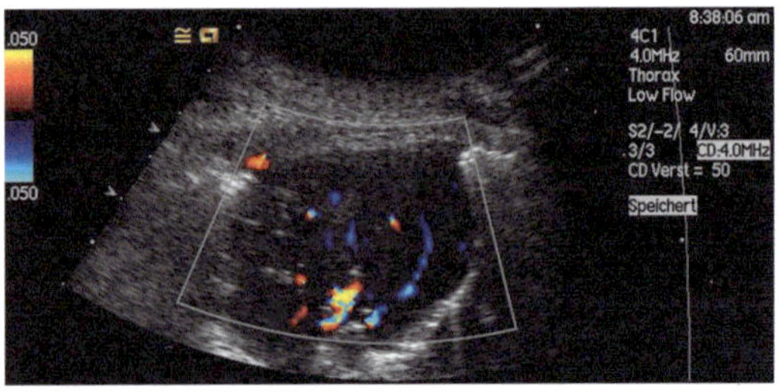

Fig. 4.13 Less or more but always irregular vascularization is a characteristic sign of malignancy

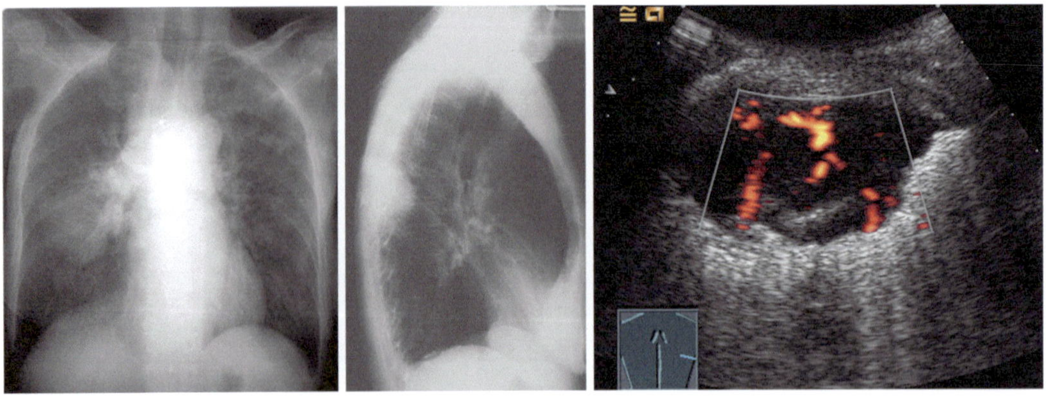

Fig. 4.12 Adenocarcinoma with irregular neovascularization—"vascular inferno"

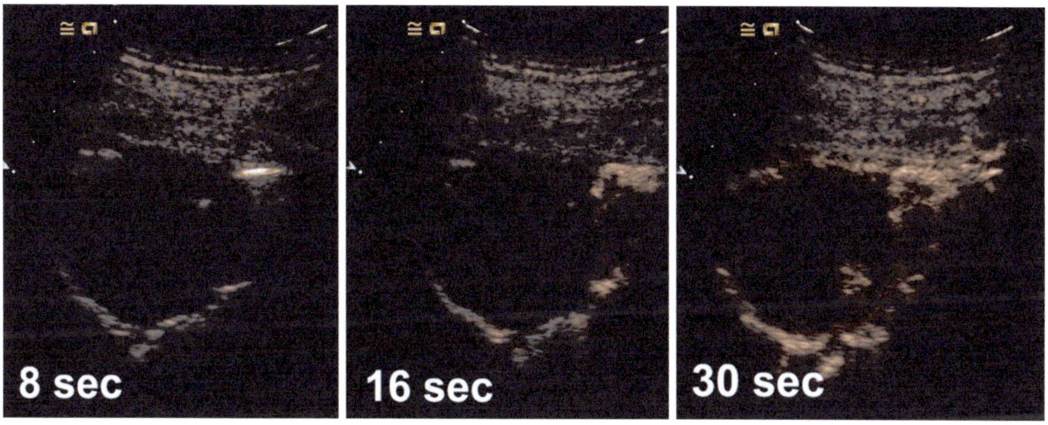

Fig. 4.14 In contrast-enhanced ultrasound (CEUS), lung cancer shows a late enhancement. This is an indicative sign for systemic circulation

Table 4.2 Sonomorphology of lung carcinomas [26]

Morphology	Echotexture	Vessels	Complex structures
Sharp margins	Inhomogeneous	Displacement of vessels	Residual ventilated areas
Rounded	Hypoechoic	Destruction of vessels	Accompanying pneumonia at the margin
Polypoid	Rarely echogenic	Interruption of vessels	Solid space-occupying lesion/pneumonia
Ramifications	Rarely anechoic	Neovascularization	Bacterial/fungal colonization
Serrated margin	Necrotic areas		Bizarre pattern in large necroses

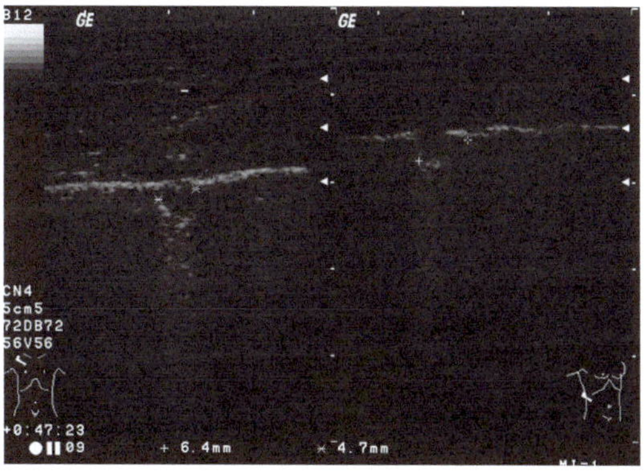

Fig. 4.15 Small metastases caused by rectal cancer, not visible in chest radiography

phy is not a suitable screening method. Metastases have no small air trappings and are usually homogeneously hypoechoic; occasionally, they have branches extending into the tissue. Pathological vessels are predominantly found at the margin (Fig. 4.15, [26]).

4.2.3 Ultrasound in Staging of Lung Cancer

Lung consolidations are seen on sonography only when no aerated tissue hinders the echo transmission. For staging of the disease and planning treatment in cases of malignant lung disease, procedures that provide sectional images such as computed tomography or magnetic resonance tomography are absolutely essential in order to obtain an overview of the entire chest. As a rule, the sonographic investigation is performed when the findings of various radiographic procedures are known. Given specific symptoms, however, a targeted symptom-oriented investigation is also meaningful (Fig. 4.16, [26]).

Thanks to ongoing scientific work, the recent international guidelines and recommendations have incorporated ultrasound as a part of the diagnostic procedure for the investigation of lung cancer. Due to its excellent resolution, ultrasound has proved equivalent to nuclear resonance tomography in the investigation of the chest wall affected by tumor invasion. Percutaneous diagnostic and therapeutic ultrasound-guided puncture is recommended and has been accepted as a reliable procedure. Endobronchial and endoesophageal ultrasound is the state of the art for staging of mediastinal lymph node involvement.

T-Staging: Invasion into adjacent structures of the chest wall is a very reliable sign of malignant growth. Therefore, the current guidelines demand a sonography for staging in lung cancer. Infiltration of the thorax wall is defined as the T3 stage and is identified in up to 6% of patients at the time of diagnosis of an NSCLC. It is important to know whether the tumor is widely fixed to the parietal pleura or is freely movable in conjunction with the lung. Quite often sonography allows better differentiation of the tumor from non-ventilated lung tissue than computed tomography (Fig. 4.17, [27, 28]). Owing to the excellent resolution and the possibility of dynamic investigation, tumor invasion of the parietal pericardium can be clearly visualized. In terms of differential diagnosis, only one disease is likely to be present here, namely, actinomycosis or nocardiosis [26].

N-Staging: Endobronchial US (EBUS) and transesophageal US (EUS) have recently been included in diagnostics at specialized centers. EUS makes it possible to biopsy paraesophageal lymph nodes in particular, and EBUS makes it possible to biopsy paratracheal, infracarinal, and hilar lymph nodes. US of the supraclavicular and lower cervical lymph nodes has a special role in the staging of bronchial carcinoma since lymph node metastases are identified in 16–26% of all patients. For NSCLC, supraclavicular lymph node metastases correspond to an N3 lymph node station, so they are an inoperable stage (Fig. 4.18, [29]).

M-Staging: The basic diagnostic procedures must include sonography of the abdomen in order

Fig. 4.16 Algorithm for ultrasound staging of lung cancer

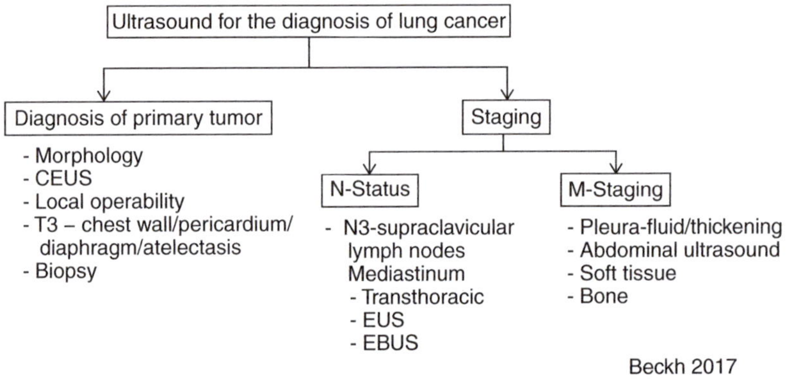

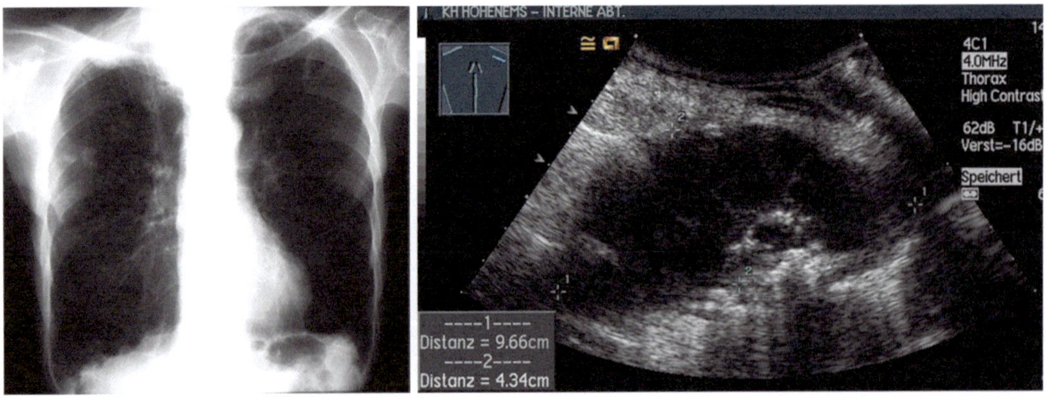

Fig. 4.17 Pancoast tumor with Horner's syndrome, infiltrating in the branchial nerve

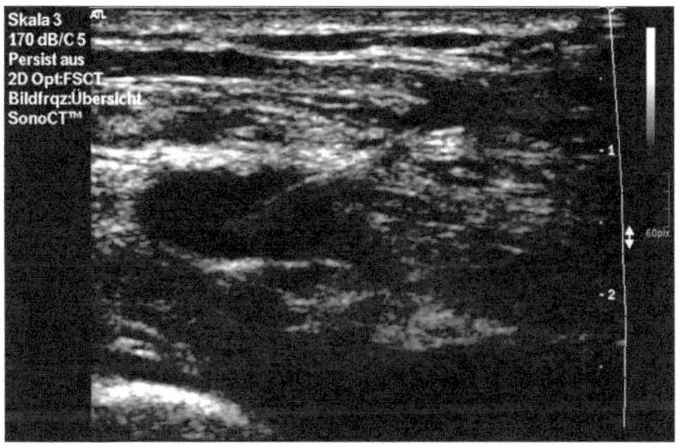

Fig. 4.18 Nonpalpable supraclavicular lymph node metastasis, secured by fine needle biopsy, not pictured in CT (Courtesy Helmut Prosch)

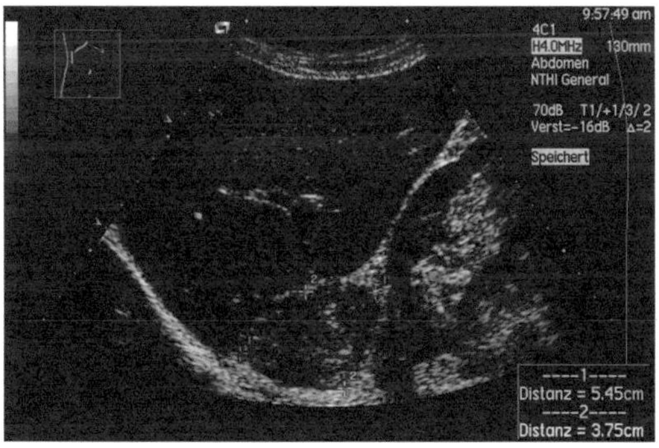

Fig. 4.19 Right adrenal metastasis in small cell lung cancer. Therefore, extensive disease is proved during the first clinical examination

to identify metastases. Distant metastases are being identified more frequently in the liver and the adrenal glands in patients with a bronchial carcinoma (Fig. 4.19). Soft-tissue metastases or metastases in the pancreas, the spleen, or the kidneys are usually only encountered in the case of very advanced tumor stages. Presumably benign lesions or lesions of an unclear nature that can be further clarified via more extensive ultrasound examination are often also identified in this process.

In all cases of ambiguous pulmonary lesions, sonography may serve as an important aid in decision-making. It helps the investigator to decide about the subsequent diagnostic procedure—either immediately in terms of a sonography-assisted biopsy or as a complementary imaging method to select the appropriate surgical procedure [24].

4.3 Pulmonary Embolism

Pulmonary embolism is the most frequent clinically non-diagnosed cause of death. Clinical symptoms are rare and tend to be quite harmless and unspecific. The chest X-ray is not very sensitive. Even in times of MSCT, one must assume that 40% of fatal pulmonary embolisms remain undiagnosed [22]. The crucial diagnostic step still is to consider the investigation procedure in the first place. The clinician is called upon to use any method that improves the diagnosis of pulmonary embolism and reduces mortality—which still is as high as 15% [30].

4.3.1 Sonomorphology of Pulmonary Embolism

4.3.1.1 Form and Echotexture

Embolism-related lung consolidations are hypoechoic and largely homogenous on ultrasound. They are largely triangular, with a pleural base, and may protrude slightly. The lesions may be rounded toward the hilum or polygonal in shape. The margin may be initially somewhat blurred but is usually sharp (Figs. 4.20 and 4.21; [22, 31, 32]).

4.3.1.2 Localization

Two-thirds of lung infarctions are located dorsally in the lower lobes of the lung, more often on the right side than on the left side. This is because of anatomical factors and because of hemodynamics: basal pulmonary arteries tend to run straight, while arteries of the upper lobe tend to branch off at a steeper angle. The dorsobasal region is particularly accessible to transcutaneous sonography [32].

4.3.1.3 Number

The improved resolution available today allows the investigator to detect more lesions than he/she could several years ago. In cases of pulmonary embolism, on average, 2.4 infarctions are seen on sonography. Given two or more lesions and the clinical likelihood of pulmonary embolism, the specificity of sonography is 97%. In

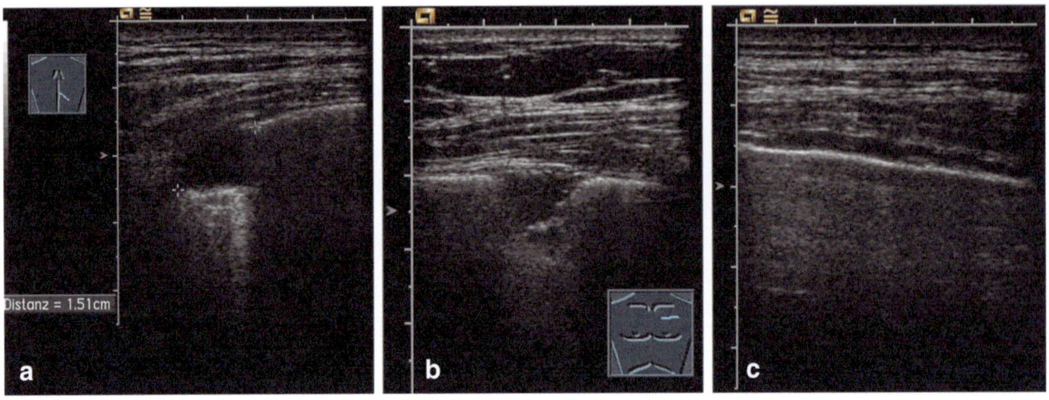

Fig. 4.20 (**a**, **b**) Triangular pulmonary infarctions of typical form and size with protrusion of the pleura. (**c**) Narrow focal pleural effusion

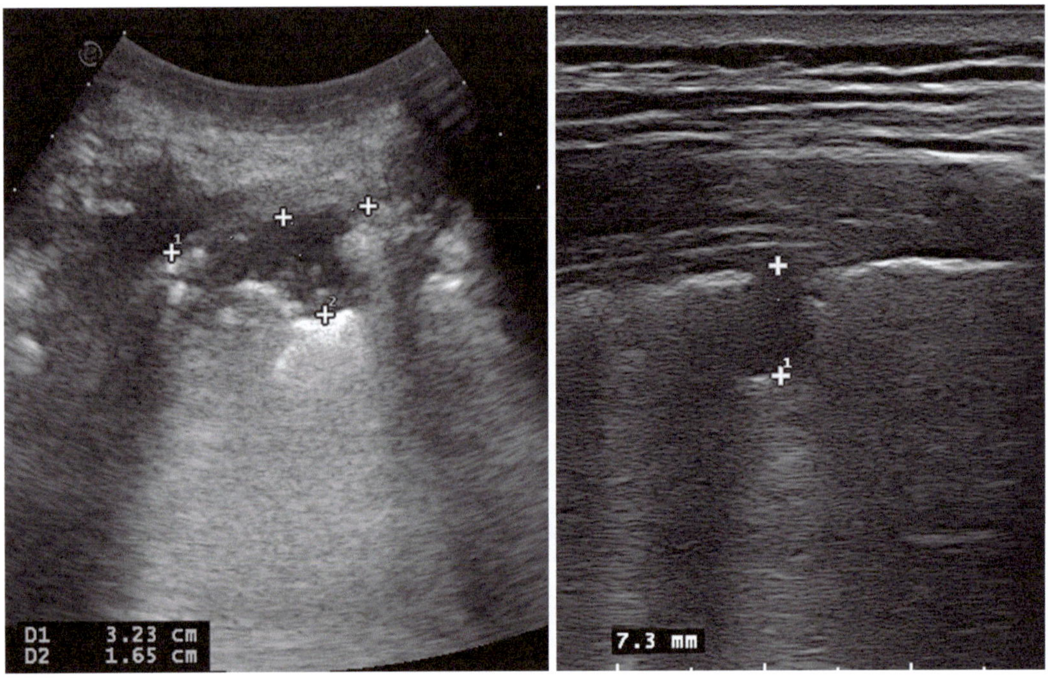

Fig. 4.21 A 52-year-old female with peritoneal liposarcoma. The patient complained dyspnea and claimed to have caught cold. Thoracic ultrasound showed a triangular and a rounded consolidation as a sign of pulmonary embolism

slim patients it would be advisable to investigate the pleural reflex with a high-frequency transducer as well (Fig. 4.22; [32]).

4.3.1.4 Size

The mean size of pulmonary infarctions is 12 mm × 16 mm (range 5–70 mm) [32]. Lesions less than 5 mm in size should not be taken into account because they might be merely scars. If at all, their progress should be monitored. Pleuritis may be marked by a similar appearance. However, pleuritis will be found at the site of pain and is usually characterized by extensive fragmentation of the pleural reflex.

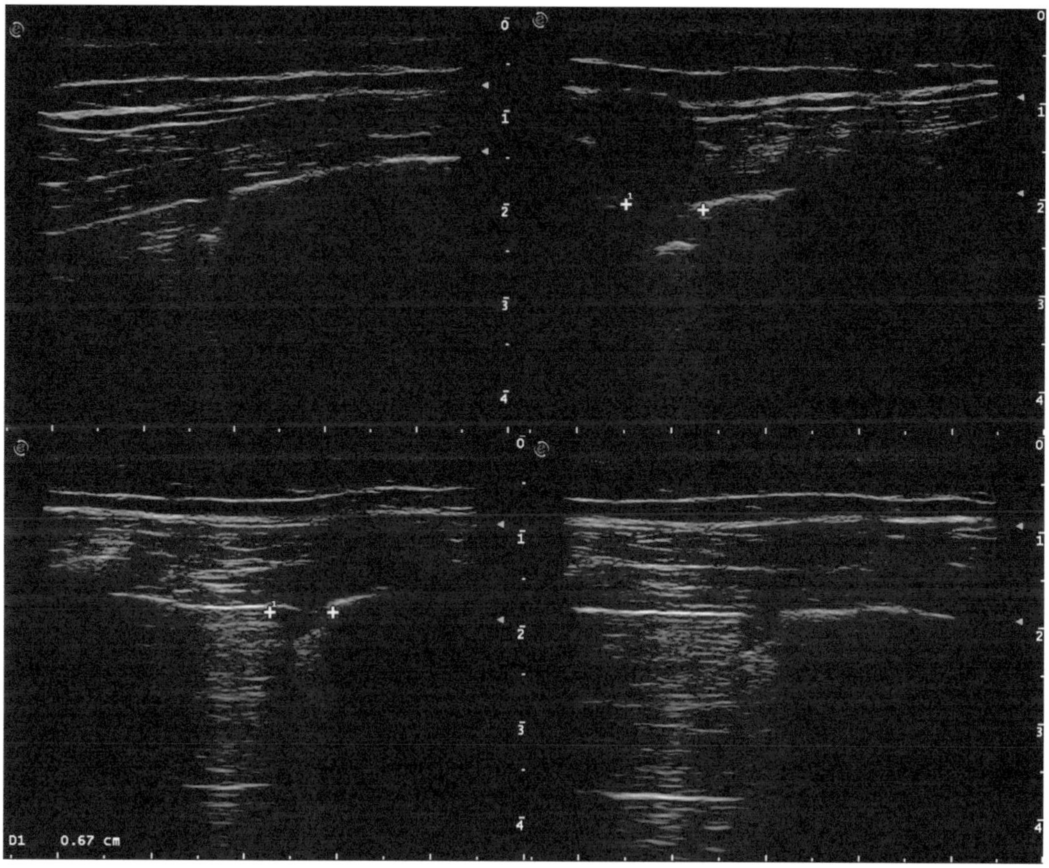

Fig. 4.22 A 24-year-old woman in pregnancy with slight dyspnea. Sonography demonstrated deep vein and pelvis thrombosis and several near 1 cm small pulmonary embolizations

4.3.1.5 Vascular Signs

In some cases one finds an anechoic band of vessels on the B-mode image. The band of vessels is oriented from the tip of the lesion to the hilum. It corresponds to the branch of the pulmonary artery congested by thromboembolism, as evidenced in computed tomography investigations as well (so-called vessel sign or vascular sign) (Fig. 4.23).

4.3.1.6 Pleural Effusion

In approximately half of cases, the investigator finds small pleural effusions either focally above the lesion or in the pleural sinuses. The effusion is largely anechoic and smaller than an infarction, which is an important criterion to distinguish this entity from compression atelectasis. ([31]; Fig. 4.20).

4.3.1.7 Signal Embolism

A massive pulmonary embolism is frequently accompanied by smaller embolic events, which then appear as signal embolisms. Such small lesions may be a precursor of an imminent pulmonary embolism or may even be present in conjunction with a massive central pulmonary embolism and thus confirm the diagnosis without the central embolus itself being demonstrated on chest sonography; it escapes detection because of air in the intervening space.

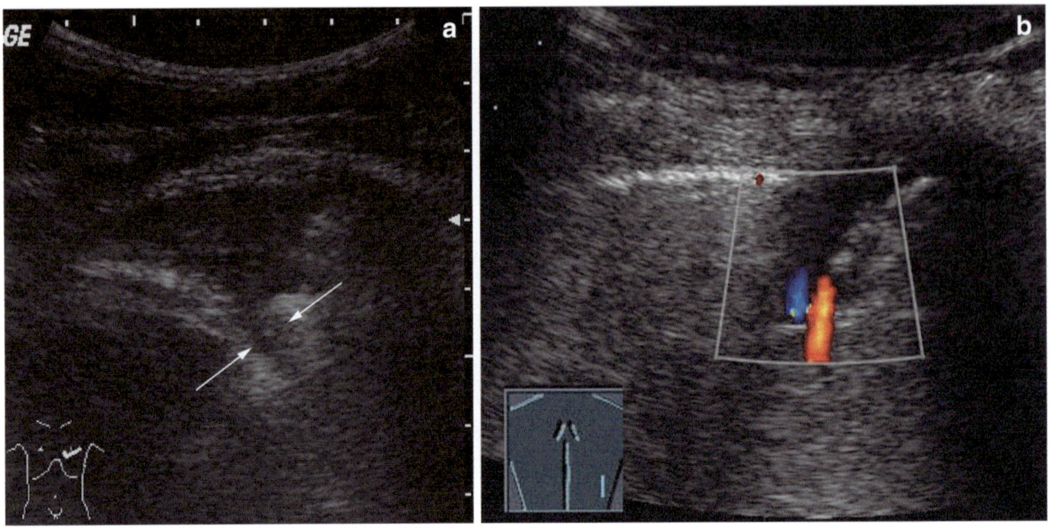

Fig. 4.23 Vascular signs in pulmonary embolism: (**a**) The thrombotic congested pulmonary artery (arrows). (**b**) Circulaton stops at the tip of the wedge-shaped pulmonary infarction

4.3.2 Color-Coded Duplex Sonography in Pulmonary Embolism

In few cases, the investigator is able to visualize, on color-coded duplex sonography, a circulation stop caused by embolism (Fig. 4.23b). This limitation has several reasons:

- Patients with dyspnea cannot hold their breath long enough.
- It is difficult to locate the supplying vessel at the right level.
- When reperfusion occurs rapidly, the lesion is revascularized early.

Nevertheless, color Doppler sonography is an important tool to differentiate subpleural pulmonary lesions [21].

4.3.3 Contrast-Assisted Sonography

Pulmonary infarctions and hemorrhage due to embolism are marked by the absence of circulation and the absence of contrast on contrast-assisted sonography as well as color Doppler sonography. At the margin of the lesion, there may be delayed or poor contrast enhancement because this area is supplied by a bronchial artery. Pleuritis and pneumonia, on the other hand, are contrasted early and strongly by a pulmonary artery supply. In case of doubt, pleural consolidations can be distinguished from embolic ones by the use of signal-enhanced ultrasound ([9, 10]; Fig. 4.24).

4.3.4 Accuracy of Chest Sonography in the Diagnosis of Pulmonary Embolism

A large multicenter study comprising 352 patients in the ordinary clinical setting round the clock, which included less experienced investigators, showed that three-fourths of patients with pulmonary embolism have typical peripheral lesions on sonography. A surprisingly high specificity of 95% was achieved in this study [32]. These figures concur with those reported for the demonstration of peripheral pulmonary embolisms in pathological studies. The results are worse, if the dorsal region is not examined.

Two recent meta-analyses of five resp 10 studies on 652/887 patients, the pooled sensitivity

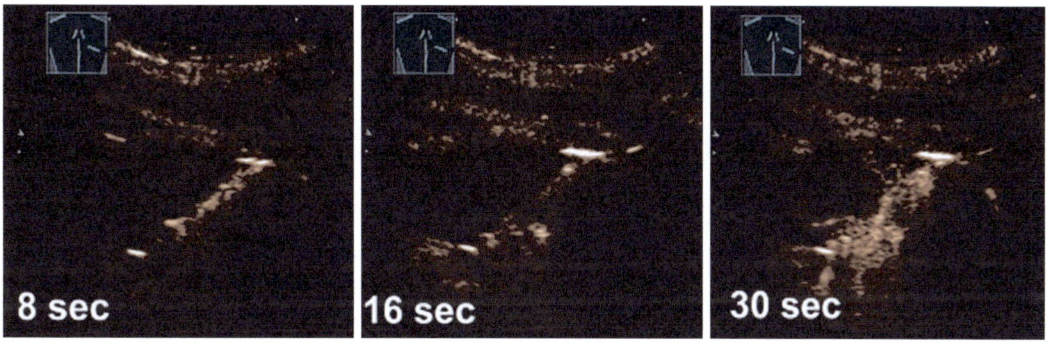

Fig. 4.24 In contrast-enhanced ultrasound, pulmonary embolism shows a very late and less intensive enhancement—very well for differentiation of inflammatory consolidations

and specificity was 80–87% and 82–93%. The authors conclude that, in view of the increasing numbers of CT investigations and the increasing collective radiation dose for specific clinical situations, such as emergency, pregnancy, renal failure, and contrast allergy, chest ultrasound serves as a diagnostic alternative to CT [33, 34]. This is recommended it actual conferences and guidelines [5, 35].

Caution: A normal chest sonogram does not exclude the presence of pulmonary embolism, as is true for a negative computed tomography or a negative D-dimer test as well [36].

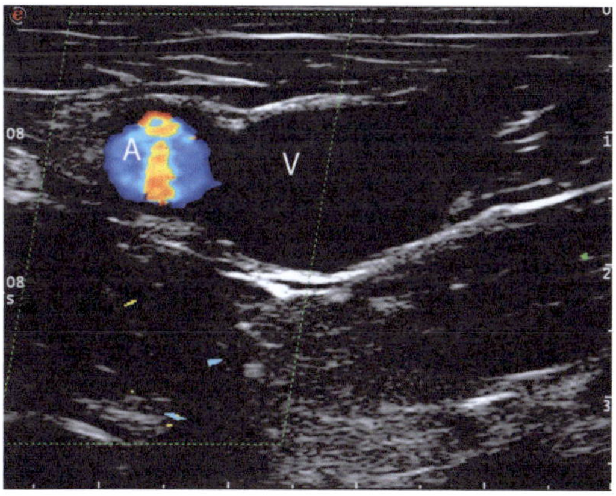

Fig. 4.25 Searching for the source of embolism: leg vein thrombosis in the femoral vein. The vein (V) is larger than the artery (A), congested with echogenic material, and cannot be compressed

4.3.5 Triple-Organ Ultrasound in Thromboembolism

In several anatomical locations, sonography has become the method of choice to diagnose thromboembolism. In a single investigation step, the experienced investigator is able to inspect several actual clinically or potentially involved regions of the body using a single imaging procedure. He/she is able to study the *source*, *pathway*, and *target* of the embolic event.

4.3.6 Duplex Sonography of Leg Veins

Much more than half of pulmonary embolisms originate from leg veins. Compression sonography is a safe procedure to confirm that an embolism is originating from a deep vein thrombosis. Patients who have anticoagulation withheld following a negative or inconclusive whole-leg compression ultrasound for suspected deep vein thrombosis have a low rate of adverse events [37].

Visualization of the thrombus and the absence of flow are direct signs of leg vein thrombosis (Fig. 4.25). Detection of the thrombus in the B-mode is indirectly improved by the application of color Doppler sonography. The thrombosed vein is not compressible or is only partially compressible, which is indicative of an occluding coagulation. However, signs of compressibility are only reliable when they are found in the inguinal or popliteal region.

4.3.7 Echocardiography

About 40% of patients with acute pulmonary embolism have a right heart load. This specifically includes patients at hemodynamic risk who have to undergo lysis or embolectomy as a lifesaving measure. The first hours after the onset of symptoms are of decisive importance for the prognosis of hemodynamically relevant pulmonary embolism. On echocardiography one can obtain a rapid overview of the degree of risk for the patient, establish the intensity of monitoring, and devise a treatment plan.

The following parameters are used to assess acute right heart load:

- Size of the right ventricle
- Contraction of the free right ventricular wall
- Movement of the interventricular septum
- Size of the right atrium
- Are embolisms seen in the right heart?
- Exclusion of atrial myxoma

Echocardiographic examination is not recommended as part of the diagnostic work-up in hemodynamically stable, normotensive patients with suspected (not high-risk) pulmonary embolism. This is in contrast to suspected high-risk PE, in which the absence of echocardiographic signs of RV overload or dysfunction practically excludes PE as the cause of hemodynamic instability. In the latter case, echocardiography may be of further help in the differential diagnosis of the cause of shock, by detecting pericardial tamponade, acute valvular dysfunction, severe global or regional LV dysfunction, aortic dissection, or hypovolemia [38].

Since the introduction of transesophageal echocardiography, the source of embolism is increasingly looked for in the heart as well. Transthoracic echocardiography may disclose sessile and floating thrombi in the right atrium. In transesophageal location, one may also find riding thrombi in the central main trunks of the pulmonary arteries.

A major advantage of sonographic investigation of embolism is its manifold applicability and its availability at the bedside, whether in the emergency department or in the intensive care unit. Lung ultrasound, echocardiography, and leg vein compression sonography according to clinical presentation yield a sensitivity of more than 90% for pulmonary embolism [32, 39].

4.4 Other Lung Consolidations

Atelectasis is defined as the absence of ventilation in portions of the lung or the entire lung. Such lack of ventilation may be transient or permanent, partially (dystelectasis) or complete, and acquired or congenital.

4.4.1 Compression Atelectasis

Sonomorphological criteria for a compression atelectasis are:

- Moderate or large pleural effusion
- Hypoechoic consolidation of the lower lung margin
- Smaller in relation to the effusion
- Uni- or biconcave
- Floating in the effusion like a winking hand
- Blurred margin to the ventilated lung
- Partial reventilation during inspiration
- Partial reventilation after aspiration of the effusion ([7, 40]; Fig. 4.26)

In the presence of exudative effusion, fibrin strands, septa, and echogenic pleural effusion, one frequently observes poor reventilation during

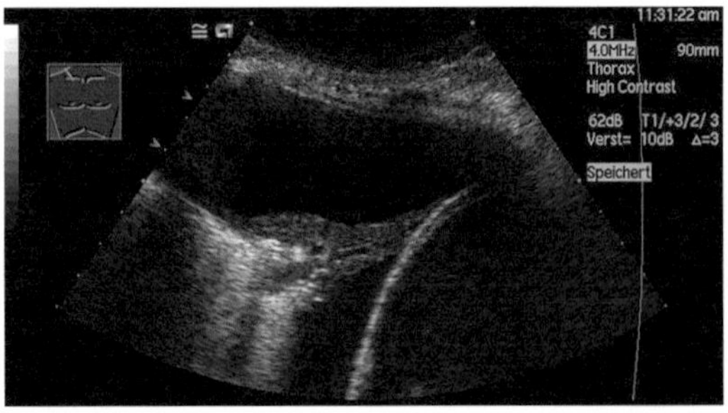

Fig. 4.26 Compression atelectasis

inspiration as a result of reduced elasticity of the lung. This condition has been described as a "trapped" lung. Concomitant inflammatory congestion restricts inspiratory ventilation. Ventilation after drainage of the effusion does not rule out an additional central space-occupying lesion.

4.4.2 Obstructive Atelectasis

Sonomorphological criteria of obstructive atelectasis are:

- Large consolidation with liver-like echotexture similar to pneumonia
- Less bronchoaerogram than pneumonia
- Hypoechoic reflexes (fluid bronchogram)
- Regular vascularization in color Doppler
- Effusion is absent or is very mild

Quite often the investigator finds focal lesions in the obturation atelectasis. As a result of dilated bronchi (due to congestion of secretion), one occasionally finds small anechoic, hypoechoic, or even echogenic lesions in the consolidated lung parenchyma. Echoic are the walls of dilated bronchi and air in the bronchi or occasionally in microabscesses. Anechoic or very hypoechoic are liquefications and microabscesses. Ultrasound-guided aspiration will allow the investigator to confirm the diagnosis and obtain material for bacteriological investigation [12]. Additional color Doppler sonography may be helpful to distinguish between central tumors and atelectatic lung tissue, as tumor tissue is characterized by poor visualization of flow signals ([40], Fig. 4.27).

4.4.3 Lung Contusion

In cases of chest trauma, particularly serial rib fractures, pulmonary contusions are visualized better on sonography than on radiographs. They are detected in 18% of blunt chest trauma. Alveolar edema and alveolar hemorrhage caused by trauma are seen as moderately hypoechoic, blurred, pale lesions with indistinct margins (Fig. 4.28). These are more pronounced in the presence of concomitant minimal pleural effusions but are also imaged on sonography in the absence of pleural effusion. In the event of any clinically relevant chest trauma, radiographs as well as sonograms should be obtained [41]. Including the presence of B-lines (85%), chest ultrasonography can accurately predict lung contusion in blunt trauma victims, in comparison to CT scan [42].

4.4.4 Congenital Pulmonary Sequestration

The very rare pulmonary sequestration underlines the value and importance of thorax sonography in neonatology and pediatrics. The neonate

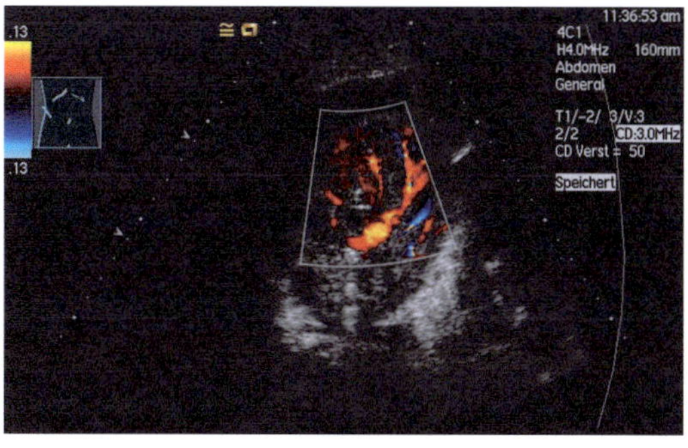

Fig. 4.27 Obturative atelectasis: liver-like echotexture, less bronchoaerogram, regular vascularization, small pleural effusion

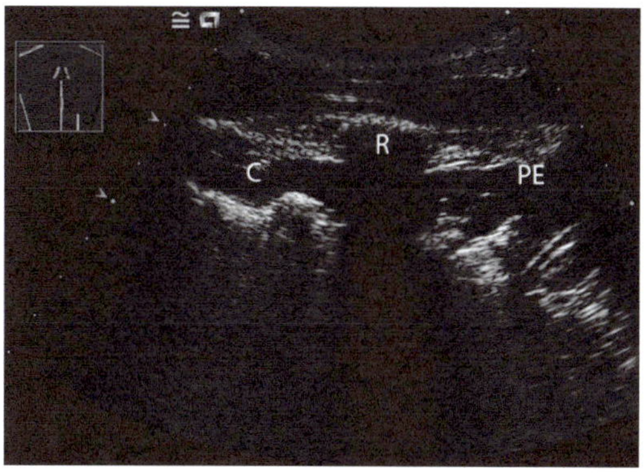

Fig. 4.28 Lung contusion. *C* Flat consolidation, *PE* small pleural effusion, *R* Rib with shadow

with this condition suffers from dyspnea and has a nonspecific systolic murmur. On chest radiograph, one may find a tumorlike shadow. On sonography, the echotexture of the pulmonary sequestration is similar to that of the liver, with wide arteries and veins. The supplying artery with the characteristic flow pattern can be identified on color-coded duplex sonography, and the diagnosis is thus confirmed. CT does not provide more information. If the lesion is imaged well on sonography, the infant can be spared the stress of angiography [12].

References

1. Gehmacher O, Mathis G, Kopf A, Scheier M. Ultrasound imaging of pneumonia. Ultrasound Med Biol. 1995;21:1119–22.
2. Mathis G, Metzler J, Fußenegger D, et al. Ultrasound findings in pneumonia. Ultraschall Klin Prax. 1992;7:45–9.
3. Reissig A, Copetti R, Mathis G, Mempel C, Schuler A, Zechner P, et al. Lung ultrasound in the diagnosis and follow-up of community-acquired pneumonia. A prospective multicentre diagnostic accuracy study. Chest. 2012;142:965–72.
4. Targhetta R, Chavagneux R, Bourgeois JM, Dauzat M, Balmes P, Pourcelot L. Sonographic approach to diagnosing pulmonary consolidation. J Ultrasound Med. 1992;11:667–72.
5. Volpicelli G, Elbarbary M, Blaivas M, et al. International evidence-based recommendations for point-of-care lung ultrasound. Intensive Care Med. 2012;38:577–91.
6. Weinberg B, Diaboumakis EE, Kass EG, et al. The air bronchogram: sonographic demonstration. AJR. 1986;147:593–5.
7. Mathis G. Thoraxsonography—part II: peripheral pulmonary consolidation. Ultrasound Med Biol. 1997;23:1141–53.
8. Lichtenstein D, Meziere G, Seitz J. The dynamic air bronchogram. A lung ultrasound sign of alveolar consolidation ruling out atelectasis. Chest. 2009;135:1421–5.
9. Bertolini FA, Gorg C, Mathis G. Echo contrast ultrasound in subpleural consolidations. Abstract ECR 2008. Eur Radiol Suppl. 2008;18:S395.
10. Görg C. Transcutaneous contrast-enhanced sonography of pleural-based pulmonary lesions. Eur J Radiol. 2007;64:213–21.
11. Yang PC, Luh KT, Lee YC. Lung abscesses: ultrasonography and ultrasound-guided transthoracic aspiration. Radiology. 1991;180:171–5.
12. Yang PC, Luh KT, Chang DB, Yu CJ, Kuo SH, Wu HD. Ultrasonographic evaluation of pulmonary consolidation. Am Rev Respir Dis. 1992;146:757–62.
13. Takayanagi N, Kagiyama N, Ishiguro T, et al. Etiology and outcome of community-acquired lung abscesses. Respiration. 2010;80:98–105.
14. Chavez MA, Shams N, Ellington LA, et al. Lung ultrasound for the diagnosis of pneumonia in adults: a systematic review and meta-analysis. Respir Res. 2014;15:50. https://doi.org/10.1186/1465-9921-15-50.
15. Hu QJ, Shen YC, Jia LQ, Guo SJ, et al. Diagnostic performance of lung ultrasound in the diagnosis of pneumonia: a bivariate meta-analysis. Int J Clin Exp Med. 2014;7:115–21.
16. Llamas-Alvarez AM, Tenza-Lozano EM, Latour-Perez J. Accuracy of lung ultrasound in the diagnosis of pneumonia in adults: systematic review and meta-analysis. Chest. 2017;151:374–82.
17. Busti C, Agnelli G, Duranti M, et al. Lung ultrasound in the diagnosis of stroke-associated pneumonia. Intern Emerg Med. 2014;9:173–8.
18. Ticinesi A, Lauretani F, Nouvenne A, et al. Lung ultrasound and chest x-ray for detecting pneumonia in an acute geriatric ward. Medicine. 2016;95(27):e4153. https://doi.org/10.1097/MD.0000000000004153.
19. Cortellaro F, Colombo S, Coen D, et al. Lung ultrasound is an accurate diagnostic tool for the diagnosis of pneumonia in the emergency department. Emerg Med J. 2012;29:19e23. https://doi.org/10.1136/emj.2010.101584.
20. Kopf A, Metzler J, Mathis G. Ultrasound in lung tuberculosis. Imaging. 1994;61(S2):12.
21. Yuan A, Yang PC, Chang DB, et al. Ultrasound guided aspiration biopsy for pulmonary tuberculosis with unusual radiographic appearances. Thorax. 1993;48:167–70.
22. Reissig A, Kroegel C. Transthoracic sonography of diffuse parenchymal lung disease: the role of comet tail artefacts. J Ultrasound Med. 2003;22:173–80.
23. Wohlgenannt S, Gehmacher O, Mathis G. Sonographic findings in interstitial lung diseases. Ultraschall Med. 2001;22:27–31.
24. Beckh S, Bölcskei PL, Lessnau KD. Real-time chest ultrasonography. A comprehensive review for the pulmonologist. Chest. 2002;122:1759–73.
25. Prosch H, Mathis G, Mostbeck GH. Perkutaner ultraschall in diagnose und staging des bronchialkarzinoms. Ultraschall Med. 2008;29:466–84.
26. Beckh S. Neoplastic consolidations in the lung: primary lung tumors and metastases. In: Mathis G, editor. Chest sonography. Berlin: Springer; 2017.
27. Bandi V, Lunn W, Ernst A, Eberhardt R, Hoffmann H, Herth FJF. Ultrasound vs CT in detecting chest wall invasion by tumor. A prospective study. Chest. 2008;133:881–6.
28. Goeckenjan G, Sitter H, Thomas M, et al. Prevention, diagnosis, therapy and follow-up of lung cancer. Interdisciplinary guideline of the German Respiratory Society and the German Cancer Society. Pneumologie. 2011;65:39–59.
29. Prosch H, Strasser G, Sonka C, Oschatz E, Mashaal S, Mohn-Staudner A, Mostbeck GH. Cervical ultrasound (US) and US-guided lymph node biopsy as a routine

procedure for staging of lung cancer. Ultraschall Med. 2007;28:598–603.
30. Özsu SS, Durmus ZG, Coskuner MB, et al. Does the incidence and mortality of pulmonary thromboembolism change over the years? Turk Thorac J. 2017;18:78–81.
31. Mathis G, Dirschmid K. Pulmonary infarction: sonographic appearance with pathologic correlation. Eur J Radiol. 1993;17:170–4.
32. Mathis G, Blank W, Reißig A, et al. Thoracic ultrasound for diagnosing pulmonary embolism. A prospective multicenter study of 352 patients. Chest. 2005;128:1531–8.
33. Niemann T, Egelhof T, Bongratz G. Transthoracic sonography for the detection of pulmonary embolism—a meta analysis. Ultraschall Med. 2009;30:150–6.
34. Squizzato A. Galli1 L, Gerdes A. Point-of-care ultrasound in the diagnosis of pulmonary embolism. Critical Ultrasound Journal. 2015;7:7–11. https://doi.org/10.1186/s13089-015-0025-5.
35. Hach-Wunderle V, Zemmmrich C. AMWF-guidelines. Thrombosis and pulmonary embolism. Vasa. 2016;90(Suppl):1–48.
36. Mathis G, Blank W, Reissig A, et al. Thoracic ultrasound for diagnosing pulmonary embolism. A prospective multicenter study of 352 patients. Chest. 2005;128:1531–8.
37. Horner D, Hogg K, Body R. et. al. K Single whole-leg compression ultrasound for exclusion of deep vein thrombosis inn symptomatic patients: a prospective observational study. Br J Haematol. 2014;164:422–30.
38. Konstantinides SV, Torbicki A, Agnelli G, et al. ESC Guidelines on the diagnosis and management of acute pulmonary embolism: the Task Force for the Diagnosis and Management of Acute Pulmonary Embolism of the European Society of Cardiology (ESC). Eur Heart J. 2014;35:3033–73.
39. Nazerian P, Vanni S, Volpicell G, et al. Accuracy of point-of-care multiorgan ultrasonography for the diagnosis of pulmonary embolism. Chest. 2014;145:950–7.
40. Görg C. Mechanical lung consolidations: atelectasis. In: Mathis G, editor. Chest sonography. Berlin: Springer; 2017.
41. Wüstner A, Gehmacher O, Hämmerle S, et al. Ultrasound diagnosis in blunt thoracic trauma. Ultraschall Med. 2005;26:285–90.
42. Soldati G, Demi M, Inchingolo R, Smargiassi A, Demi L. On the Physical Basis of Pulmonary Sonographic Interstitial Syndrome. J Ultrasound Med. 2016;35:2075–86.

Interstitial Lung Diseases

5

M. Sperandeo and G. Rea

5.1 Introduction

In the last years, transthoracic ultrasound (TUS) has regained a growing interest from both clinicians and radiologists as a useful and noninvasive diagnostic tool for the study of many pleuropulmonary conditions, including interstitial lung diseases. The main advantages of this imaging technique are that US allows real-time examination and can be performed without the use of ionizing radiation. The performance is strongly limited by the anatomy of the rib cage and by the constant presence of air-related artifacts. Only ≈70% of the pleural surface can be assessed through TUS [1]; therefore, only alterations or lesions involving this pleural portion can be visualized [2, 3].

B-lines and other artifacts may be present in association with lung or pleural modifications in many interstitial lung diseases and other diffuse parenchymal lung diseases, including idiopathic pulmonary fibrosis (IPF), systemic sclerosis, interstitial pneumonia, rheumatoid arthritis, nephrotic syndrome, ARDS, and radiation fibrosis [4–9].

M. Sperandeo (✉)
Unit of Diagnostic and Interventional Ultrasound, Department of Internal Medicine, "Casa Sollievo della Sofferenza" Hospital, IRCCS, San Giovanni Rotondo, Italy
e-mail: m.sperandeo@operapadrepio.it

G. Rea
Ultrasound Diagnostic Unit, Department of Radiology, Monaldi Hospital, AORN, Naples, Italy

5.2 From the Anatomy to the Artifacts

The visceral and parietal pleurae are each 30–40 μm thick [10]. They both have similar histologic features and are separated by a thin pleural space containing pleural fluid. Each pleura is made of two layers, a mesothelial layer (from 16.4 ± 6.8 to 41.9 ± 9.5 μm in size) facing the pleura space and a connective tissue layer (10 μm in size). The connective tissue itself consists of four layers: submesothelial connective tissue; a superficial elastic layer; a thick, loose subpleural connective tissue layer, containing a variety of cells, lymphatics, and blood vessels; finally a deep fibroelastic layer [11, 12].

5.2.1 Hyperechoic "Pleural Line"

US scanner machines are calibrated at a homogeneous and constant sound speed in soft tissue (≈1540 m/s). However, the US propagation speed is 330 m/s in air and it is about 440 m/s in lungs, because of interstitium interposition [13]. Therefore, the large difference in acoustic

F. Feletti et al. (eds.), *Thoracic Ultrasound and Integrated Imaging*,
https://doi.org/10.1007/978-3-319-93055-8_5

impedance between the chest wall and pulmonary air generates artifacts [14]. More than 96% of the US beam is reflected by the tissue/air interface, so it is not available for further imaging [15, 77]. The result is the hyperechoic "pleural line" that moves during respiration (gliding or sliding sign) [16]. The pleural line in US is a hyperechoic artifact inside which there is the sum of the parietal pleura, visceral pleural, virtual space, a mesothelial layer, and a connective tissue layer and, because of the difference in acoustic impedance, is thicker than its actual anatomic size (≈200–250 μm, equivalent to 0.2–0.25 mm) [17–20].

The pleural line is a continuous sharp line, well-defined, and highly hyperechoic [21].

The thickness of pleural line in the healthy subject, using the machine settings for thoracic ultrasound (gain control: 40–50%; harmonic imaging; electronic focus: pleural line), is 0.7–1.8 mm (sd ± 0.2 mm) using a high-frequency probe (8–12 MHz) (Fig. 5.1a) and 1.2–2.8 mm (sd ± 0.2 mm) with a 3.5–5 MHz convex probe (Fig. 5.1b). This happens because the hyperechoic "pleural" line does not correspond to anatomical structure of the normal lungs [22–25].

5.2.2 B-Line Artifacts

First of all, the artifacts present in normal pulmonary parenchyma may be also visible in the post-pneumonectomy space, which contains residual air, liquid films and/or edema, and scar tissue [26, 27] (Fig. 5.1c, d).

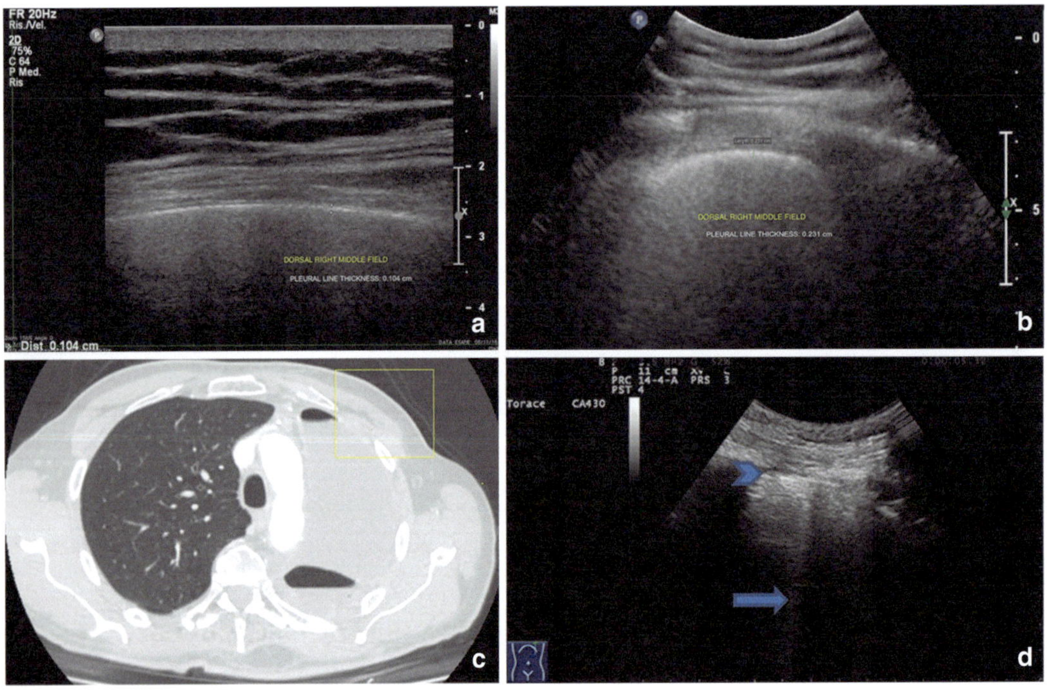

Fig. 5.1 (**a**) US using a L12-5 linear probe (upper segment of the right lower lobe) shows a curvilinear, regular, hyperechoic aspect of the pleural line. The thickness of the pleural line is 0.104 cm (≈1 mm, sd ± 0.2 mm), which is a normal value if a linear probe is used. (**b**) US using a C1–6 convex probe (same anatomic level as that evaluated with a linear probe) shows an increase in the thickness of the pleural line with a slight "coarse aspect" compared with that obtained with a linear probe. The thickness of the pleural line is 0.231 (≈2 mm, sd ± 0.2 mm), which is a normal value if a convex probe is used. (**c**) Corresponding CT of the patient (after pneumonectomy) (**d**) US left anterior scan in a patient undergone pneumonectomy reveals one B-line (arrow) and fixed "hyperechoic pleural line," resembling the pleural line, but motionless during respiration (arrow head). The physical explanation for this hyperechoic line is a substantial difference in acoustic impedance between soft tissues and an air-containing cavity

The terms "comet tail," "B-lines," and "ring down" are used in the literature in different ways to define the same physical artifacts [28–30]. Lichtenstein et al. [31] stated that B-lines originate from the thickened subpleural interlobular septa (a low-impedance structure bounded on all sides by air with a high acoustic mismatch), which would reflect the ultrasound beam, giving birth to comet-like artifacts. On the other hand, Kohzaki et al. [32] address the origin of these artifacts to a different mechanism, namely, the resonance among clusters of air bubbles and liquid, called "ring down." Well-designed experiments by Soldati et al. [33–35] and Spinelli et al. [36] seem to confirm that B-lines are reverberations, originating most often from volumetric variations in the relationship between the aerated and tissue/fluid-filled parts of the lung and rarely from the thickened interlobular septa. However, visualization and the number of B-lines can be influenced by the machine settings and signal processing, including the use of compound [37, 38]. In our experience [39], the number of B-lines was higher when using a low–medium-frequency (3.5–5.0 MHz) convex probe than with a high-frequency (8.0–12.5 MHz) linear probe.

All these elements must be considered very carefully to understand the role of B-lines. B-lines have limited specificity; edematous B-lines cannot be readily differentiated from fibrotic B-lines related to interstitial pulmonary fibrosis, as found (for example) in systemic sclerosis [40].

Moreover, subcutaneous emphysema or morbid obesity can reduce the quality of images [41].

Despite many recent attempts of counting artifacts for the diagnosis of pulmonary edema, or any extravascular lung water, have been proposed, these artifacts lack any disease specificity [42].

This is the main reason why the diagnosis of pleuropulmonary diseases using US must remain strictly complementary to chest X-ray and/or CT. In particular, HRCT is the "gold standard" for the appropriate detection, characterization, follow-up, and management of ILDs in a multidisciplinary setting as sanctioned by world guidelines [43, 44].

5.3 TUS in Fibrosis: Future Perspectives

The feasibility of TUS is opening up new areas of application day after day.

For example, it should be considered a valuable complementary tool for early detection of pulmonary fibrosis in systemic sclerosis (SSc) patients. In SSc, pulmonary fibrosis generally starts from the peripheral and inferior/posterior sites of the interstitial lung tissue, spreading upward and outward as the disease progresses.

Those areas of the lung are largely accessible to ultrasound, despite some limitations. For instance, in cases of pleuritis, blebs, emphysema, obesity, and other cardiopulmonary comorbidity, the capacity of this technique to successfully diagnose pulmonary fibrosis at an early stage is much reduced [45].

Our previous studies [46] investigated the role of US in interstitial lung diseases. Patients with pulmonary fibrosis have typical, although not specific, signs such as diffuse and/or irregular thickening of the pleural line and subpleural nodules.

We recently [47] compared the findings of chest US to those of HRCT scan in 175 consecutive patients with systemic sclerosis, diagnosed according to ACR/EULAR criteria. In all patients without HRCT signs of interstitial involvement, pleural line thickness was lower than 3.0 mm. Moreover, among the 95 asymptomatic patients with normal pulmonary function tests and single-breath diffusing capacity for carbon monoxide (DLCO), 26 patients had normal HRCT features and pleural line thickness ≤ 3 mm, while the 69 patients with pleural line thickening had reticular or reticular-nodular HRCT pattern limited to basal area. The sensitivity of pleural line thickness (Fig. 5.2a, b) to identify HRCT-detected interstitial lesions ranged from 74.3% for reticular-nodular if the width was >3.5 mm, to 80.0% for reticular pattern with a width of >3.0 to ≤ 5 mm, and to 90.1% for honeycombing if width was higher than 5.0 mm.

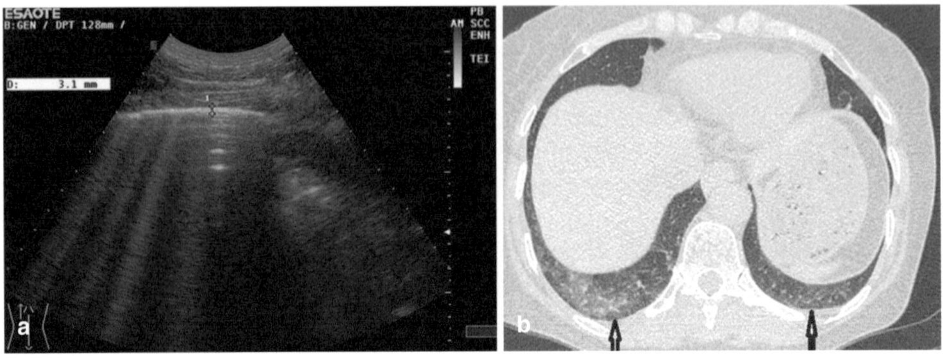

Fig. 5.2 (**a**) Postero-basal TUS scan show B-lines and the thickening of the pleural line (3.1 mm) in a patient with initial pulmonary fibrosis secondary to systemic sclerosis. (**b**) HRCT corresponding of the patient: early fibrosis postero-basal, bilateral (black arrows)

5.4 Infiltrative Disorders: HRCT Versus Chest Ultrasound

Infiltrative disorders of the lung (which include the strictly defined ILDs) are a large group of diseases, most of which are limited to the lung. Frequently the possible presence of overlapping diseases (e.g., smoking-related ILDs) may cause difficulties in interpretation of radiologic findings [48].

The chest radiograph is the first examination in a chest study. However, it has a low sensitivity and specificity for the detection of subtle interstitial changes. HRCT is an extremely valuable diagnostic solution for ILDs. HRCT can be used to resolve interstitial alterations efficiently by identifying (if pathologic and thickened) interlobular septa that measure 0.1 mm and are not visible if they are unaffected by alterations of a different nature (e.g., liquid or fibrotic changes. Furthermore, volumetric sampling allows reconstructions in all planes of space (multiparametric acquisition), permitting following of bronchial structures correctly, and providing optimal differential-diagnostic evaluation between traction bronchiolectasis and honeycombing in patients with advanced fibrotic changes [49].

Apart from the obvious advantages achieved with such an investigation, however, there is growing concern of the clinical risk associated with the use of ionizing radiation required for this imaging method, despite the significant reduction of the dose delivered to the patient (≤50% with low-dose and ultra-low-dose HRCT) [50].

Despite the limitations, we will try to clarify the artifactual elements of TUS that may be linked to diffuse infiltrative diseases so that subsequent study with HRCT can elicit a confident diagnosis for appropriate management of disease [51].

The 2013 update of guidelines, an official American Thoracic Society/European Respiratory Society statement: Update of the international multidisciplinary classification of the idiopathic interstitial pneumonias [52], includes reclassification of idiopathic interstitial pneumonias (IIPs) into four main groups: chronic fibrosing IIPs (IPF and NSIP); smoking-related IIPs (desquamative interstitial pneumonias (DIP), respiratory bronchiolitis-interstitial lung disease (RB-ILD)); acute and subacute IIPs (cryptogenic organizing pneumonia, acute interstitial pneumonia); and rare IIPs (lymphoid interstitial pneumonia, idiopathic pleuroparenchymal fibroelastosis (IPPFE)) [53]. An additional consideration is the recent introduction of an ILD category called "unclassifiable" because of the inability in some cases to reach a consistent clinical and radiologic diagnosis. The 2013 revision suggests that management of ILDs, much more than for other conditions, requires careful clinical and radiologic evaluation and, in some cases, cannot be resolved. Therefore, we wish to provide an assessment of the main and most common diseases of high clinical–radiologic–pathologic interest related to the interstitial compartment and main diffuse infiltrative diseases. We wish to provide a close correlation between US evaluation and HRCT evaluation to allow the reader to understand the limitations and diagnostic possibilities derived from this correlation of the subpleural lung surface. Most of the clinical images will, therefore, be correlated with a matrix linear multifrequency transducer, linear multifrequency probe, and convex multifrequency probe. Hence, readers can check the correlation with HRCT images the differences related to the use of different transducers in the same patient and obvious differences in US patterns [54].

5.5 Chronic Fibrosing IIPs (IPF, NSIP)

5.5.1 Idiopathic Pulmonary Fibrosis (IPF)

IPF is characterized by clinical and radiologic markers of disease that are well-defined by HRCT. The patient (often male, >65 years, former/current smoker) usually presents with an alteration in pulmonary function tests (PFTs) with reduction of forced vital capacity (FVC) and mild, moderate, or severe reduction in the diffusing capacity of the lungs for carbon monoxide (DLCO) [55].The most relevant symptom is dyspnea upon exertion or rest (when the condition is in an advanced stage). The typical auscultation findings are crackles in lower chest fields ("velcro sounds"). These findings arise in subpleural regions and are mainly due to reticulations that proceed to honeycombing through traction bronchiolectasis. IPF involves the peripheral portion of secondary lobules (septal compartment), and its progression determines the overall structural alteration of the entire lobule, creating deformations of segmental and subsegmental bronchioles (with a predominance of the lower lobes) leading to small structures similar to lung cysts in a final framework called "honeycomb lung" [56] (Figs. 5.3, 5.4, 5.5, 5.6, 5.7, and 5.8).

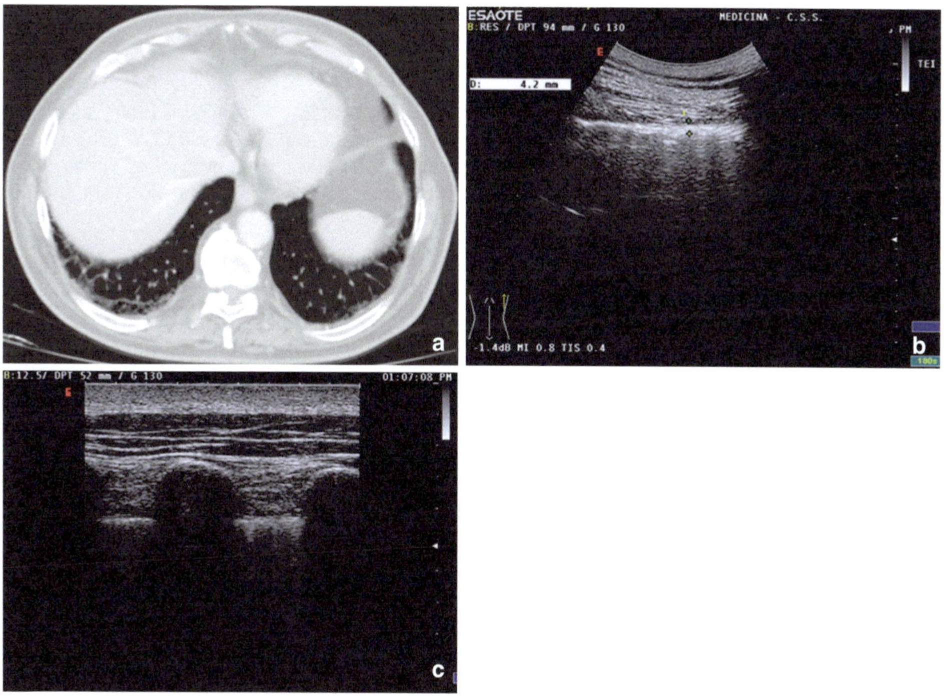

Fig. 5.3 (**a**) HRCT shows a fibrotic scar in the subpleural region with mild reticular subpleural thickening of interlobular septa. (**b**) US using a convex probe (at the same level as the HRCT image at lower lobe) shows irregularity and increased thickness (>4 mm) of the pleural line. B-lines are also visible. (**c**) US using a linear probe (at the same level as the convex probe image) provides a better view of slight irregularity and increased thickness of the pleural line. The visibility of artifacts is poor

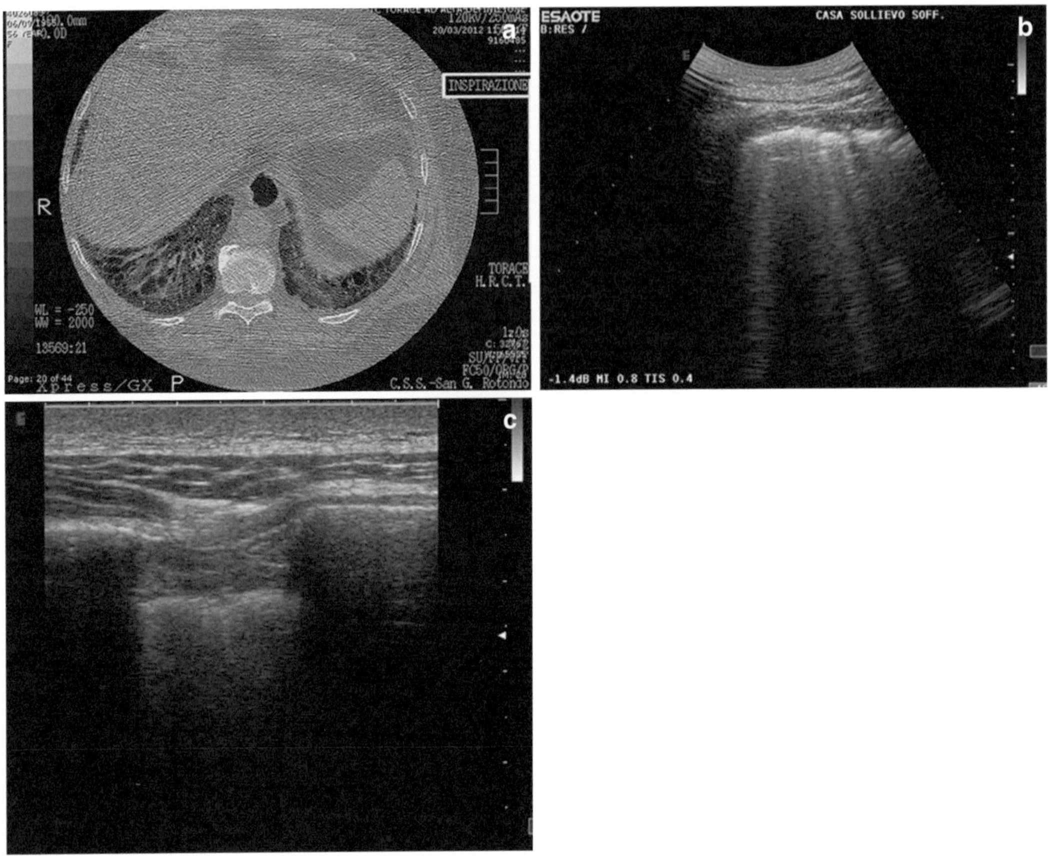

Fig. 5.4 (**a**) HRCT (basal/posterior segment of lower lobes) shows small subpleural cysts. These are typical findings discovered predominantly in the subpleural space in patients with definite UIP. (**b**) US using a convex probe (same level as the HRCT image on the lower lobe) shows marked irregularity and increased thickness (>3 mm) of the pleural line with B-lines. (**c**) US using a linear probe (same level as the convex probe image on the lower lobe) view irregularity of the pleural line with an increase in thickness (>2 mm)

Take-Home Messages

As evident from the cases showing a HRCT pattern of "possible UIP" with a pathologic-conclusive diagnosis (video-assisted thoracoscopic surgery) of UIP and in the clinical context of IPF, understanding what US can show in relation to HRCT (as well as the limitations and traps in trying to make a US diagnosis without precise correlation with HRCT) is important. Some crucial considerations are:

- Fibrotic changes can be observed with US as an irregular and increased thickness of the hyperechoic pleural line. These effects are not observed in healthy individuals [57].
- Irregularity of the pleural line seems pronounced and visible in the areas of greatest distorted fibrotic changes. The pleural line is often blurred, thickened, and fragmented [58].
- Areas of honeycombing and areas with traction bronchiolectasis or with interstitial intralobular thickening and intralobular GGO changes cannot be discriminated only with US. These areas can produce the same artifactual alterations, more or less severe, depending on the degrees of severity of the distortion, but without enabling discrimination of one pathologic finding from another: this is possible only with HRCT.
- A US convex probe shows the worst spatial resolution of more superficial structures. It also shows an increase in the pleural line.
- Artifacts in fibrotic conditions are sometimes poorly discriminable from each other. Hence,

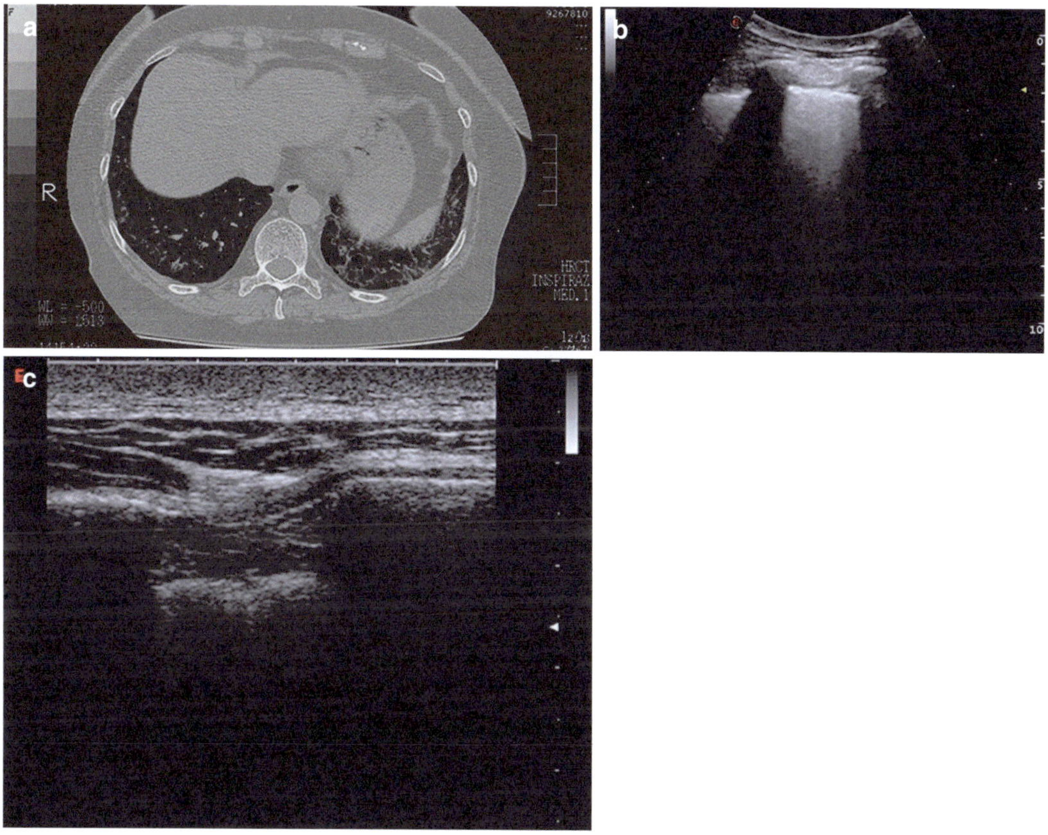

Fig. 5.5 (**a**) HRCT (basal/posterior segment of the lower lobes) shows (on the left) a small traction subsegmental bronchiolectasis, with a reticular pattern and intralobular thickening. (**b**) US using convex probe (same level as the HRCT image on the left lower lobe) shows mild irregularity and an increased thickness of the pleural line. Also visible are B-line artifacts. (**c**) US using a linear probe (same level as the convex probe image on the right lower lobe) provides a better view of marked irregularity of the pleural line with an increase in thickness in some parts

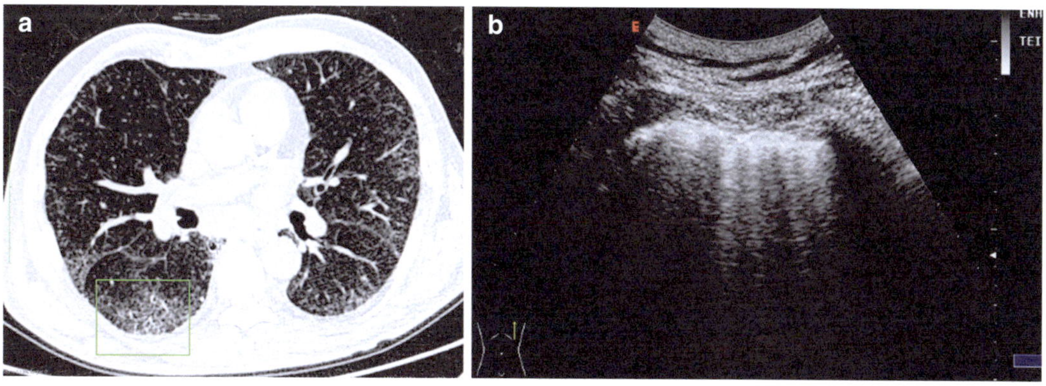

Fig. 5.6 (**a**) HRCT (upper segment of lower lobes) shows (on the right) mild subpleural intralobular/interlobular interstitial thickening with slight traction subsegmental bronchiolectasis without honeycombing. (**b**) Use of a convex probe (same level as the HRCT image on the right lower lobe) shows irregularity and an increase in thickness of the pleural line (>4 mm) in some parts. B-lines are also visible

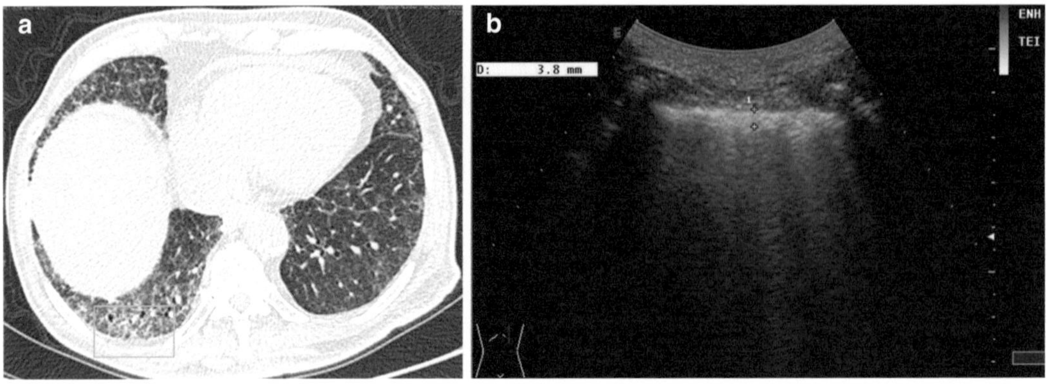

Fig. 5.7 (**a**) HRCT (posterior segment of lower lobes) shows (on the right) very mild subpleural intralobular/interlobular interstitial thickening without honeycombing and slight fibrotic ground-glass opacities. (**b**) US using a convex probe (same level as the HRCT image on the right lower lobe) shows mild irregularity, fragmentation, and increased thickness (>2 mm) of a blurred pleural line with an increase in the number of blurred artifacts

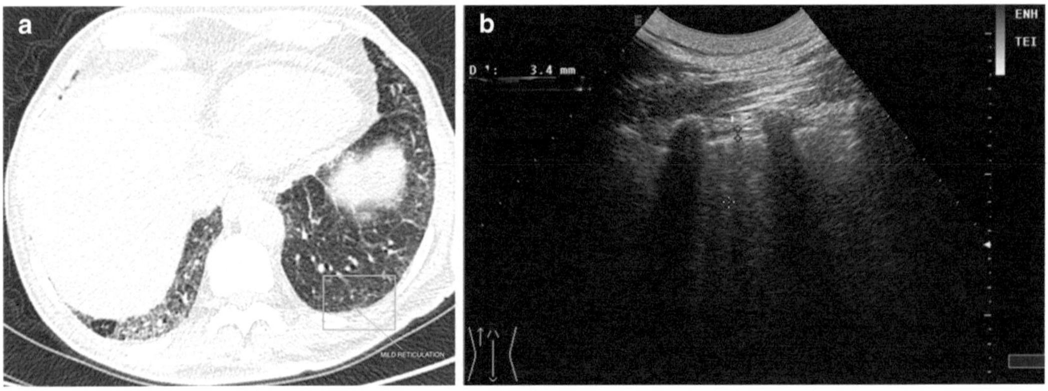

Fig. 5.8 (**a**) HRCT (posterior segment of lower lobes) shows (on the left) slight focal interlobular thickening without traction bronchiolectasis and/or honeycombing. (**b**) US convex probe (same level as the HRCT image on the right lower lobe) shows mild irregularity and increased thickness (>3 mm) of the pleural line. B-line artifacts are also visible

there could be many artifacts, but they are not identifiable or quantifiable with high accuracy. Therefore, UIP must be assessed with extreme caution.

5.6 NSIP

NSIP is the potential evolution of several fibrotic ILDs. Its differential diagnosis is mainly with UIP/IPF, and it can be of a primitive nature (i-NSIP) or secondary (connective tissue diseases, CHP, drug toxicity). NSIP usually has a favorable prognosis (lymphocytosis prevailing according to bronchoalveolar lavage fluid (BALF) [59]. NSIP is very sensitive to therapy and, therefore, is potentially reversible with corticosteroids. However, the aggressive form of NSIP (BALF showing dominant neutrophilia) is refractory to corticosteroid therapy and has a poor prognosis, similar to that of UIP/IPF [60].

NSIP was described first by Katzeinstein and Fiorelli in 1994 [61]. The histology of NSIP is characterized by inflammation and fibrosis of different degrees and entities in the lung, with prevalent involvement of the alveolar walls. Typical characteristics compared with a UIP/IPF pattern shown by HRCT are:

- Temporal and spatial homogeneity of alterations.
- GGO-dominant pattern in the "cellular" rather than "fibrosing" form of the disease.
- Widespread extension into central and subpleural lung areas.
- Anatomic gradient in the cranio-caudal plane shows invariably predominant alterations in the lower lobes. These alterations may be confined to the lower portions of both lungs.
- In the axial plane, slight subpleural sparing is observed in 20–40% of cases [62].

It is difficult to distinguish between the aggressive form of NSIP and the classic forms of UIP/IPF based on pathology. Mild GGOs, severe interstitial thickening, reticulation, bronchiolectasis, and honeycombing are responsible for severe forms of lung fibrosis that carry a poor prognosis.

Auscultation is characterized by crackles and "velcro sounds" that are less intense than the classic forms of UIP/IPF. Spirometry is characterized by a restriction more or less severe with reduced FVC and DLCO. Upon longitudinal evaluation, the extent of GGOs can decrease with disease evolution, but the extent of reticular abnormalities can persist or increase (until a UIP pattern is reached). Patients with HRCT-pathologic findings of NSIP have longer survival than those with the HRCT aspects of UIP. HRCT is the gold standard for detection, characterization, and longitudinal evaluation of NSIP. However, the conclusive diagnosis of i-NSIP requires careful clinical–radiologic–pathologic evaluation by a multidisciplinary team [63].

Take-Home Messages

As evident from the case of cellular NSIP presented, understanding what US can show in relation to HRCT, as well as the limitations and traps in trying to make a US diagnosis without precise correlation with HRCT, is important. Some crucial considerations are:

- Areas of extensive GGO changes show only moderate increases in thickness of the pleural line with a US convex probe (more evident in lower lobes).
- Compared with distorting and fibrotic changes, the GGO area does not determine frank irregularities or fragmentations of the pleural line (which looks fairly linear).
- Despite the pathologic changes of GGO, a large number of artifacts may not be detected.
- In this respect more research should be important to clarify or reconsider a possible role of TUS in the early diagnosis of this condition.
- Alterations despite definite alveolar-interstitial involvement that is clearly visible on HRCT.

5.7 CHP (Chronic Hypersensitivity Pneumonia)

CHP is a complex chronic inflammatory disease that affects alveolar/interstitial and small-airway compartments of the lungs. It is caused by recurrent exposure factors, environmental or otherwise (e.g., mites, mold, dust), capable of determining antigenic activation. CHP is divided into acute, subacute, and chronic. The chronic form is characterized by fibrotic changes of more or less severe pathologic entities with elements that can "remember" the previous stages of CHP (centrilobular nodules, areas of air-trapping, lung cysts). In a consistent clinical–radiologic context and with BALF showing significant (>30%) lymphocytosis, a diagnosis of CHP is out of the question. Fundamental for the diagnosis is the prevalence of alterations detected in the upper lobes, axial/peribronchial fibrosis, and areas of air-trapping. If there are at least three areas of air-trapping in a single lobe and this pattern occurs in at least four lobes, together with coexisting fibrotic changes, then a diagnosis of CHP is highly probable (and, in some cases, pathognomonic). If there is predominance for the lower lobes and in the absence of significant and multiple areas of air-trapping, then it is often difficult to discriminate UIP in CHP from UIP in IPF [64].

Key findings of CHP using HRCT are:

- Predominance of alterations in the upper–middle areas of the lungs
- Peribronchial distribution
- Air-trapping

- Traction bronchiolectasis
- Honeycombing (at the late stage) (Figs. 5.9 and 5.10)

Take-Home Messages

- In US, fibrotic changes can be observed as an irregular, thickened hyperechoic pleural line. These features are not observed in healthy individuals.
- Irregularity of the pleural line is more pronounced and visible in areas of greatest distorted fibrotic changes. The pleural line is often blurred, thickened, and fragmented.
- Areas of honeycombing, traction bronchiolectasis and/or interstitial intralobular thickening, and GGO changes cannot be discriminated in CHP using US only. US can produce the same artifactual alterations, more or less severe, depending on the degree of severity of the distortion, but without the ability to discriminate one pathologic finding from another; this is possible only with HRCT.

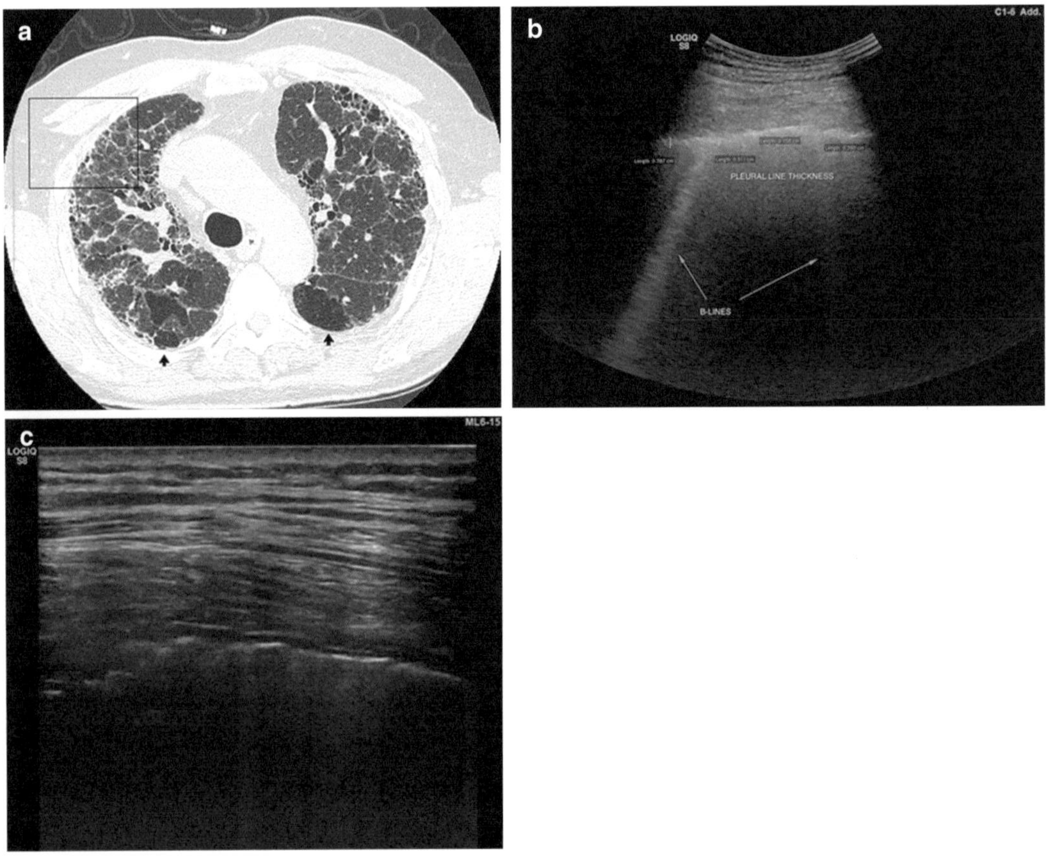

Fig. 5.9 (**a**) HRCT (upper lobes) shows, on the right (box), a reticular pattern with septal thickening, intralobular thickening with superimposed mild fibrotic areas of ground-glass opacities, and sporadic small cysts in subpleural areas. Small areas of decreased attenuation density are also visible, which are typical findings of air-trapping (black arrows). (**b**) US using a S8 C1-6 convex probe (same level as the HRCT image on the right upper lobe, anterior segment) shows a blurred, mildly irregular pleural line with a small increase in thickness. A small number of B-line artifacts are also present. (**c**) US using a ML6-15 matrix linear probe (same level as the HRCT image on the right upper lobe) provides a better view of the markedly irregular and multi-fragmented pleural line with a slight increase in thickness in some parts. There is very poor visibility of blurred artifacts and a complete absence of discrimination between intralobular/interlobular thickening and subpleural cysts; these features are visible only on HRCT

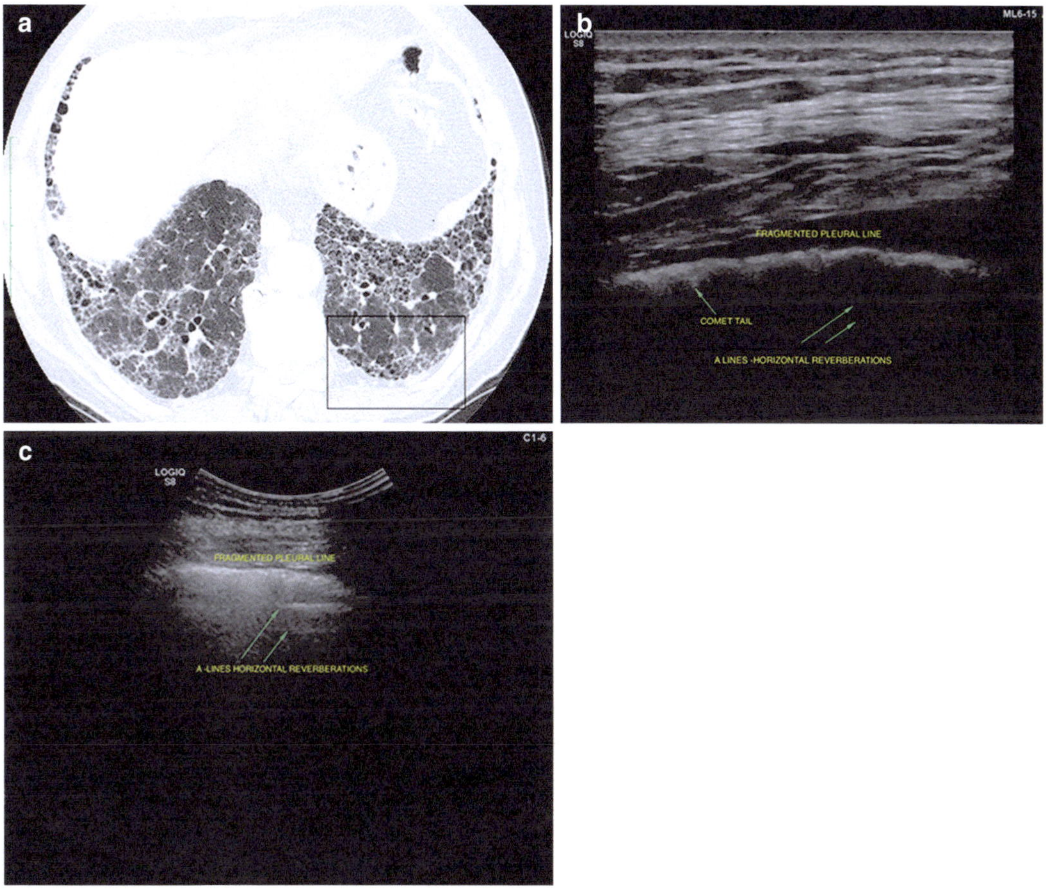

Fig. 5.10 (**a**) HRCT (lower lobes) shows, on the left (box), a severe reticular pattern with septal thickening, intralobular thickening with superimposed fibrotic areas of ground-glass opacities, traction bronchiolectasis, and slight honeycombing in subpleural areas. Small areas of decreased attenuation density (air-trapping) are also visible. (**b**) US using a ML6-15 matrix linear probe (same level as HRCT image on the right lower lobe) provides a better view of the markedly irregular, slightly thickened (>2 mm) pleural line (**c**) Us using a C1-6 convex probe (same level as the HRCT image on the left lower lobe) shows a blurred and thickened pleural line (>3 mm). B-line artifacts are absent, but A-line artifacts can be seen on the right of the screen

- A US linear probe allows better and more defined evaluation of the pleural line, but in some circumstances, it may lead to the detriment of display of artifacts (which are less defined and less well represented than in UIP/IPF).
- A US convex probe shows the worst spatial resolution of more superficial structures. It shows an unreal and paradoxical increase in thickness of the pleural line, which appears coarser and is less well discriminated. In areas of marked distortion in the left lower lobe, US may also detect reverberation artifacts (A-lines) which are not correlated with the HRCT pattern of fibrotic alterations.

5.8 DIP (Desquamative Interstitial Pneumonia)

In the classification of IIPs, DIP is a smoking-related ILD characterized by accumulation in the alveolar compartment of pigment-laden macrophages. DIP-like alterations are also observed in acute intoxication by irritating/chemical fumes. HRCT findings are characterized by:

- Extensive GGO pattern
- Septal thickening
- Lower-zone predominance in 75%, subpleural distribution in 60%, and random distribution in 25% of cases
- Scattered lung cysts (20%)
- Linear and reticular opacities
- Traction bronchiolectasis and honeycombing (end-stage DIP in <10% of cases)

The differential diagnosis is NSIP, in which traction bronchiolectasis and volume loss are often visible. A history of tobacco smoking and macrophages in BALF supports the diagnosis of DIP [65] (Fig. 5.11).

Take-Home Messages

TUS has to be strictly related with HRCT to make a correct diagnosis. Some crucial considerations are:

- Areas of extensive GGO on HRCT can be related to an increased thickness of the pleural line in some parts.
- The US linear probe allows a better and more defined evaluation of the pleural line because of its power of resolution.
- The use of an US convex probe highlights the increased in thickness of the pleural line that is not well-defined and has a coarse pattern.

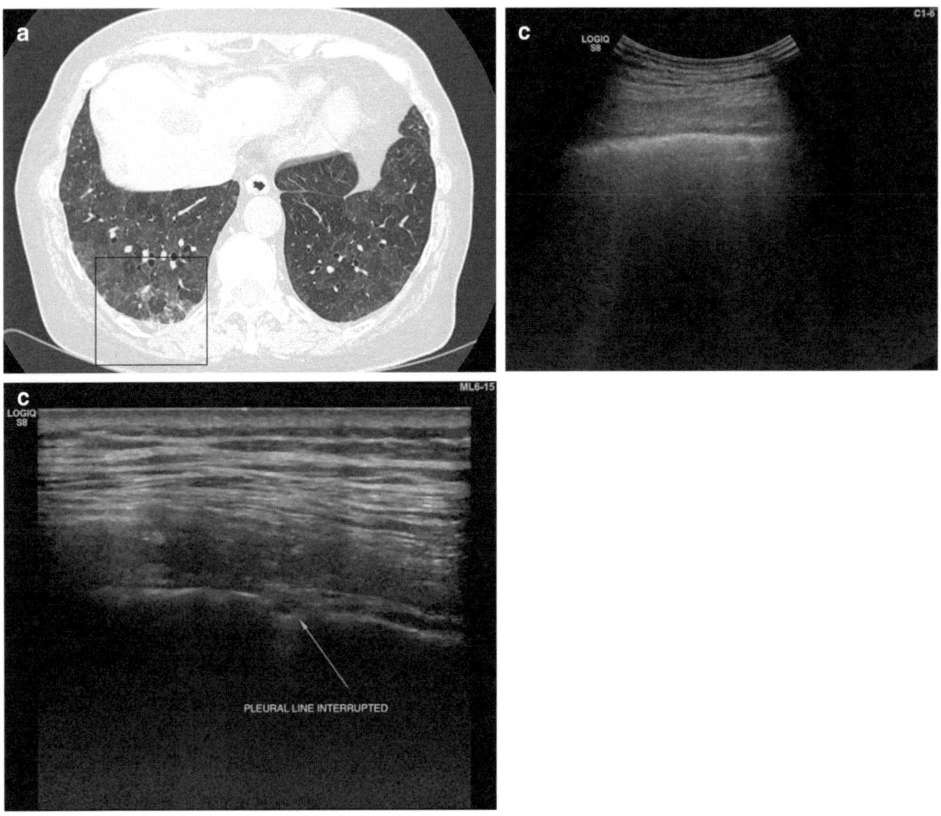

Fig. 5.11 (**a**) HRCT (lower lobes) with, on the right (box), extensive areas of ground-glass opacities in both lungs with predominance in the right lung. There is mild reticulation with interstitial thickening but without traction bronchiolectasis or honeycombing. Small areas of mildly decreased attenuation may be related to smoking. Focal irregular pleural thickening in the posterior segment of the right lower lobe can be observed. (**b**) US using a C1-6 convex probe (at the same level as the HRCT image on the left lower lobe) shows a mildly blurred and thickened (>3 mm) pleural line in some parts. A mildly irregular hypoechoic area can be observed in the right part of the screen. A small number of B-lines are also present. (**c**) US using a ML6-15 matrix linear probe (at the same level as the HRCT image on the left lower lobe) provides a better view of a pleural line that is mildly irregular, blurred, fragmented, and slightly thickened (>2 mm) in some parts

5.9 Other Infiltrative Lung Disorders

5.9.1 Sarcoidosis

Sarcoidosis is a systemic idiopathic disease mainly affecting the lung. The pathologic "key finding" is the non-necrotic granuloma, which develops in many organs and may disappear or may progress to fibrotic alterations resulting in end-stage lung fibrosis.

The classic symptoms are fatigue, night sweats, and progressive weight loss. Two-thirds of patients can experience remission, whereas in one-third of patients, the disease can worsen determining damage to the lungs, brain, heart, skin, liver, or spleen. Despite disease staging (I–IV) is based on chest radiography. HRCT of the chest is the gold standard for the diagnosis because sarcoidosis is characterized by a particular tropism and "greed" for lymphatic tissue (lymph nodes, fissures, interlobular septa, pleural compartment). Hence, nodules localize next to these structures (classic perilymphatic distribution). Differential diagnoses are CHP, IPPFE, radiation pneumonia, tuberculosis, talcosis, and silicosis. At end-stage sarcoidosis, honeycombing with large cysts is evident [66].

Key Findings:

- Small nodules with perilymphatic distribution and dominance for upper/middle lung regions along with fissures and interlobular septa with a central distribution
- Mediastinal lymph nodes involvement, sometimes with calcifications
- Coalescence of gross nodules and or/galaxy sign
- Numerous small nodules that determine the characteristics of the GGO pattern (atypical finding) (Figs. 5.12 and 5.13)

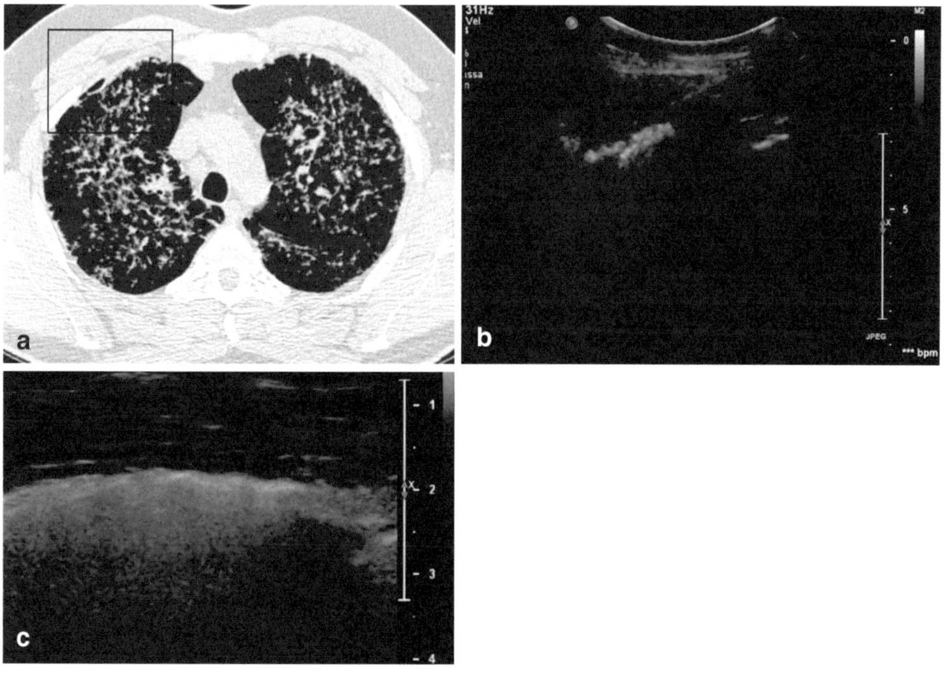

Fig. 5.12 (**a**) HRCT (upper lobes) with, on the right (box), marked septal thickening and small nodules with a perilymphatic distribution. Coarse and irregular reticular opacities are evident next to subpleural areas of the upper lung lobes (anterior segment of the right upper lobe). (**b**) At the same level of the HRCT image, US using a C1-5 convex probe highlights a multi-fragmented, irregular, and thickened (>3 mm) pleural line. This US pattern is not specific for sarcoidosis. (**c**) At the same level as the HRCT image, a L12-5 linear probe points out irregular, blurred, fragmented, and thickened (>2 mm) pleural line

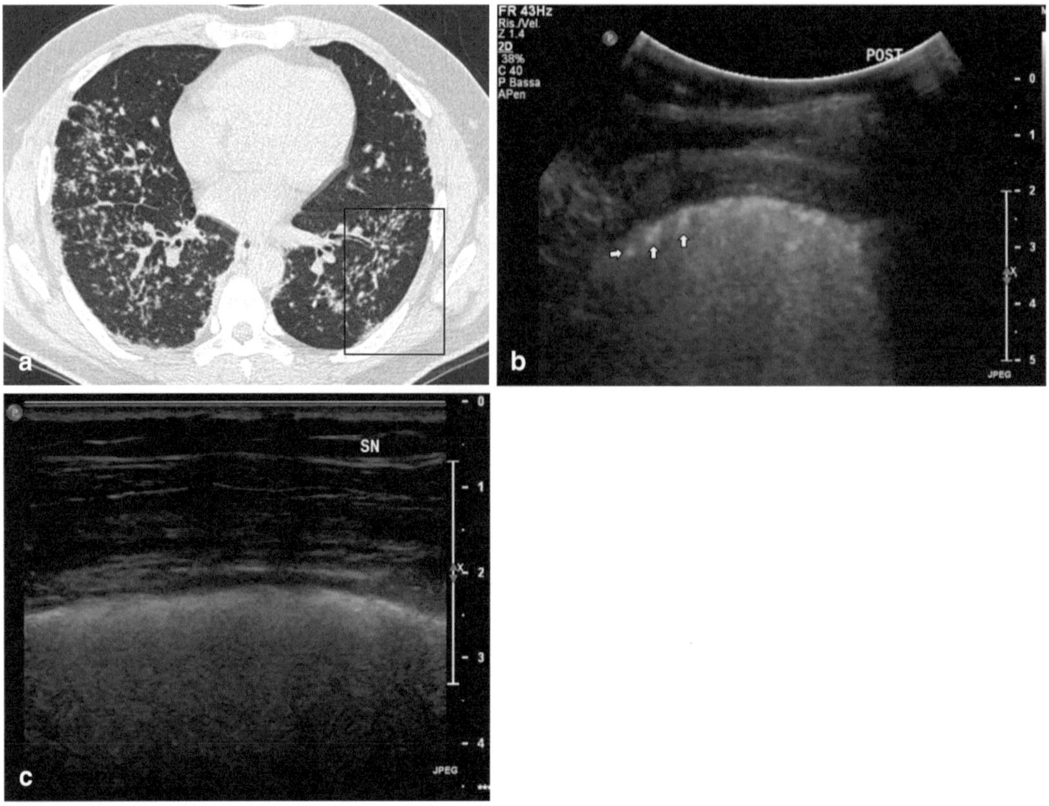

Fig. 5.13 (**a**) HRCT (lower lobes) with, at the left (box), small nodules with a perilymphatic distribution. Coarse and irregular reticular opacities and few nodules are visible in the subpleural compartment of the left lung lobes. A symmetric distribution of alterations and some evidence of a few, undefined artifacts are evident. (**b**) At the same level as the HRCT image, US using a C1-5 convex probe highlights a slight increase in thickness (>3 mm) at some parts of a fragmented pleural line. This US pattern is not specific for sarcoidosis. Comet tails (arrows) and some undefined B-line artifacts are evident. (**c**) At the same level as the HRCT image, a L12-5 linear probe points out an irregular, blurred, fragmented, and thickened (>2 mm) pleural line

Take-Home Messages

- Sarcoidosis is characterized by reticular (septal compartment and perilymphatic tropism) and nodular alterations of the lung and pleural compartments. Hence, US can highlight a slight or marked irregularity of the pleural line with a blurred appearance, fragmentation, and thickening especially at the upper and middle third of the chest.
- Using both a convex and a linear probe, a focal increased thickness of the pleural line could be evident.

5.10 Tuberculosis

Tuberculosis is a particularly severe, infectious disease. The clinical and radiologic manifestations of tuberculosis depend on immunologic status, age, and previous exposure to *Mycobacterium tuberculosis*. The primary form of tuberculosis develops in individuals with a normal immunity. Postprimary tuberculosis may develop in those with acquired specific immunity.

Clinical and radiologic manifestations are pyrexia, cough, asthenia, weight loss, hemoptysis, bronchopneumonic infiltrates, pleural effusion, cavitary consolidations, nodules, as well as alterations in the small airways and mediastinal lymph nodes. Postprimary tuberculosis usually involves upper lobes. Compared with primary tuberculosis (which is an acute/subacute disease), postprimary tuberculosis is typically chronic, slowly progressive and associated with high morbidity and mortality if not treated appropriately. Pleural effusion is more common in postprimary tuberculosis and is usually unilateral. Sequelae of postprimary tuberculosis may be localized lung fibrosis (fibrothorax); bronchiolectasis; cavitations; calcified granulomas; dense fibrotic bands; and areas of air-trapping due to constrictive bronchiolitis, bronchopleural fistulae, or lung cancer [67].

5.11 Miliary Tuberculosis

Miliary tuberculosis is characterized by multiple, small nodules (diameter, 3–5 mm) with defined margins and distributed in more than two-thirds of the lung with a random distribution. This pattern is caused by the massive hematogenous dissemination tuberculosis (Figs. 5.14 and 5.15).

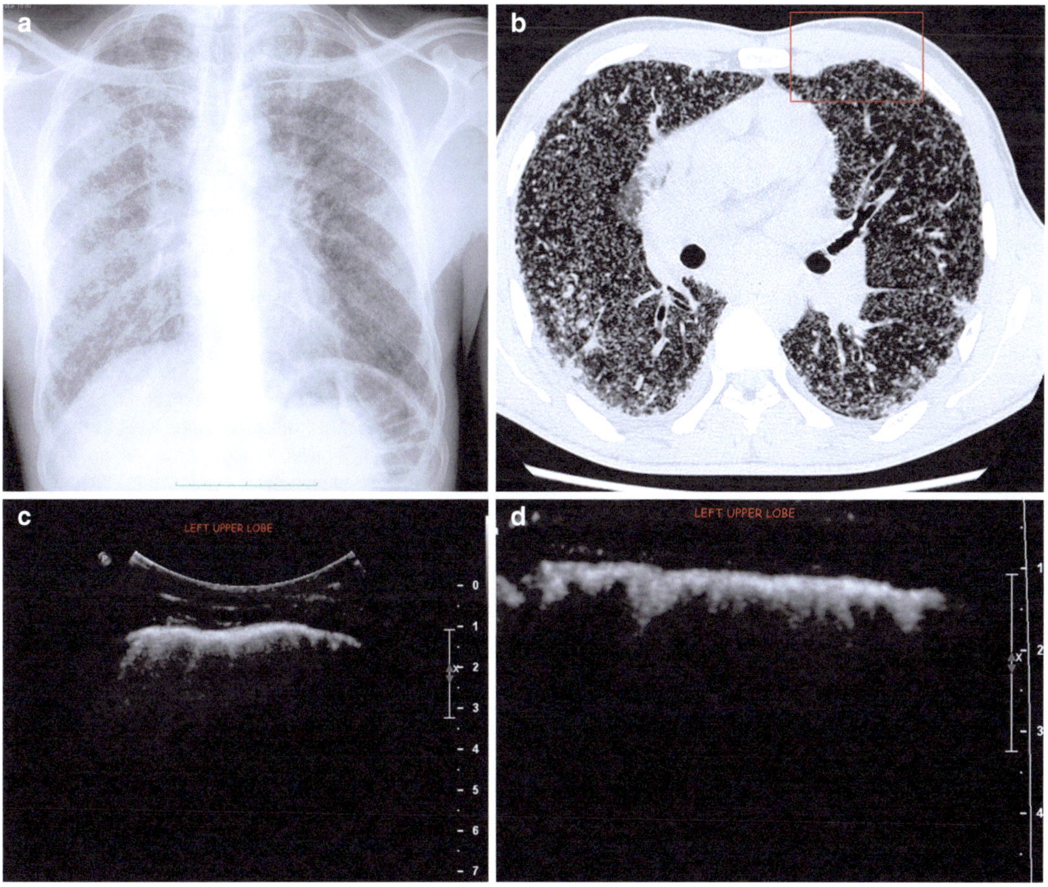

Fig. 5.14 (**a**) Chest radiography (posteroanterior view) with hundreds of minute nodules and the classic "snowstorm" miliary pattern. (**b**) HRCT (upper lobes) shows, on the left (box), evidence of multiple nodules with a random distribution clearly evident until the pleural line. (**c**) At the same level as the HRCT image, US using a C1-5 convex probe highlights a thickened pleural line (>3 mm) that is not related to a real increase in pleural layers (as visible on HRCT). Multiple (some divergent) comet-tail and B-line/ring down artifacts are visible. (**d**) At the same level as the HRCT image, a L12-5 linear probe points out an irregular, blurred, fragmented, and thickened (>2 mm) pleural line. It is, therefore, impossible to differentiate miliary tuberculosis with another pattern (e.g., reticular in pulmonary fibrosis or nodular in sarcoidosis)

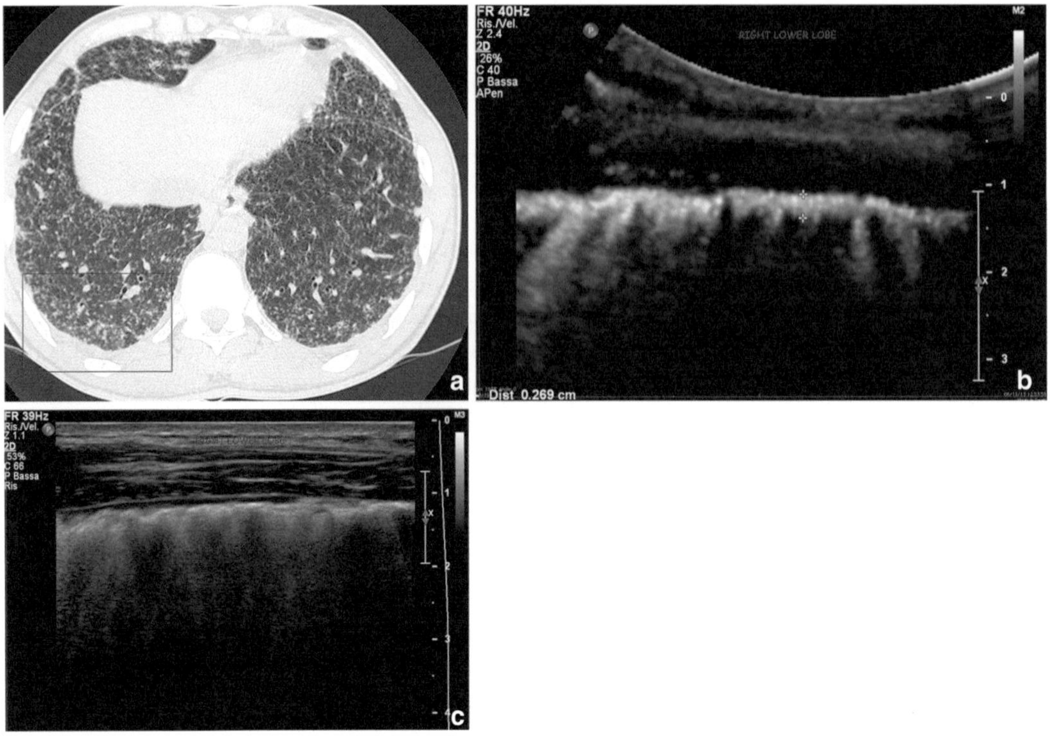

Fig. 5.15 (**a**) HRCT (upper lobes) shows, on the right (box), multiple minute nodules with a random distribution until the pleural line. (**b**) At the same level as the HRCT image, US using a C1-5 convex probe highlights multiple (some divergent) irregular, coalesced, blurred, comet-tail, and B-line artifacts. Both a normal hyperechoic pleural line (0.28 mm) and thickened (>3 mm, in some parts) pleural line are clearly visible. As seen clearly from HRCT, nodules adhering to the pleura are not differentiable from possible fibrotic changes (as in the patterns for UIP, NSIP, DIP, or CHP) analyzed previously. Also nodules can produce comet tail, ring down, and blurred/coalescence of coexisting artifacts, with the same US presentation of many other conditions. (**c**) At the same level as the HRCT image, US 12-5L linear probe points out an irregular, blurred, fragmented, and thickened (>2 mm) pleural line

Take-Home Messages

- Miliary tuberculosis is characterized by hundreds of minute nodules with a random distribution in both lungs. Many are close to fissures and pleural layers. Hence, US can highlight a slight or marked irregularity of the hyperechoic pleural line characterized by a blurred appearance, fragmentation, and thickening from the apex to the base of the lung.
- Comparing US and HRCT scans, it is clear that nodules adhering to the pleura are not differentiable by US from fibrotic changes (as in the patterns for UIP, NSIP, DIP, and CHP) analyzed previously. Moreover nodules can determine B-lines and blurred/coalescence of coexisting artifacts with a nonspecific pattern.
- In US, significant changes in the pleural line, with a blurred and fragmented appearance, might suggest an aggressive- or advanced-stage fibrotic disease. Therefore, the US pattern could be a confounding factor. Only clinical evaluation, laboratory data, and HRCT allow a correct diagnosis of miliary tuberculosis.

5.12 Pulmonary Alveolar Microlithiasis (PAM)

PAM is a very rare idiopathic disease. It is characterized by multiple minute calcium deposits localized diffusely within the alveoli. HRCT of the chest is considered to be the gold standard for PAM diagnosis.

HRCT revealed hundreds of minute nodules, with calcific aspects, in a miliary-type distribution with a "sandstorm aspect." Nodules showed a high prevalence in the middle, right middle, and lower lobes. Other findings were septal thickening, GGO, and, in some areas, a "crazy paving" pattern. Sometimes, calcification of pleura was present. On The TUS examination, A- and B-line artifacts were not detected despite the severity of interstitial/alveolar involvement. The only TUS finding was an increased thickness and irregular profile (more evident in the dorsal lower lung regions) of the hyperechoic pleural line [68] (Figs. 5.16 and 5.17).

Take-Home Messages

PAM is characterized by small nodules with a random distribution in both lungs. US can produce slight or marked irregularity of a hyperechoic pleural line characterized by a blurred and thickened appearance in both lungs.

- No horizontal reverberations (A-lines) or vertical artifacts (B-lines) were observed despite the severity of interstitial/alveolar involvement. The only TUS finding was an increased thickness and irregular profile (more evident in the dorsal lower lung regions) of the hyperechoic pleural line (evident only with a convex transducer). This finding may have been due

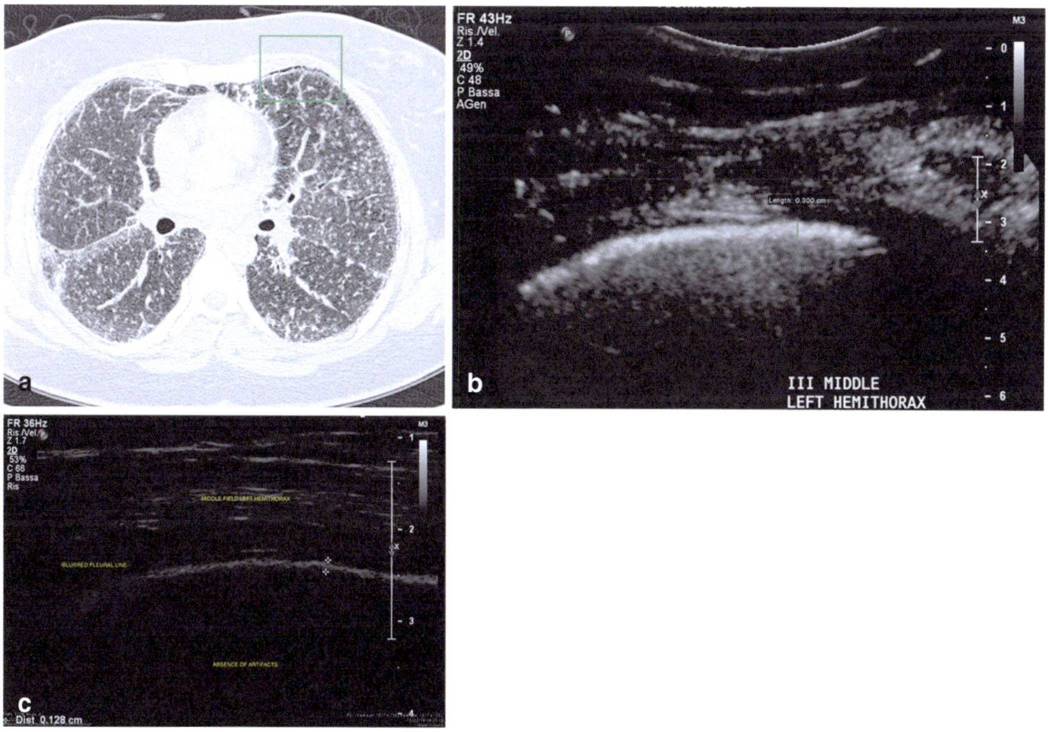

Fig. 5.16 (**a**) HRCT of the chest shows a diffuse random distribution of multiple minute nodules and ground-glass opacities (sandstorm pattern) that is highly suggestive of PAM in the clinical context in the upper lung lobes. Subtle cystic changes are also depicted bilaterally in the subpleural ventral region and identified as a dark pleural line. Also, multiple minute nodules and smooth interlobular septal thickening are present in both lungs. (**b**) US using a C1-5 convex probe (at the same level as the HRCT image) shows the maximum limit of the normal value of a hyperechoic pleural line: 3 mm (this is not related to the real increase of pleural layers as shown on HRCT). There is an unexplained absence of artifacts compared with the evidence of gross pathology (nodular and interstitial) evident on HRCT. (**c**) US using a L12-5 linear probe (at the same level as the HRCT image) provides a better view of the blurred pleural line. Also, there is an undefined absence of artifacts below the pleural line

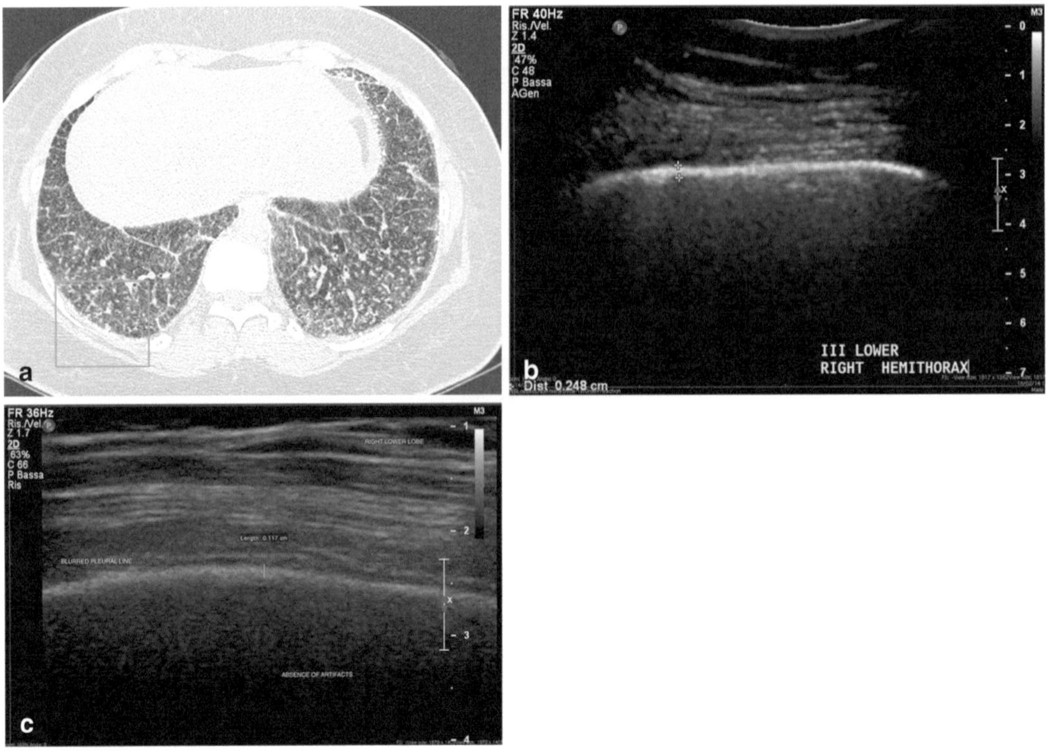

Fig. 5.17 (**a**) HRCT of the chest shows a diffuse, random distribution of multiple minute nodules and ground-glass opacities (sandstorm pattern) that is highly suggestive for PAM in the upper lung lobes. Subtle cystic changes are also depicted bilaterally in the subpleural ventral region and identified as a dark pleural line. Also, multiple minute nodules and smooth interlobular septal thickening are present in both lungs. (**b**) US using a C1-5 convex probe (at the same level as the HRCT image) shows a normal hyperechoic pleural line: 2.4 mm (this is related to the pleural layers shown on HRCT). There is an absence of artifacts compared with the evidence of a mixed-pattern (nodular and interstitial) disease, evident on HRCT. (**c**) US using a L12-5 linear probe (at the same level as the HRCT image) shows an absence of artifacts with a blurred aspect below the pleural line

to microcystic changes ("micro-honeycombing") immediately underlying the thickened pleura. Nodules adhering to the pleura (seen from HRCT) are not differentiable from possible fibrotic changes (as seen in the patterns for UIP, NSIP, DIP, and CHP).

5.13 Lung Involvement in Connective Tissue Disease

Lung involvement is one the most common extra-articular features of connective tissue diseases. ILD is quite common in systemic sclerosis (SSc). In SSc, pulmonary fibrosis, generally, starts in the peripheral lower subpleural sites of the lung [69]. This fibrotic reaction in interstitial tissue usually follows (within a variable timeframe) an acute alveolitis [70].

The most common HRCT pattern in SSc patients is NSIP with a greater proportion of GGOs and a lower degree of coarse reticulation. However, in rare cases, a UIP pattern can also be seen. Honeycomb cysts can be seen in up to one-third of patients with SSc–ILD and are more common in patients with limited cutaneous-SSc. The HRCT pattern predicts the underlying histopathology, with reticulation representing the underlying fibrosis on biopsy and consolidation representing inflammation [71].

In SSc patients, pulmonary fibrosis initially involves the lower posterior subpleural regions of the lung, which are largely accessible to US, despite some limitations (see page 5, TUS in fibrosis: future perspective [42, 43]). Scholars have investigated employment of US in interstitial lung diseases. TUS could be a useful complementary method in SSc management, because it is more sensitive than PFTs as a screening tool for interstitial lung involvement. Consequently, we believe that, at least in patients without lung and heart comorbidities, US could be a valuable tool to select patients for HRCT of the chest in the early phases of disease and follow-up of treatment with sensible savings in terms of cost and radiation exposure [72].

Take-Home Messages

- In SSc, pulmonary fibrosis usually starts from the peripheral and lower-posterior sites of subpleural lung tissue and spreads upward and outward as the disease progresses.
- TUS could be a useful complementary method in SSc management, because it is more sensitive than PFTs as a screening tool for interstitial lung involvement.
- The HRCT pattern seen in SSc patients is, in general, NSIP, with a greater proportion of GGOs and a lower degree of coarse reticulation in the early and mid-phase of SSc. When the disease progresses, there is an increase in reticulation and distortion with septal/interlobular/intralobular thickening leading to traction bronchiolectasis and, finally, in rare cases, to honeycombing.
- The pattern seen on HRCT can predict the underlying histopathology, with reticulation representing underlying fibrosis on biopsy and consolidation often representing inflammation.
- HRCT is the gold standard for the diagnosis of connective tissue diseases related lung involvement.

5.14 Conclusions

Some of TUS findings are sensitive (but not specific) for interstitial lung diseases. ILDs can be diagnosed with the aid of HRCT at an early stage [73]. TUS is a useful complementary tool to HRTC and conventional radiology for the study of pleural and interstitial lung diseases. On the other hand, TUS signs presumably visible in ILD are not yet cited in the most important scientific societies' guidelines [52, 74–76]. Moreover, a deep knowledge of the physical principles of US, of the machine settings, and of the general principles of US-based anatomy and US artifacts and a long-term experience in general TUS are mandatory to perform TUS in order to avoid dangerous misdiagnosis.

References

1. Mathis G. Thorax sonography—part I: chest wall and pleura. Ultrasound Med Biol. 1997;23:1131–9.
2. Reissig A, Görg C, Mathis G. Transthoracic sonography in the diagnosis of pulmonary diseases: a systematic approach. Ultraschall Med. 2009;30:438–54.
3. Sperandeo M, Filabozzi P, Varriale A, et al. Role of thoracic ultrasound in the assessment of pleural and pulmonary diseases. J Ultrasound. 2008;11(2):39–46.
4. Tsai CL, Wang HP, Lien WC, et al. B-lines artefacts on abdominal sonography to predict pulmonary abnormalities in the emergency department. Emerg Med J. 2005;22:747–8.
5. Trovato GM, Sperandeo M, Catalano D. Thoracic ultrasound: possible complementary criteria for the assessment of pulmonary fibrosis. Ann Thorac Med. 2014;9:179.
6. Marino F, Martorano C, Tripepi R, et al. Subclinical pulmonary congestion is prevalent in nephrotic syndrome. Kidney Int. 2016;89:421–8.
7. Zhang YK, Li J, Yang JP, Zhan Y, Chen J. Lung ultrasonography for the diagnosis of 11 patients with acute respiratory distress syndrome due to bird flu H7N9 infection. Virol J. 2015;12:176.
8. Davidsen JR, Bendstrup E, Henriksen DP, Graumann O, Laursen CB. Lung ultrasound has limited diagnostic value in rare cystic lung diseases: a cross-sectional study. Eur Clin Respir J. 2017;4(1):13301111.
9. Petruzzelli MF, Vasti MP, Tramacere F, et al. The potential role of lung ultrasound B-lines for detection of lung radio-induced toxicity in breast cancer patients after radiation therapy. Echocardiography. 2016;33:1374–80.
10. Francis Lee K, Olak J. Anatomy and physiology of the pleural space. Chest Surg Clin N Am. 1994;4(3):391–403.
11. Michailova KN. Ultrastructural observation on the human visceral pleura. Eur J Morphol. 1997;35(2):125–35.
12. Falaschi F. Anatomy of pleural, chest wall and diaphragm. Radiol Med. 2000;5(Suppl 2):29–35.

13. Aldrich JE. Basic physics of ultrasound imaging. Crit Care Med. 2007;35(Suppl 5):S131–7.
14. Wells PNT. Ultrasonic imaging of the human body. Rep Prog Phys. 1999;62:671–722.
15. Kossoff G. Basic physics and imaging characteristics of ultrasound. World J Surg. 2000;24(2):134–42.
16. Dunn F, Fry WJ. Ultrasonic absorption and reflection by lung tissue. Phys Med Biol. 1961;5:401–10.
17. Reuter KL, Bogdan A. Physics of diagnostic ultrasound creating the image. In: Bolliger CT, FJF H, Mayo PH, Miyazawa T, Beamis JF, editors. Clinical chest ultrasound: from the ICU to the bronchoscopy suite. Prog respir res, vol. 37. Basel: Karger; 2009. p. 2–10.
18. Sagar KB, Rhyne TL, Myers GS, Lees RS. Characterization of normal and abnormal pulmonary surface by reflected ultrasound. Chest. 1978;74:29–33.
19. Corrin B, Addis BJ. Histopathology of the pleura. Respiration. 1990;5:160–75.
20. Murali R, Park K, Leslie KO. The pleura in health and disease. Semin Respir Crit Care Med. 2010;31(6):649–73.
21. Dietrich CF, Hirche TO, Schreiber D, Wagner TO. Sonographie von pleura and lunge. Ultraschall Med. 2003;24:303–11.
22. Sperandeo M, Rotondo A, Guglielmi G, Catalano D, Feragalli B, Trovato GM. Transthoracic ultrasound in the assessment of pleural and pulmonary diseases: use and limitations. Radiol Med. 2014;119(10):729–40.
23. Soldati G, Smargiassi A, Inchingolo R, Sher S, Nenna R, Valente S, Inchingolo CD, Corbo GM. Lung ultrasonography may provide an indirect estimation of lung porosity and airspace geometry. Respiration. 2014;88:458–68.
24. Trovato GM, Sperandeo M. The resistible rise of B-line lung ultrasound artefacts. Respiration. 2015;89(2):175–6.
25. Trovato GM, Catalano D, Sperandeo M, Graziano P. Artifacts, noise and interference: much ado about ultrasound. Respiration. 2015;90(1):8.
26. Sperandeo M, Varriale A, Sperandeo G, et al. Characterization of the normal pulmonary surface and pneumonectomy space by reflected ultrasound. J Ultrasound. 2011;14:22–7.
27. Cavaliere F, Zamparelli R, Soave MP, Gargaruti R, Scapigliati A, De Pauli S. Ultrasound artifacts mimicking pleural sliding after pneumonectomy. J Clin Anesth. 2014;26:131–5.
28. Dietrich CF, Mathis G, Blaivas M, et al. Lung B line artifacts and their use. J Thorac Dis. 2016;8:1356–65.
29. Kirberger RM. Imaging artefact in diagnostic ultrasound: a review. Vet Radiol Ultrasound. 1995;36:297–306.
30. Louvet A, Bourgeois JM. Lung ring down artefact a sign of pulmonary alveolar-interstitial disease. Vet Radiol Ultrasound. 2008;49:344–77.
31. Licthenstein D, Meziere G, Biderman P, Gepner A, Barre O. The comet tail artefact. An ultrasound sign of alveolar interstitial syndrome. Am J Respir Crit Care Med. 1997;58:1640–6.
32. Kohazaki S, Tsuruski K, Uetani M, Nakanishi K, Hayashi K. The aurora sign: an ultrasonographic sign suggesting parenchymal lung disease. Br J Radiol. 2003;76:437–43.
33. Soldati G, Copetti R, Sher S. Sonographic interstitial syndrome: the sound of lung water. J Ultrasound Med. 2009;28:163–74.
34. Zanforlin A, Smargiassi A, Inchingolo R, Sher S, Ramazzina E, Corbo GM, Soldati G. B-lines: to count or not to count? JACC Cardiovasc Imaging. 2014;7:635–6.
35. Soldati G, Copetti R, Sher S. Can lung comets be counted as "objects"? JACC Cardiovasc Imaging. 2011;4:438–9.
36. Spinelli A, Vinci B, Tirella A, et al. Realization of a poro-elastic ultrasound replica of pulmonary tissue. Biomatter. 2012;2:37–42.
37. Trovato GM, Sperandeo M. Objectively measuring the ghost in the machine: B-lines as uncertain measures on which to base clinical assessment. JACC Cardiovasc Imaging. 2015;8(12):1470.
38. Trovato GM, Sperandeo M. Sounds, ultrasounds, and artifacts: which clinical role for lung imaging? Am J Respir Crit Care Med. 2013;187:780–1.
39. Sperandeo M, Varriale A, Sperandeo G, Polverino E, Feragalli B, et al. Assessment of ultrasound acoustic artifacts in patients with acute dyspnea: a multicenter study. Acta Radiol. 2012;53:885–92.
40. Tinti MG, Rea G, Mirijello A, Frongillo E, Sperandeo M. Is there any role for thoracic ultrasound for interstitial lung disease underlying rheumatologic conditions? Comment. Intern Emerg Med. 2017;12(6):903–4.
41. Trovato GM, Catalano D, Sperandeo M, Graziano P. Artifacts, noise and interference: much ado about ultrasound. Respiration. 2015;90(1):85.
42. Covic A, Siriopol D, Voroneanu L. Use of lung ultrasound for the assessment of volume status in CKD. Am J Kidney Dis. 2018;71(3):412–22. https://doi.org/10.1053/j.ajkd.2017.10.009. pii:S0272-6386(17)31039-9. Epub ahead of print.
43. Raghu G, Collard HR, Egan JJ, et al. An official ATS/ERS/JRS/ALAT statement: idiopathic pulmonary fibrosis: evidence-based guidelines for diagnosis and management. Am J Respir Crit Care Med. 2011;183:788–824.
44. Frauenfelder T, Winklehner A, Nguyen TD, et al. Screening for interstitial lung disease in systemic sclerosis: performance of high-resolution CT with limited number of slices: a prospective study. Ann Rheum Dis. 2014;73(12):2069–73.
45. Sperandeo M, Carnevale V, Arcangela Grimaldi M. Chest ultrasonography as a screening tool for high-resolution computed tomography referral in patients with systemic sclerosis-a future perspective: comment on the article by Suliman et al. Arthritis Rheumatol. 2016;68(9):2345–6.
46. Sperandeo M, Varriale A, Sperandeo G, et al. Transthoracic ultrasound in the evaluation of pulmo-

nary fibrosis: our experience. Ultrasound Med Biol. 2009;35:723–9.
47. Sperandeo M, De Cata A, Molinaro F, Trovato FM, Catalano D, Simeone A, Varriale A, Martines GF, Trovato G. Ultrasound signs of pulmonary fibrosis in systemic sclerosis as timely indicators for chest computed tomography. Scand J Rheumatol. 2015;44(5):389–98.
48. Rea G, Valente T, Marchiori E. HRCT in smoking-related interstitial lung diseases: a kaleidoscopic overlap of patterns. J Bras Pneumol. 2016;42(2):157.
49. Bouros D, Wells AU, Nicholson AG, et al. Histopathologic subsets of fibrosing alveolitis in patients with systemic sclerosis and their relationship to outcome. Am J Respir Crit Care Med. 2002;165(12):1581–6.
50. Othman AE, Brockmann C, Yang Z, et al. Impact of image denoising on image quality, quantitative parameters and sensitivity of ultra-low-dose volume perfusion CT imaging. Eur Radiol. 2016;26(1):167–74.
51. Palmucci S, Roccasalva F, Puglisi S, et al. Clinical and radiological features of idiopathic interstitial pneumonias (IIPs): a pictorial review. Insights Imaging. 2014;5(3):347–64.
52. Travis WD, et al. An official American Thoracic Society/European Respiratory Society statement: update of the international multidisciplinary classification of the idiopathic interstitial pneumonias. Am J Respir Crit Care Med. 2013;188(6):733–48.
53. Rea G, Poletti V, Iadevaia, et al. Idiopathic pleuroparenchymal fibroelastosis: incidental findings in a patient with suspected pneumonia. J Bras Pneumol. 2015;41(5):478–9.
54. Sperandeo M, Carnevale V, Muscarella S, et al. Clinical application of transthoracic ultrasonography in inpatients with pneumonia. Eur J Clin Investig. 2011;41(1):1–7.
55. Tominaga J, Sakai F, Johkoh T, Noma S, et al. Diagnostic certainty of idiopathic pulmonary fibrosis/usual interstitial pneumonia: the effect of the integrated clinico-radiological assessment. Eur J Radiol. 2015;84(12):2640–5.
56. Schmidt SL, Sundaram B, Flaherty KR. Diagnosing fibrotic lung disease: when is high-resolution computed tomography sufficient to make a diagnosis of idiopathic pulmonary fibrosis? Respirology. 2009;14(7):934–9.
57. Rea G, Trovato GMA. Farewell to B-lines: ageing and disappearance of ultrasound artifacts as a diagnostic tool. Respiration. 2015;90(6):522.
58. Soldati G, Demi M. The use of lung ultrasound images for the differential diagnosis of pulmonary and cardiac interstitial pathology. J Ultrasound. 2017;20(2):91–6.
59. Akira M, Inoue Y, Kitaichi M, et al. Usual interstitial pneumonia and nonspecific interstitial pneumonia with and without concurrent emphysema: thin-section CT findings. Radiology. 2009;251(1):271–9.
60. MacDonald SL, Rubens MB, Hansell DM, et al. Nonspecific interstitial pneumonia and usual interstitial pneumonia: comparative appearances at and diagnostic accuracy of thin-section CT. Radiology. 2001;2221(3):600–5.
61. Katzenstein AL, Fiorelli RF. Nonspecific interstitial pneumonia/fibrosis. Histologic features and clinical significance. Am J Surg Pathol. 1994;18(2):136–47.
62. Sumikawa H, Johkoh T, Ichikado K, et al. Usual interstitial pneumonia and chronic idiopathic interstitial pneumonia: analysis of CT appearance in 92 patients. Radiology. 2006;241(1):258–66.
63. White ES, Borok Z, Brown KK, Eickelberg O et al. on behalf of the American Thoracic Society Respiratory Cell and Molecular Biology Assembly Working Group on Pulmonary Fibrosis. An American Thoracic Society official research statement: future directions in lung fibrosis research. Am J Respir Crit Care Med. 2016;193(7):792–800.
64. Vasakova M, Morell F, Walsh S, Leslie K, Raghu G. Hypersensitivity pneumonitis: perspectives in diagnosis and management. Am J Respir Crit Care Med. 2017;196(6):680–9.
65. Bak SH, Lee HY. Overlaps and uncertainties of smoking-related idiopathic interstitial pneumonias. Int J Chron Obstruct Pulmon Dis. 2017;1(12):3221–9.
66. Dhagat PK, Singh S, Jain M, Singh SN, Sharma RK. Thoracic sarcoidosis: imaging with high resolution computed tomography. J Clin Diagn Res. 2017;11(2):15–8.
67. Rea G, D'Amato M. The imaging spectrum of pulmonary tuberculosis: a critical appraisal. Acta Radiol. 2015;56(1):1–2.
68. Rea G, Sperandeo M, Sorrentino, et al. Chest ultrasound findings in pulmonary alveolar lithiasis. J Med Ultrason. 2015;42:591–4.
69. Vivero M, Padera RF. Histopathology of lung disease in the connective tissue diseases. Rheum Dis Clin N Am. 2015;41(2):197–211.
70. Desai SR, Veeraraghavan S, Hansell DM, et al. CT features of lung disease in patients with systemic sclerosis: comparison with idiopathic pulmonary fibrosis and nonspecific interstitial pneumonia. Radiology. 2004;232:560–7.
71. Goldin JG, Lynch DA, Strollo DC, et al. High-resolution CT scan findings in patients with symptomatic scleroderma-related interstitial lung disease. Chest. 2008;134:358–67.
72. Sperandeo M, Trovato GM, Catalano D. Quantifying B-lines on lung sonography: insufficient evidence as an objective, constructive, and educational tool. J Ultrasound Med. 2014;33(2):362–5.
73. NICE Clinical Guidelines, No. 163 National Clinical Guideline Centre (UK). London: Royal College of Physicians (UK). Diagnosis and management of suspected idiopathic pulmonary fibrosis; 2013. https://www.ncbi.nlm.nih.gov/pubmedhealth/PMH0068972/
74. Wells AU, Hirani N, British Thoracic Society Interstitial Lung Disease Guideline Group, et al.

Guidelines on interstitial lung disease. Thorax. 2008;63(Suppl 5):v1–58.
75. Tzilas V, Bouros E, Tzouvelekis A, Bouros D. Guidelines for idiopathic pulmonary fibrosis: everything flows. Respiration. 2017;93(6):401–3.
76. Wells AU. The revised ATS/ERS/JRS/ALAT diagnostic criteria for idiopathic pulmonary fibrosis (IPF)-practical implications. Respir Res. 2013;14(Suppl 1):S2.
77. Lee RK. Grayscale ultrasound artifacts. In: Dogra V, Rubens DJ, editors. Ultrasound secrets. Philadelphia: Elsevier; 2005. p. 8–13.

6 Pleural Conditions

Francesco Feletti, Bruna Malta,
and Andrea Aliverti

6.1 Introduction

Thoracic Ultrasound (TUS) permits the identification, evaluation, and control of pleural effusion and pneumothorax and can also provide useful information in inflammatory and neoplastic pleural processes.

Using ultrasound to investigate pleural conditions requires a clear understanding of ultrasound semeiotics and normal finds.

Electronic Supplementary Material The online version of this chapter (https://doi.org/10.1007/978-3-319-93055-8_6) contains supplementary material, which is available to authorized users.

F. Feletti (✉)
Dipartimento di Diagnostica per Immagini, Ausl della Romagna, Ospedale S. Maria delle Croci, Ravenna, Italy

Dipartimento di Elettronica, Informazione e Bioingegneria, Politecnico di Milano, Milan, Italy
e-mail: francesco.feletti@auslromagna.it

B. Malta
Dipartimento di Diagnostica per Immagini, Ausl di Ferrara, Ospedale Universitario di Ferrara, Ferrara, Italy
e-mail: mltbrn@unife.it

A. Aliverti
Dipartimento di Elettronica, Informazione e Bioingegneria, Politecnico di Milano, Milan, Italy
e-mail: andrea.aliverti@polimi.it

6.1.1 Pleural Line

The pleura is made up of a single layer of mesothelial cells, and a thin supportive scaffold that accompanies the capillary tributary network of the systemic circus, lymphatic vessels, and nerve endings; the latter is present in the parietal pleura alone.

Under normal conditions, the leaflet visceral tissue and the parietal surface of the pleura are indistinguishable in TUS and appear as a single hyperechogenic linear imaging, called the "pleural line" (Fig. 6.1).

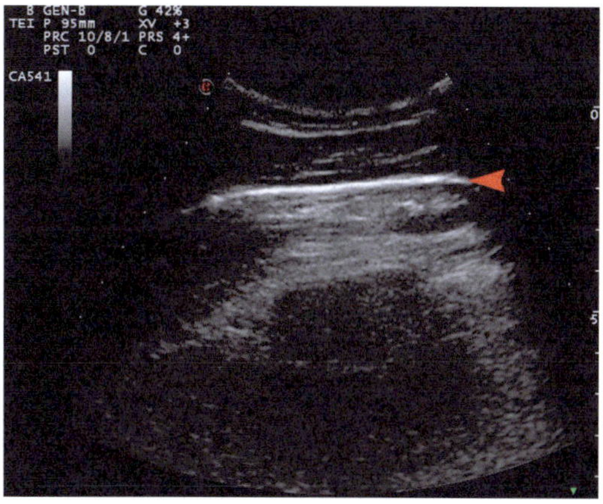

Fig. 6.1 Pleural line. The visceral pleura and the parietal pleura in physiological conditions are not distinguishable from each other with TUS and appear as a single and clear hyperechogenic line (arrow)

F. Feletti et al. (eds.), *Thoracic Ultrasound and Integrated Imaging*,
https://doi.org/10.1007/978-3-319-93055-8_6

6.1.2 Lung Sliding

During respiratory movements, the sliding of visceral pleura against the parietal pleura along the pleural line is visible; this normal finding is called "lung sliding" or "gliding sign" (Video 6.1).

If the two pleural layers cannot move over each other, as is the case with cicatricle adhesions, atelectasis lungs, or during apnoea, there is no pulmonary sliding.

Furthermore, lung sliding is not visible when the visceral pleura is missing below the parietal pleura, i.e. pneumothorax [1] or pneumonectomy [2].

6.1.3 A-Lines

A-lines are typical reverberations present in physiological conditions, when the permeability to ultrasound abruptly changes at the pleural line, passing from soft tissues (average acoustic impedance of about 1.5 g/cm^2) to air (acoustic impedance of 42.8 g/cm^2) [3].

The ultrasound beam is strongly reflected and returned to the transducer, and the monitor shows the image of the pleural line.

The transducer reflects the main part of the beam which propagates again to the pleura line, where the reflection is repeated giving rise to a second representation of the pleural line.

This second representation is shown on the screen at double the depth relative to the first, based on the time between the first emission of the beam and this second echo signal (refer to Chaps. 1 and 2 for a more detailed explanation).

The ultrasonic waves bounce between the ultrasound probe and the pleural line until they are completely absorbed, generating a sequence of weaker and deeper ultrasound signals.

These linear images parallel to the pleural line decrease in intensity while they increase in-depth, and are called A-lines (Fig. 6.2a, b).

Under certain conditions, the interfaces between the tissue layers that make up the thoracic wall also contribute to the formation of A-lines.

6.1.4 Z-Lines

Z-lines are downward vertical lines and start at the pleural line.

Z-lines are short, with a length ranging from 1 to 3 cm, are fixed relative to pleural flow, and may coexist with A-lines.

Thanks to these characteristics, Z-lines are easily distinguishable from B-lines, which are much longer, move with lung sliding, and generally replace A-lines.

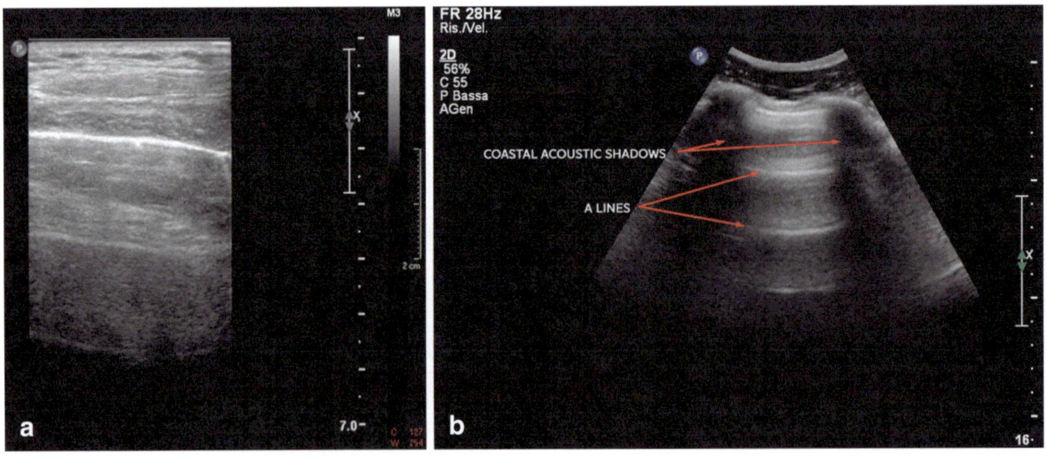

Fig. 6.2 Lines A. Normal findings. These depend on the reverberation generated by the different acoustic impedance of soft tissues and air. They appear as linear images parallel to the pleural line and progressively diminish in depth. Ultrasound image with linear (**a**) and convex (**b**) probes

Although they have an uncertain origin [4], they are part of the normal findings; are shaped like comet tails and are likely associated with internal reverberation due to microcalcifications or small adipose tissue thickening of the parietal pleura.

6.2 Pleural Effusion

Under normal physiological conditions, the presence of a thin fluid film between the two pleural sheets guarantees their mutual flow by creating a mechanical coupling system between lung and chest wall.

Generally, the pleural space contains approximately 5 mL of liquid [5], produced mainly by the parietal pleura, due to the gradient between hydrostatic capillary pressure and the negative pressure of the pleural space [6].

The parietal pleura is responsible for about 75% of the drainage of the pleural cavity.

Its lymph vessels may increase their absorption capacity up to 20 times and vary locally if necessary, ensuring a significant margin of safety against the formation of pleural effusion [7].

The amount of pleural fluid is adjusted based on the equilibrium between hydrostatic and oncotic pressure (Starling's law).

The increased production of pleural fluid may cause a pleural effusion.

It may depend on the increase in capillary permeability, as in the case of inflammatory exudate in phlogistic diseases, or the increase in hydrostatic pressure as in the case of exudates in cardiac failure.

Pleural effusion can also be caused by a reduction in reabsorption, such as obstruction of the parietal pleural vessels due to neoplastic infiltration, or a reduction in lymphatic drainage due to increased systemic venous pressure [7, 8].

A rare cause of pleural effusion is hyponatremia [7, 9]; instead, atelectasis may increase the negative pressure of the pleural space causing higher production of pleural fluid [5].

Finally, pleural effusion may have a peritoneal origin and reach the pleura through the discontinuity of the diaphragm or the diaphragmatic lymph vessels.

6.2.1 Ultrasound Aspects

Pleural effusion may have the same echographic appearance regardless of its genesis and the chemical-physical composition.

In TUS, pleural effusion appears as a quadrangular, fusiform, semilunar, or circular shape image with a profound side represented by the visceral pleura that is called the *lung line* [2].

When the lung underneath the effusion is aired, there is no posterior reinforcement because the beam reflects completely. Instead, if the lung is consolidated, there is a variable degree of posterior reinforcement [10].

The respiratory cycle often modifies the distribution of the effusion, causing the pleural layers to move; in M-mode, this generates a sinusoidal graph, also called the *sinusoid sign* [11].

With TUS, in order to best visualize small effusions in the posterior costophrenic sinus, the patient may be asked to assume a sitting position or bend over slightly.

In this way, the effusion is collected in a descending position and can be more easily documented.

Sometimes, Doppler colour may be of further help for small pleural effusions, since it can detect small fluid displacements synchronous with respiratory cycles or the heartbeat: this is the *fluid colour sign* (Video 6.2), and it has a sensitivity of 89.2% and a 100% specificity [12, 13].

In the ultrasound study, serum-pleural effusion generally appears as a non-echogenic space, and with respiratory movements, it quickly changes its spatial arrangement.

Most pleural effusions of an inflammatory nature (Fig. 6.3a–c) are often associated with pleural thickening or pulmonary consolidation and may contain corpusculous suspended material which may also confer a full hypoechoic appearance or present septations (Fig. 6.4a–d).

Neoplastic effusions are almost always rich in suspended corpuscular material and often have fibrin seams or branches.

The hemothorax (Fig. 6.5a–d) and empyema typically show homogeneously distributed echoes; however, they may also appear ultimately as a non-echogenic space.

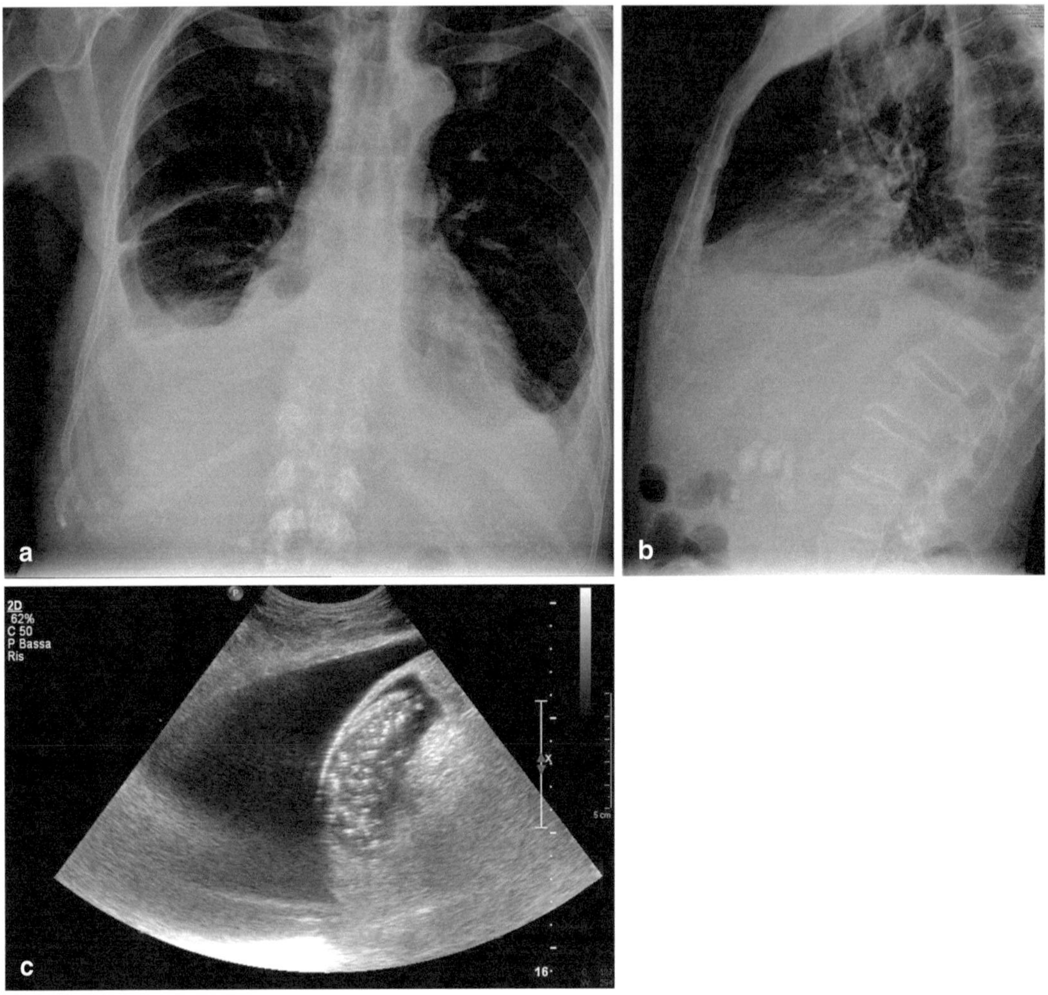

Fig. 6.3 Exudation of the pleural effusion in a 54-year-old patient with miliary Tuberculosis (TB). X-rays (**a**, **b**) and ultrasound (**c**): the right basal pleural effusion appears anechogenic. Small scattered splenic calcifications testify to the consequences of the previous pathology. In the past, the patient had also been subjected to right nephrectomy surgery for TB

Although an exudate is invariably anechogenic, a non-echogenic effusion can also be exudate [5];, in fact, with ultrasound, we can demonstrate the presence of materials in the effusion but not its chemical composition, and the differential diagnosis requires the aspiration of a sample with an ultrasound-guided thoracentesis to attain the amount of protein LDH in the effusion [14] (Table 6.1).

Based on these criteria, about a quarter of transudates are misdiagnosed as exudates in patients who are on diuretics or have chronic thoracentesis.

Therefore, in uncertain cases, it may be useful to examine the serum-pleural fluid protein gradient [18].

In addition to the Light's criteria listed in the table, routine dosage of the following biomarkers may be useful in diagnosis of the nature of the effusion: protein C reactive in bacterial infectious forms; natriuretic peptides in heart failure; adenosine deaminase in tuberculosis; and mesothelium, immunocytochemical stains, and fibulin-3 in neoplasms [17].

Determining any compartments of the effusion is crucial in programming a thoracentesis evacuation manoeuvre.

Indeed, the presence of chambers may hinder or render it unsuitable, limiting suction to the contents of one or more cells.

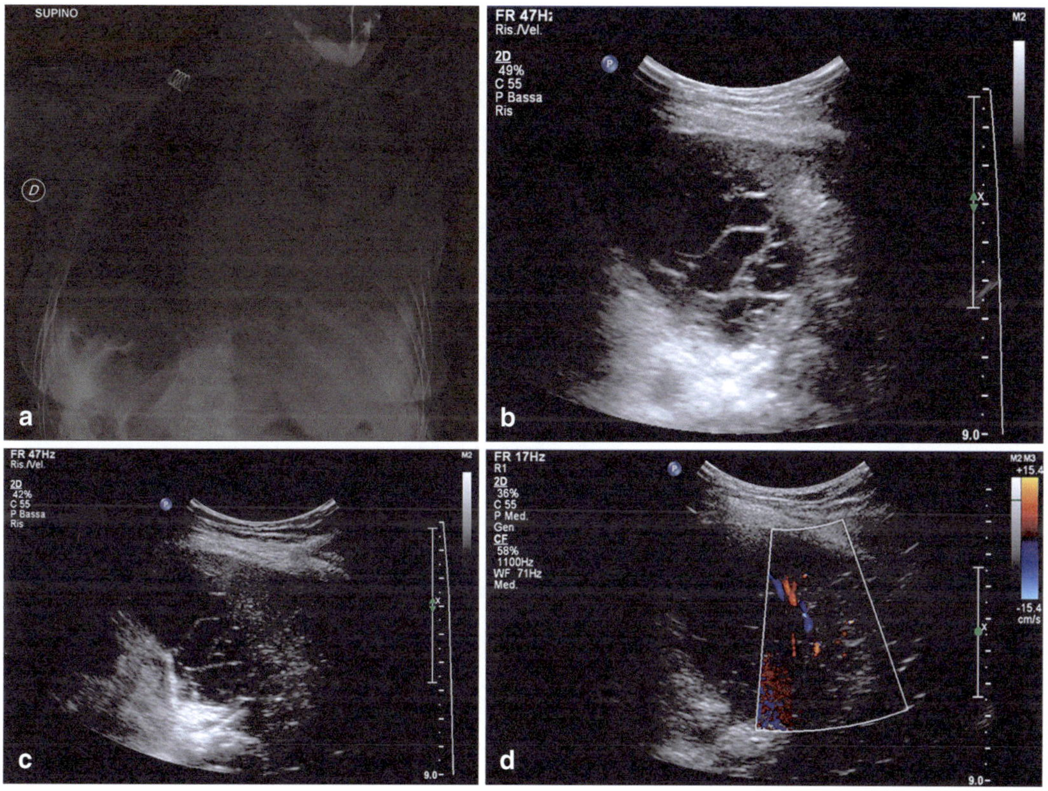

Fig. 6.4 Abundant pleural effusion. In this case of white hemithorax to the left of the X-ray (**a**), the ultrasound scan showed the loculated nature of the spill (**b**) and allowed distinction between the effusion and the associated atelectatic component (**c**). In an atelectatic lung, the vessels, better visualized with colour Doppler (**d**), arrange themselves in parallel, testifying to the loss of volume

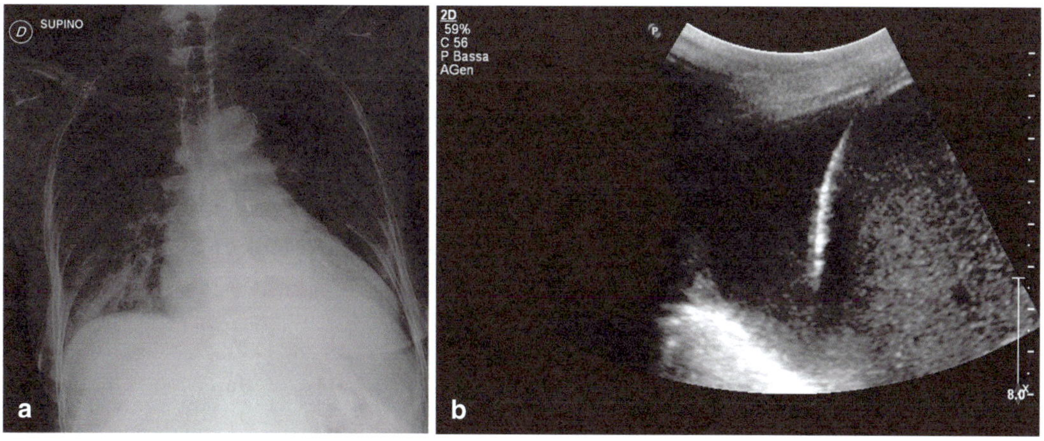

Fig. 6.5 Correlation of X-ray (**a**) and TUS (**b–d**) of hemothorax. The patient, who was affected by metastatic melanoma, came to our attention for costal trauma. The effusion had a corpuscular component and hyperechogenic elements on the TUS, some of which fluctuated with respiratory movements and decubitus changes, indicating fibrous shoots and clots

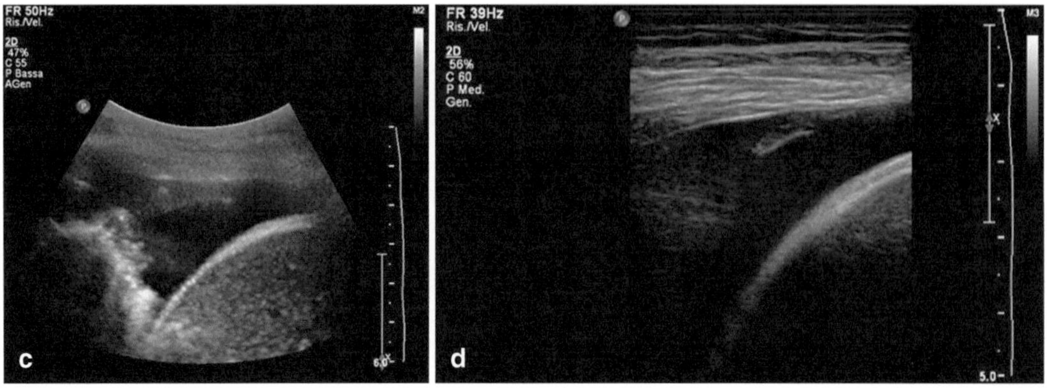

Fig. 6.5 (continued)

Table 6.1 Criteria for exudate diagnosis [15–17]

Criteria for the exudate diagnosis		Sensitivity (%)	Specificity (%)
Light's criteria	At least one of the following three criteria	98	83
Total protein concentration in pleural fluid/serum proteins	>0.5	86	84
Pleural LDH (absolute value)	>2/3 of the upper limit of the normal range of the LDH serum or >200μL	90	82
LDH concentration in serum pleurisy/ LDH serum	>0.6	82	89

Ultrasound is the most sensitive imaging method in highlighting septa and chambers, since the liquid/septum interface represents a mirror reflection surface.

In traditional radiology, the diagnosis of loculated effusions is impossible because of the low resolution of the method and the silhouette effect, which eliminates the image of different structures that are in contact with each other.

Even CT, due to partial volume effects or low densitometry gradient, may not provide a true image of the thinner branches.

6.2.2 The Role of Thoracic Ultrasound

The accuracy of clinical examination in the diagnosis of pleural effusion is limited, with sensitivity and specificity values of 69% and 77%, respectively [19].

TUS is, therefore, an advantageous method to support clinical examination.

It allows the detection of 3–5 mL [20] effusions, which is far more sensitive than conventional radiology [21, 22].

At least 200 mL is needed for radiograms taken in orthostasis in order to obtain images of a meniscus in chest radiography and to obscure the lateral costophrenic spaces [4].

If the effusion is small, even a radiogram in the lateral decubitus may be insufficient.

Furthermore, TUS is more sensitive than chest radiography in orthostasis for the diagnosis of abundant but sub-pulmonary effusions [4], that is, effusions between the diaphragm and lower lung surfaces.

In this case, radiography in orthostasis lacks the meniscus image, and the profile of the effusion is convex in its upper section and indistinguishable from the hemidiaphragm.

If the effusion is free-flowing, radiographic diagnosis may be possible through a further radiogram in lateral decubitus [21].

However, the effusion can also be loculated.

Besides, not all patients can assume lateral decubitus (Fig. 6.6a–d); for example, it is not

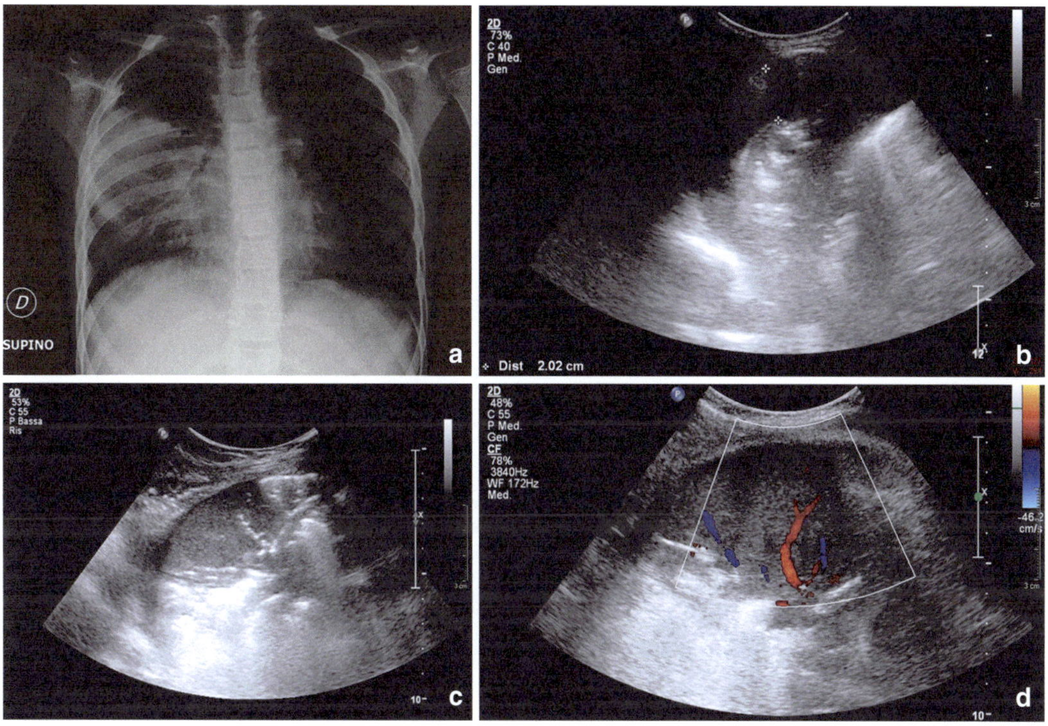

Fig. 6.6 X-ray (**a**) and TUS (**b–d**) aspects in an 8-year-old girl with a high fever and productive cough. With an X-ray performed in supine decubitus, a large area of parenchymal hypodiaphany with contextual aerial bronchogram was seen, involving a large part of the right middle-basal lung. TUS showed the concomitance of a discreet pleural layer with a thickness of 2 cm, less visible radiologically

possible in trauma patients or most patients in intensive care [23].

In conclusion, TUS is, therefore, a sensitive method for diagnosing pleural effusion as well as being versatile and useful in uncooperative, traumatized, or hospitalized patients in intensive care [23].

6.2.3 Radiological Correlations

From a radiological point of view, a free-flowing pleural effusion can mimic pneumonia or a lobar collapse.

Also, when the effusion is around a lobe, or if trapped at the level of a scissure or between two pulmonary lobes, it can create uninterpretable images in traditional radiology.

Likewise, it may be impossible to distinguish a confined effusion from a pleural thickening on a chest radiogram; generally, the effusion causes a convex shadow toward the lung, but this sign is neither constant nor specific.

Even in orthostasis, a small free-flowing effusion may be collected along the side chest wall or remain along one of the cardiac margins, simulating an enlargement of the cardiac silhouette.

In these situations, TUS can quickly and safely demonstrate the liquid nature of dubious radiological opacity; it is also better for differentiating loculated pleural effusions from pleural thickening, allowing identification of the most suitable draining point even for the smallest sizes.

However, the identification of a loculated or scissural effusion in ultrasonography can only be achieved if the collection is peripheral or if the neighbouring atelectasis or thickened parenchyma creates a suitable acoustic window [24].

For these reasons, in TUS it is crucial to look for effusions from different access points over the entire thoracic surface since it is not possible to exclude the presence of effusion only because it is absent from the pulmonary bases or the lateral costophrenic space.

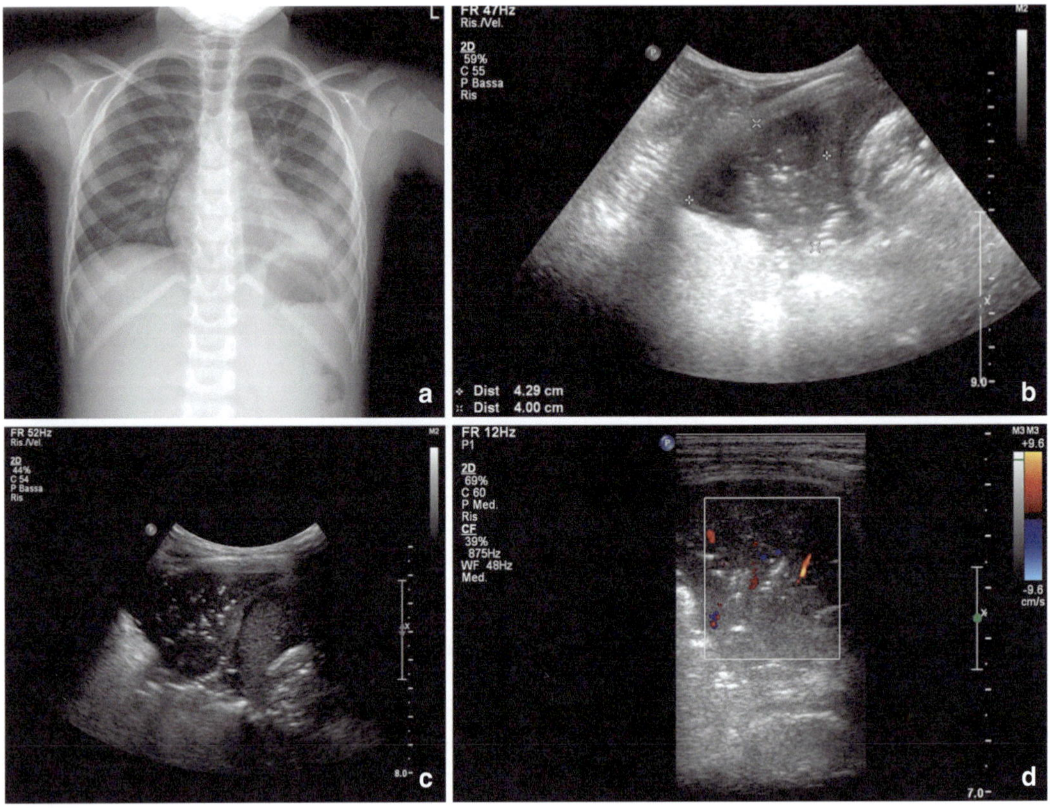

Fig. 6.7 X-ray (**a**) and ultrasound (**b–d**) aspects in a young girl with pneumonia. From this X-ray performed in orthostasis (**a**) in a single PA projection for radioprotection reasons, there is an area of hypodiaphany with triangular-shaped morphology in the lingual seat. TUS made it possible to distinguish the parenchymal component from the pleurogenic component, evaluating its relative contribution in determining radiological opacity. Subsequently, the pleuropulmonary picture was analyzed by TUS alone

When interpreting opaque hemithorax radiological images is difficult due to different and sometimes concomitant conditions, ultrasound permits distinction between pulmonary consolidation and pleural effusion (Fig. 6.7a–d).

In opaque hemithorax, TUS also shows the characteristics of the effusion and may suggest its possible causes (Video 6.3), for example it may identify an underlying pneumonia.

6.2.4 Quantification of Pleural Effusion

From a radiographic viewpoint, it is not possible to differentiate an effusion from a consolidated area or atelectasis, much less quantify, even in very general terms, the pleural fluid component.

TUS, on the other hand, allows immediate quantification of pleural effusion [25], either because it makes it possible to distinguish between the liquid and the collapsed lung or because it allows direct measurements of the thickness of the effusion (Fig. 6.8a–f).

It is worthwhile remembering that measuring a loculated pleural effusion, especially when its size is fully explored, can be simple; however, it is not possible to accurately quantify free-flowing pleural effusions, due to the complex geometry of the pleural cavity.

The estimate of the effusion, therefore, depends on the operator's approximate visual-

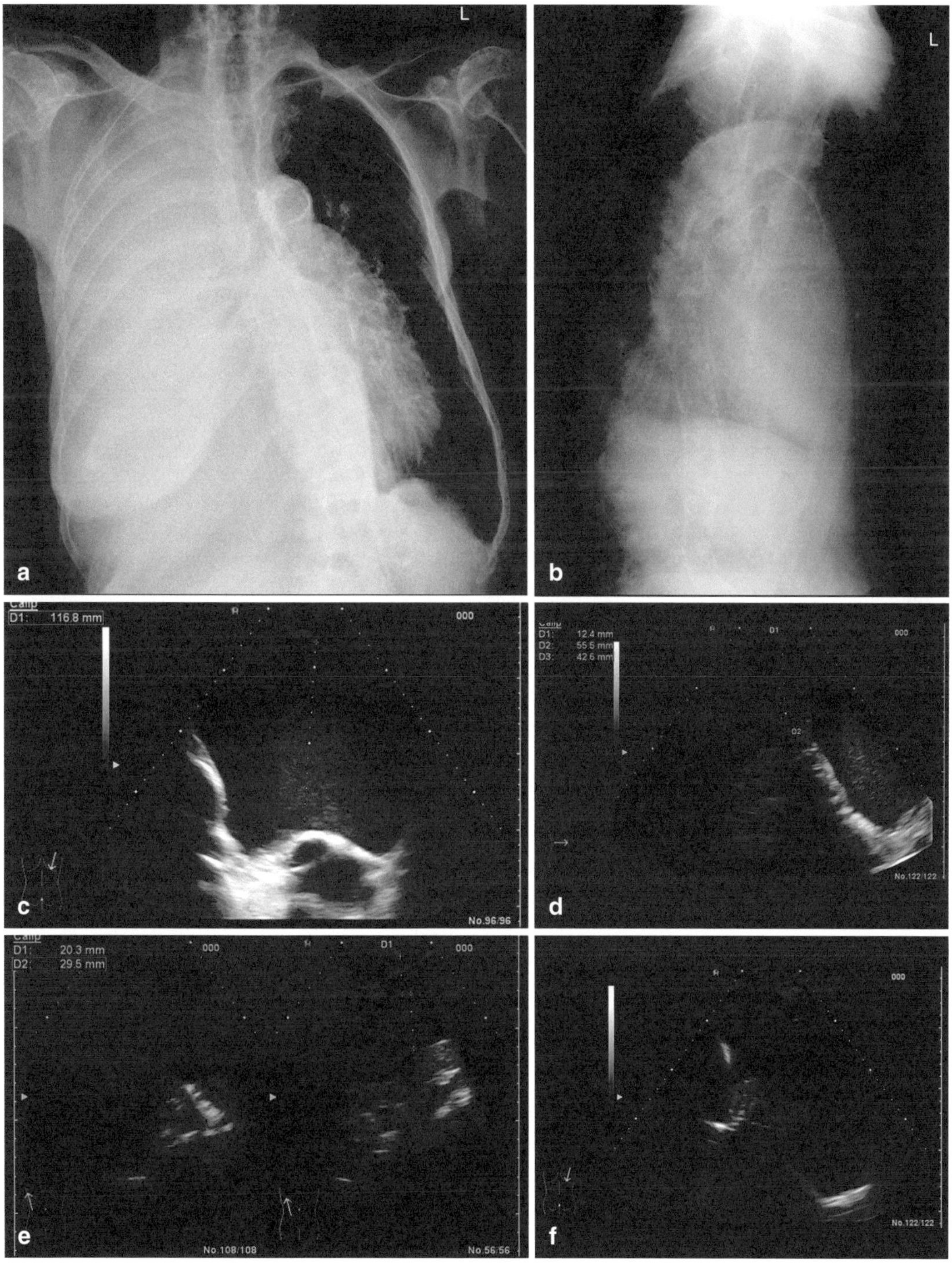

Fig. 6.8 X-ray hemithorax opaque in X-ray (**a**, **b**). TUS (**c**–**f**) allowed identification of a massive pleural effusion and therefore allowed quantitative measurements of the effusion (explanation in the text)

ization; alternatively, it is possible to measure the depth of the effusion or its longitudinal diameter, which often correlates with the amount of liquid [26, 27].

To be as accurate and repeatable as possible, the quantitative evaluations of the effusion, should always be performed with the probe in the same position and orientation.

At the same time, to avoid any redistribution of the liquid, the patient must always assume the same decubitus.

Usually, the effusion is measured while the patient is supine, since this is the obligatory position for most patients during TUS examination.

In this position, free-flowing effusions are distributed in the posterior costophrenic recess and in a transverse scan they appear as sickles.

Despite the limits described above, some authors have tried to standardize the quantification of pleural effusion.

The method proposed by Eibenberger et al. is based on measurement of the distance between the thoracic wall and the posterior pulmonary profile [28].

This evaluation is carried out on a supine patient using a transverse scan that simultaneously displays both the chest wall and the pulmonary base, trying to keep the probe orthogonal to the chest wall in order not to overestimate the effusion.

With this approach, the volume of the effusion is calculated as follows:

$$V = 47.6A \times 837,$$

where V is the volume of the effusion in mL and A represents the thickness in millimetres (measured as described above).

The authors report a calculation of the actual volume that is more accurate than the data obtainable with radiology (r = 0.80 vs. r = 0.58, $p < 0.05$) [28].

For patients undergoing mechanical ventilation, Roch et al. proposed performing transverse scans on the supine patient and measuring the distance from the lung to the posterior chest wall, about 3 cm from the lung base.

The authors reported that a thickness exceeding 5 cm was significantly related to a pleural effusion >500 mL (sensitivity of 83%, specificity of 90%, positive predictive value of 91%, and negative predictive value of 82%) [29] and that drainage of effusion with a thickness >5 cm significantly increases the PaO_2/fraction of the inspired oxygen ratio ($p < 0.01$) [29].

Goecke and Schwerk [30] have instead proposed the following formula to accurately estimate ($r = 0.68$) effusions with the patient in the sitting position:

$$V = H \times 90,$$

where V is the volume of the effusion in mL and H is the thickness of the effusion in cm at the lateral chest wall, while 90 is an empirical factor.

However, some limitations of these techniques have to be considered.

In tall patients they lead to an underestimation of the volume when the patient is in a supine position and an overestimation when the patient is seated.

Inaccuracies of the opposite kind can occur in endomorphic patients or in the presence of diaphragmatic elevations.

These limits are mainly due to the execution of a single measurement and, for this reason, methods where multiple measurements were proposed.

Goecke et al. have proposed a system based on two measurements with the patient in the sitting position.

This method is more accurate ($r = 0.87$), especially for small effusions that would otherwise be overestimated by methods based on a single measurement.

The calculation is summarized in the following formula [31]:

$$V = \left(H + S\right) \times 70,$$

where V is the volume of the effusion in mL, H is the maximum lateral height of the effusion in cm, and S is the maximum distance between the pulmonary base and the diaphragm.

In clinical practice, according to our experience, it is often sufficient to measure the longitudinal and transverse diameters by scanning the scapular line adopting a field of view that includes the diaphragm, together with the indication of the most cranial level reached by the effusion, with the patient in the sitting position.

With a supine patient, it may be suitable to measure the distance between the thoracic wall and the pulmonary profile from the back.

This trouble-free approach allows a sufficiently reproducible evaluation in the same patient and therefore of practical utility for follow-up after draining or undergoing medical treatment.

6.2.5 Role of Ultrasound Guidance for Thoracentesis

Ultrasound is an accurate and safe instrument, especially if the effusion is minor or if the patient is not very collaborative, both in guiding drains with a thin needle and in executing thoracentesis, because in real-time it helps prevent aerated lungs and large veins, thus minimizing complications [32, 33].

Ultrasound can highlight the presence of septations in the effusion and avoid unsuccessful thoracentesis attempts or guide the targeted puncture of larger loculations.

In the case of a septated effusion, contrasting opinions remain on the possibility of associating intrapleural fibrinolytic therapy with urokinase or streptokinase, with the purpose of dissolving the loculations and the strands, thus simplifying the drainage procedure and avoiding the need to resort to further surgical procedures [34–36].

There have been controversial findings in medical studies [37], especially regarding the effectiveness of fibrinolytic therapy and its possible side effects [38].

Recent studies focused on the efficacy of intrapleural fibrinolytic therapy in reducing the period of hospital stay, without increasing the incidence of side effects [39].

Other studies have highlighted that urokinase is more effective than other fibrinolytic agents (e.g., alteplase) and is burdened by fewer adverse reactions [40], allowing it to be used as a therapy in pleural empyema in infants [41].

6.2.6 Pleural Empyema

Pleural empyema is the buildup of purulent exudate in the pleural cavity, characterized by a prevalence of polymorphonucleates and a leukocyte count higher than 5000/mm^3.

Although there are different causes, the onset of an infectious effusion is more frequent in the course of pyogenic pneumonia.

Pleural empyema generally has a moderate echogenicity, nearly homogeneous and with near-still or fixed internal echoes; the nearby pleura is generally thicker.

In TUS the differential diagnosis between a pleural empyema and a subpleural pulmonary abscess may be challenging.

Empyema can be differentiated from peripheral pulmonary empyema because it has a regular, usually lenticular shape.

Scans in both sitting and prone positions or lateral decubitus can demonstrate morphological changes and the mobility of the pleural collection.

Empyema, unlike the abscess, has walls of quite uniform thickness, with smooth and regular profiles.

The *lung line*, represented by the visceral pleura, separates the lung from the collection.

The underlying pulmonary parenchyma is generally compressed, resulting in the displacement of vessels and bronchi that typically assume an arched arrangement.

In these cases, the use of Doppler colour can easily demonstrate the curvilinear course of the lung veins; on the contrary, in a lung abscess, vessels and the bronchi may stop at the lesion.

Finally, the treatment of choice for empyema is often ultrasound-guided transthoracic drainage.

6.3 Pleurisy

Pleuritic pain is characteristic of pleurisy; it is an intense thoracic pain generated by respiratory movements. Sounds from pleural friction, fever, as well as signs and symptoms of any associated pathologies may be present.

Ultrasound examination is useful because it quickly shows the following signs: pleural irregularity, small (thickness <2 cm) subpleural pulmonary consolidations, and pleural effusions that are free-flowing or localized in variable quantities [42] (Fig. 6.9a–d).

However, TUS has a low specificity because these signs are common to many conditions, including pneumonia, pulmonary infarction, and malignant neoplasms.

Rarely does Doppler colour show a signal increase [42].

Görg et al. described the use of contrast media in patients with clinical and ultrasound signs of pleurisy to confirm or deny infective aetiology [43].

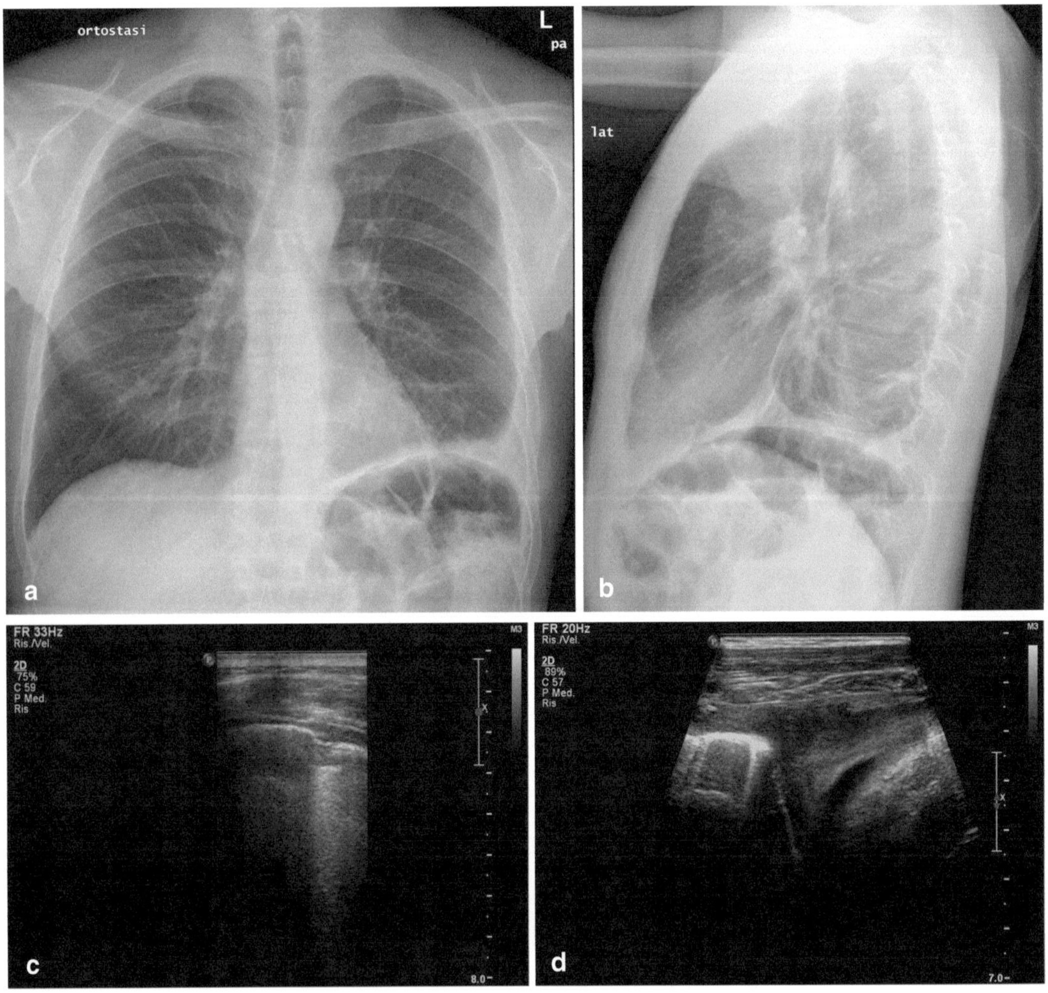

Fig. 6.9 Pleurisy in a 35-year-old male patient, with opacification of the left costophrenic sinus in the X-ray (**a**, **b**). A slightly echogenic effusion in TUS (**c**, **d**)

6.4 Pneumothorax

In chest radiograms, appropriate orthostatic projections in either expiratory or lateral positioning are required to visualize pneumothorax [1, 44].

Usually, in critical or bedridden patients, radiography is performed on a supine patient, with the limit that only massive pneumothoraxes can be excluded.

Ultrasonography, however, allows the identification of pneumothoraxes of the smallest size, even in a supine position [1].

6.4.1 Ultrasound Scans for Pneumothorax

During the ultrasound examination, the pneumothorax should be searched for in the antigravity-dependent portion of the pleural space. Consequently, if the patient is supine, the probe should be positioned on the front chest wall, both in the parasternal area and just below the sternum.

It should be considered that, in supine decubitus, small pneumothoraxes tend to settle in the juxtacardiac area and along the diaphragm, corresponding to the radiological image of hypertransparency, known as the *deep sulcus sign* [45].

In collaborative patients, smaller pneumothoraxes are identifiable by placing the probe along the axillary line with a patient in decubitus on the contralateral side.

If the patient is instead seated, a small apical pneumothorax may be located in the upper lungs with a supraclavicular approach.

Beyond diagnosis, TUS is suitable for monitoring the evolution of small pneumothoraxes that do not require the positioning of a chest drain.

6.4.2 Abolition of Lung Sliding

When present, lung sliding safety excludes (100% negative predictive value) the presence of pneumothorax [1] at the chest point being examined.

Table 6.2 Other causes for the abolition of lung sliding

Causes of abolition of lung sliding different from pneumothorax
Apnea
Atelectasis
Inflammatory adhesions between pleural leaflets
Congenital pleural symphysis
Pulmonary fibrosis with loss of lung expansion [45]
Pneumonectomy
Pulmonary talcosis

However, the absence of this sign is not specific to a pneumothorax (Table 6.2).

In anaesthesia or asthma, the pleural excursion may be reduced, and lung sliding needs to be carefully examined because it becomes less evident.

Under normal conditions, a study in M-mode shows a *seashore* appearance, while in pneumothorax the pattern is called *barcode*; in fact, in M-mode, the lack of lung sliding gives the appearance of parallel lines in the pulmonary field, hence the comparison to a barcode.

6.4.3 A-Lines, B-Lines, and Pneumothorax

If TUS detects B-lines or pleural thickening, there is no pneumothorax at that site.

The acoustic barrier caused by air in the pleural space makes it impossible to visualize any anatomical structure beneath the parietal pleura, including the B-lines generated at the lung surface.

A-lines are also present in the pneumothorax, where they tend to be more intense and more regular (Fig. 6.10a–c).

The air contained in the pleural cavity reflects the ultrasounds in the same way as lung air does in a healthy patient.

6.4.4 Lung Points

In the partial pneumothorax, the lung remains partially attached to the parietal pleura.

So, while in areas affected by pneumothorax lung sliding is not present, it usually is pres-

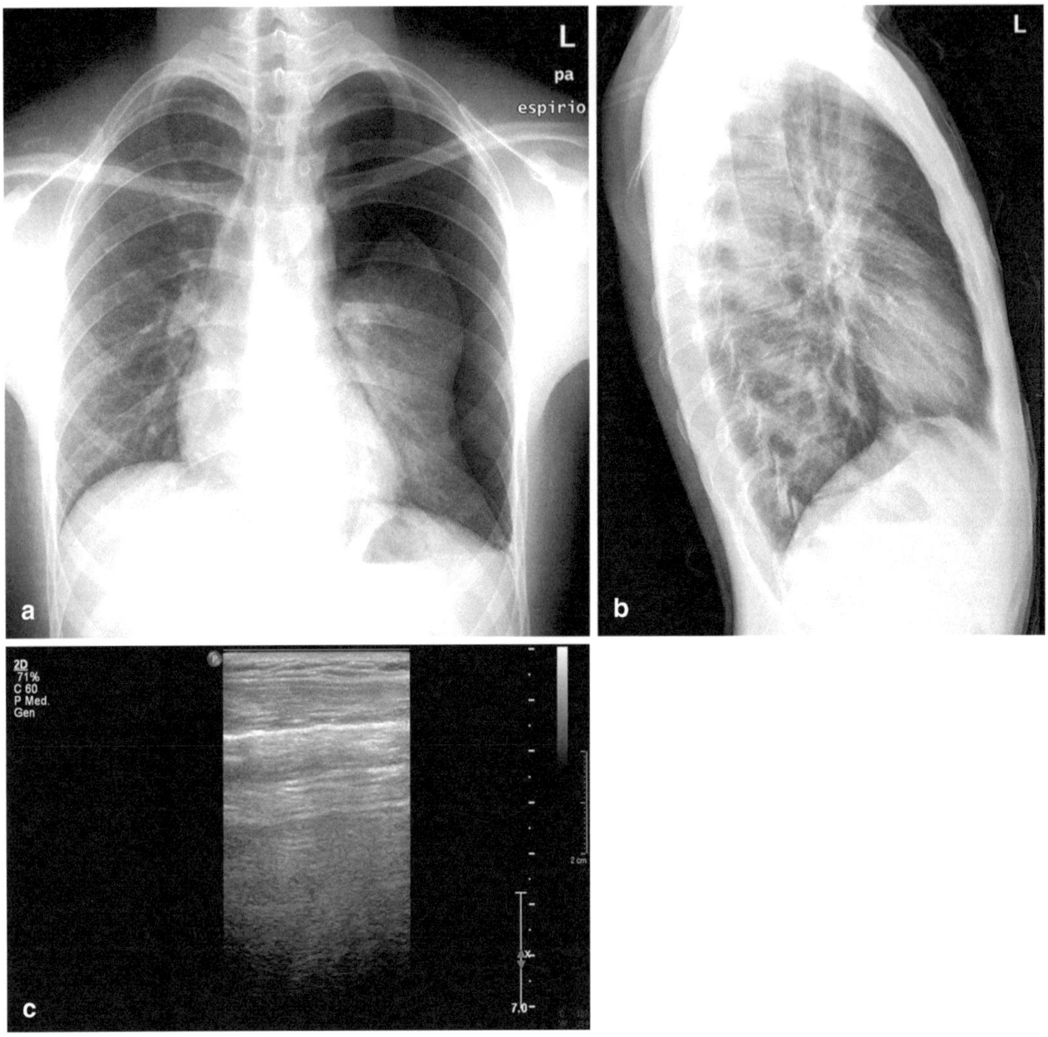

Fig. 6.10 X-ray (**a**, **b**) of a massive left pneumothorax in an 18-year-old male. In TUS, A-lines (**c**) were visible; lung sliding was not visible

ent where the visceral pleura and parietal pleura are regularly coupled.

Lung points are defined as the points that show the passage from the appearance to the absence of lung sliding (Fig. 6.11a, b) (Video 6.4).

With atelectasis, lung sliding may be missing; in this context, the equivalent of the lung point will be the abrupt transition from an ultrasound pattern of the atelectasis-affected lung to the pneumothorax [1] with A lines.

The lung point is, therefore, a specific sign of pneumothorax [46], but it is not highly sensitive (sensitivity range, 66%–79%) [47].

6.4.5 Algorithm for Ultrasound Diagnosis of Pneumothorax

When lung sliding is absent, and there are one or more lung points, pneumothorax can be diagnosed.

If lung sliding is absent, but there are no lung points, the diagnosis of massive pneumothorax is likely.

It is essential to recognise that the presence of B-lines, lung sliding, and other lung finds allows for the exclusion of pneumothorax limited to that particular area of the chest.

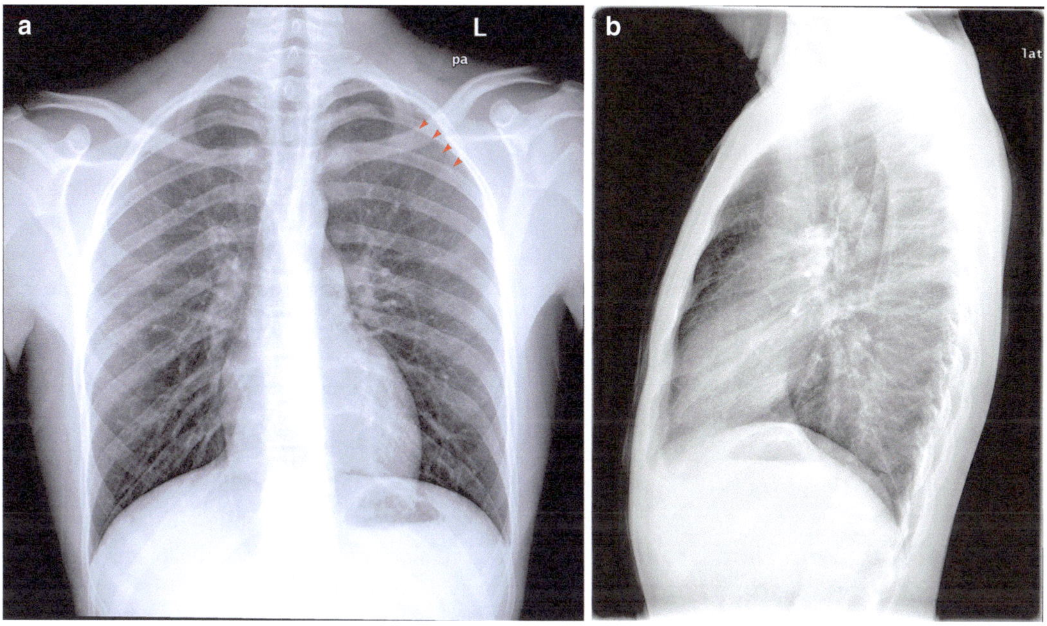

Fig. 6.11 Small pneumothorax. A pneumothorax like this must be detected very carefully on the chest radiogram (arrows). TUS allows an immediate diagnosis because lung sliding is absent where the pneumothorax is present. Sonographically, the point at which the lung returns to being received at the wall is called the lung point

6.4.6 Quantification of the Pneumothorax

Ultrasound examination can estimate the size and extension of pneumothorax via identification of the lung points [46].

To facilitate this task, one can also mark the lung points on the patient's chest with a dermographic pen.

Soldati et al. support the use of ultrasound in therapeutic planning for pneumothorax [46].

In particular, conservative therapy and clinical-ultrasound monitoring may be the best choice in patients who are not candidates for mechanical ventilation and with anterior only pneumothorax in a supine patient.

Instead, thoracic drainage is the right choice in patients who, in a supine position, show laterally extended pneumothorax [46].

In general, TUS, thanks to rapid execution in the supine position and the elevated sensitivity for diagnosing pneumothorax, is increasingly effective in initial evaluations of chest trauma [46, 48].

TUS is also an excellent tool for continuous monitoring of pneumothorax, avoiding further use of radiological examinations with logistical, economic, and radioprotection benefits.

In the ultrasound study of pneumothorax, the main obstacle is subcutaneous emphysema (as is the case with most pleural and pulmonary diseases) [1].

6.4.7 Pneumothorax in Ultrasound-guided Interventional Manoeuvres

Ultrasound is sufficient to exclude the appearance of a possible pneumothorax during interventional manoeuvres on the chest.

However, when performing ultrasound-guided manoeuvres, the appearance of a pneumothorax prevents operators from continuing ultrasound assistance because it affects the display of any anatomical structure below the parietal pleura.

6.4.8 Hydropneumothorax

Hydropneumothorax is characterized by the presence of air bubbles in a pleural effusion.

The gaseous component is hyper-reflective in TUS, creating posterior dirty shadows.

The gaseous component may consist of sporadic gas bubbles or be abundant, giving rise to a veritable air-liquid level, which moves with respiratory acts.

Since the gaseous component masks the underlying structures, while the pleural effusion provides an optimal acoustic window, in TUS an air-liquid level looks like the lower edge of a curtain which, descending with inspiration, obscures any underlying detail [45].

6.5 Pleural Cancers

6.5.1 Mesothelioma and Other Signs of Asbestos Exposure

Pleural mesothelioma is notoriously associated with exposure to asbestos, while other causative factors are exposure to other mineral fibres (zeolite, erionite), infection from SV40 (simian virus 40), chronic inflammation such as tuberculosis and empyema, certain organic chemical substances (polysilicon, polyurethane, ethylene oxide), or exposure to ionizing radiation, including radiation therapy [49].

However, 80% of the cases of pleural mesothelioma is attributed to asbestos, and the latency period for the appearance of the disease varies from a few years to more than 40 [50].

Under TUS examination, mesothelioma appears as an irregular thickening of the pleura, with a nodular appearance and often massive pleural effusions (Fig. 6.12a–h).

The pleura and subpleural perilesional fat is often thickened, while pleura that is incorporated and eroded by the tumour may appear as a hyperechoic line that, from the surface, deepens into the tumour mass [51, 52].

The diagnosis of pleural mesothelioma commonly involves cytological analysis and pleural biopsy.

Since the disease often begins with a pleural effusion, cytological analysis of the pleural effusion is frequently the first step.

The cytology has a sensitivity range from 32 to 67% [53]; diagnostic accuracy increases if a generous sample of the effusion is collected and with the addition of immunohistochemistry [54].

The diagnostic sensitivity of thoracoscopy varies between 94 and 98% [55–57], while a percutaneous image-guided cutting needle biopsy has an 86% sensitivity [58].

Pleural plaques are among the consequences of asbestos exposure, of which they are considered a marker [51, 59].

Plaques are also associated with an increased risk of neoplasia compared to asbestos exposure alone, identifying a high-risk subgroup of malignancy [59].

Made up of agglomerates of collagen fibres and coated by mesothelial cells, plaques are relatively acellular and avascular [59].

Isolated pleural plaques can be found in tuberculosis, after hemothorax or chest trauma, but multiple plaques in typical sites are almost always associated with exposure to asbestos [59].

Ultrasound examination can effectively detect pleural plaques without the interpretational errors typical of chest radiography, where rib fractures, subpleural fat deposits, and serratus anterior and external oblique muscles can be confused with pleural plaques [60, 61].

In ultrasound, plaques appear as areas of pleural thickening of intermediate echogenicity, unevenly distributed in the parietal pleura, where the visceral pleura flows regularly; if calcifications are present, they appear as hyper-reflective thickenings with posterior acoustic shadowing.

Ultrasound can also show signs of other conditions related to asbestos exposure, such as round atelectasis and asbestosis.

Round atelectasis is determined by the consolidation of the lung parenchyma as a result of pleural fibrosis and affects posterior lower lobes.

Under TUS, it shows up as a hepatized, hypoechoic pleurally based mass with posterior reinforcement; the eroded and invaginated pleural line extends from the pleura in the mass in 86% of cases.

Concomitant is the thickening of the adjacent pleural and extrapleural fat [52].

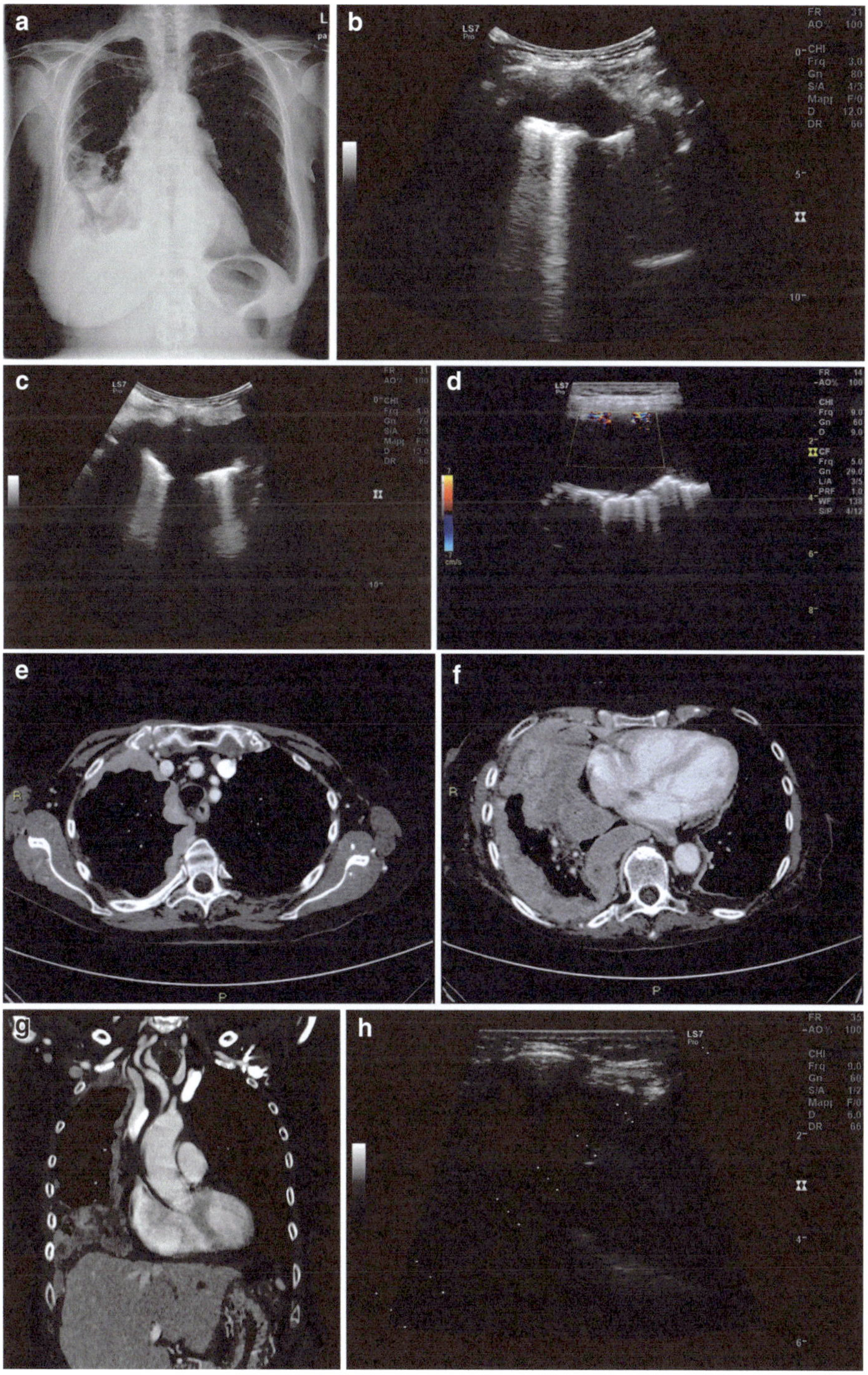

Fig. 6.12 Pleural mesothelioma. Chest X-ray (**a**) shows extensive pleuroparenchymal opacity in the right mid-baseline. TUS with convex (**b**, **c**) and linear (**d**) probes showed the presence of coarse tissue thickening of the pleura, mamelonated, and of variable thickness, as well as the presence of pleural effusion. The CT in axial (**e**, **f**) and coronal (**g**) scanning, after administration of contrast medium, confirmed the marked "rind-like" pleural thickening, almost entirely involving the right hemithorax, with sub-atelectatic areas of the parenchyma at the base. Echo-guided biopsy (**h**) allowed for tissue characterization and diagnosis of epithelioid cell mesothelioma

Asbestosis is diffuse pulmonary fibrosis prevalently located in peripheral regions and lower segments and under TUS examination gives rise to B-lines prevailing in the basal region [62].

Thanks to high levels of sensitivity, specificity, and positive and negative predictive values compared to with CT, TUS can be considered an additional tool in the follow-up of pleural plaques and interstitial thickening in subjects occupationally exposed to asbestos, after the initial CT assessment [63].

6.5.2 Pleural Metastasis

When TUS identifies pleural thickening, the differential diagnosis is mainly between inflammatory and neoplastic processes.

In general, neoplastic infiltration more often determines a widespread and irregular thickening of the pleura.

Pleural metastasis may appear as hypoechoic nodules [64], or they can appear as rounded or polypoid formations with variable echogenicity, sometimes even hyperechoic [65].

TUS does not allow in any way a differential diagnosis between metastatic lesions and a peripheral primitive neoplastic lesion [28], although multiple pleural nodules concurrently of a pleural effusion, in a patient with a known primitive malignancy, can indicate metastasis from serous carcinomas [66, 67].

However, limitations related to the weak panoramic nature of TUS, the difficulties of visualizing pleural lesions of smaller sizes [60], and the inability to display lesions of visceral pleura in the presence of reflecting elements along the pleural line must always be considered [28].

6.6 Conclusions

TUS offers a simple, practical approach to the study of pleural disease, in many cases resulting complementary to traditional radiography; it is also useful as a support for interventional procedures with both diagnostic and therapeutic purposes.

The absence of ionizing radiation, the low cost and the lack of invasiveness make this method particularly useful in the diagnosis and follow-up of common conditions, such as pleural effusion and pneumothorax.

References

1. Lichtenstein DA, Menu Y. A bedside ultrasound sign ruling out pneumothorax in the critically ill. Lung sliding. Chest. 1995;108(5):1345–8.
2. Lichtenstein D, Mezière G. Relevance of lung ultrasound in the diagnosis of acute respiratory failure. Chest. 2008;134:117–25.
3. Sasso A. Fisica degli ultrasuoni. In: Bazzocchi M, et al., editors. Ecografia. Napoli: Idelson-Gnocchi; 2002. p. 3–17.
4. Soldati G, Copetti R. Ecografia toracica. Torino: C.G. Edizioni Medico Scientifiche; 2006.
5. Müller NL. Imaging of the pleura. Radiology. 1993;186(2):297–309.
6. Pistolesi M, Miniati M, Giuntini C. Pleural liquid and solute exchange. Am Rev Respir Dis. 1989;140:825–47.
7. Fabbri M. Cooperativa Libraria Universitaria Editrice Bologna CLUEB Malattie dell'Apparato Respiratorio; 2003. p. 137–8.
8. Allen SJ, Laine GA, Drake RE, Gabel JC. Superior vena caval pressure elevation causes pleural effusion formation in sheep. Am J Phys. 1988;255:492–5.
9. Eid AA, Keddissi JI, Kinasewitz GT. Hypoalbuminemia as a cause of pleural effusions. Chest. 1999;115:1066–9.
10. McLoud TC, Flower CD. Imaging the pleura: sonography, CT, and MR imaging. AJR Am J Roentgenol. 1991;156:1145–53.
11. Lichtenstein D. Lung ultrasound in the critically ill. Clin Intensive Care. Chest. 2005;16:79–87.
12. Wu RG, Yuan A, Liaw YS, et al. Image comparison of real-time gray-scale ultrasound and color Doppler ultrasound for use in diagnosis of minimal pleural effusion. Am J Respir Crit Care Med. 1994;150(2):510–414.
13. Wu RG, Yang PC, Kuo SH, Luh KT. "Fluid color" sign: a useful indicator for discrimination between pleural thickening and pleural effusion. J Ultrasound Med. 1995;14:767–9.
14. Light RW, Macgregor MI, Luchsinger PC, et al. Pleural effusions: the diagnostic separation of transudates and exudates. Ann Intern Med. 1972;77:507–13.
15. Burges LJ, Maritz FJ, Taljaard JJ. Comparative analysis of the biochemical parameters used to distinguish between pleural transudates and exudates. Chest. 1995;107:1604–9.
16. Light RW. Pleural effusion. N Engl J Med. 2002;346:1971–7.

17. Porcel JM. Pleural fluid biomarkers: beyond the Light criteria. Clin Chest Med. 2013;34(1):27–37.
18. Light RW. The Light criteria: the beginning and why they are useful 40 years later. Clin Chest Med. 2013;34(1):21–6.
19. Piccoli M, Trambaiolo P, Salustri A, et al. Bedside diagnosis and follow-up of patients with pleural effusion by a hand-carried ultrasound device early after cardiac surgery. Chest. 2005;128:3413–20.
20. Gryminski J, Krakowka, Lypacewicz G. The diagnosis of pleural effusion by ultrasonic and radiologic techniques. Chest. 1976;70:33–7.
21. Felson B. Chest roentgenology. Philadelphia: WB Saunders; 1973. p. 361.
22. Moskowitz H, Platt RT, Schachar R, Mellins H. Roentgen visualization of minute pleural effusion. An experimental study to determine the minimum amount of pleural fluid visible on a radiograph. Radiology. 1973;109:33.
23. Gardelli G, Feletti F, Nanni A, et al. Chest ultrasonography in the ICU. Respir Care. 2012;57(5):773–81.
24. Battista G, Ghigi G, Zompatori M, Salizzoni E, Canini R. Torace. In: Bazzocchi M, et al., editors. Ecografia. Napoli: Idelson-Gnocchi; 2002. p. 297–318.
25. Eibenberger WI, Dock ME, Ammann, et al. Quantification of pleural effusion: sonography versus radiography. Radiology. 1994;191(3):681–4.
26. Vignon P, Chastagner C, Berkane V. Quantitative assessment of pleural effusion in critically ill patients by means of ultrasonography. Crit Care Med. 2005;33:1757–63.
27. Krackov R, Rizzolo D. Real-time ultrasound-guided thoracentesis. JAAPA. 2017 Apr;30(4):32–7. https://doi.org/10.1097/01.JAA.0000508210.40675.09.
28. Beckh S, Bölcskei PL, Lessnau KD. Real-time chest ultrasonography a comprehensive review for the pulmonologist. Chest. 2002;122:1759–73.
29. Roch A, Bojan M, Michelet P, et al. Usefulness of ultrasonography in predicting pleural effusions >500 mL in patients receiving mechanical ventilation. Chest. 2005;127:224–32.
30. Goecke W, Schwerk WB. Chapter 12: Die Real-Time Sonographie in der Diagnostik von Pleuraergüssen. In: Gebhardt J, et al., editors. Ultraschalldiagnostik, vol. 89. Berlin: Springer; 1990. p. 385–7.
31. Reuss J. Sonographic imaging of the pleura: nearly 30 years experience. Eur J Ultrasound. 1996;3:125–39.
32. Yu CJ, Yang PC, Chang DB, Luh KT. Diagnostic and therapeutic use of chest sonography: value in critically ill patients. Am J Roentgenol. 1992;159:695–701.
33. Izumi S, Tamaki S, Natori H, Kira S. Ultrasonically guided aspiration needle biopsy in diseases of the chest. Am Rev Respir Dis. 1982;125:460–4.
34. Diacon AH, Theron J, Schuurmans MM, et al. Intrapleural streptokinase for empyema and complicated parapneumonic effusions. Am J Respir Crit Care Med. 2004;170:49–53.
35. Davies RJ, Traill ZC, Gleeson FV. Randomised controlled trial of intrapleural streptokinase in community acquired pleural infection. Thorax. 1997;52:416–21.
36. Bouros D, Schiza S, Tzanakis N, et al. Intrapleural urokinase versus normal saline in the treatment of complicated parapneumonic effusions and empyema: a randomized, double-blind study. Am J Respir Crit Care Med. 1999;159:37–42.
37. Maskell NA, Davies CW, Nunn AJ, et al. U.K. controlled trial of intrapleural streptokinase for pleural infection. N Engl J Med. 2005;352:865–74.
38. Cameron R, Davies HR. Intra-pleural fibrinolytic therapy versus conservative management in the treatment of adult parapneumonic effusions and empyema. Cochrane Database Syst Rev. 2008;(2):1.
39. Nie W, Liu Y, Ye J, Shi L, Shao F, Ying K, Zhang R. Efficacy of intrapleural instillation of fibrinolytics for treating pleural empyema and parapneumonic effusion: a meta-analysis of randomized control trials. Clin Respir J. 2014;8(3):281–91.
40. Alemán C, Porcel JM, Alegre J, Ruiz E, Bielsa S, Andreu J, Deu M, Suñé P, Martínez-Sogués M, López I, Pallisa E, Schoenenberger JA, Bruno Montoro J, de Sevilla TF. Intrapleural fibrinolysis with urokinase versus alteplase in complicated parapneumonic pleural effusions and empyemas: a prospective randomized study. Lung. 2015;193(6):993–1000.
41. Cha LM, Choi S, Kim T, Yoon SW. Intrapleural urokinase therapy in a neonate with pleural empyema. Pediatr Int. 2016;58(7):616–9.
42. Gehmacher O, Kopf A, Scheier M. Can pleurisy be detected with ultrasound? Ultraschall Med. 1997;18(5):214–9.
43. Görg C, Bert T, Görg K. Contrast-enhanced sonography for differential diagnosis of pleurisy and focal pleural lesions of unknown cause. Chest. 2005;128(6):3894–9.
44. Holzapfel L, Demingeon G, Benarbia S, et al. Diagnostic du pneumothorax chez le malade presentant une insuffisance respiratoire aigue. Rean Soins Intens Med Urg. 1990;6:38–41.
45. Gordon R. The deep sulcus sign. Radiology. 1980;136:25–7.
46. Soldati G, Testa A, Sher S, et al. Occult traumatic pneumothorax: accuracy of lung ultrasonography in the emergency department. Chest. 2008;133:204–11.
47. Oveland NP. Lung point: Response. Chest. 2013; 143(6):1838–9.
48. Feletti F, Mucci V, Aliverti A. Chest ultrasonography in modern day extreme settings: From military setting and natural disasters to space flights and extreme sports. Can Respir J. 2018 Mar 15;2018:8739704. https://doi.org/10.1155/2018/8739704.
49. Yang H, Testa JR, Carbone M. Mesothelioma epidemiology, carcinogenesis, and pathogenesis. Curr Treat Options in Oncol. 2008;9:147–57.
50. Wechsler RJ, Steiner RM, Conant EF. Occupationally induced neoplasm of the lung and pleura. Radiol Clin N Am. 1992;30:1245–68.
51. Koh DM, Burke S, Davies N, Padley SP. Transthoracic US of the chest: clinical uses and applications. Radiographics. 2002;22(1):1.
52. Marchbank ND, Wilson AG, Joseph AE. Ultrasound features of folded lung. Clin Radiol. 1996;51(6):433–7.

53. Husain AN, Colby T. Guidelines for pathologic diagnosis of malignant mesothelioma. Arch Pathol Lab Med. 2013;137:647–67.
54. Patel SC, Dowell JE. Modern management of malignant pleural mesothelioma. Lung Cancer (Auckl). 2016;7:63–72.
55. Boutin C, Rey F. Thoracoscopy in pleural malignant mesothelioma: a prospective study of 188 consecutive patients. Cancer. 1993;72(2):389–93.
56. Loddenkemper R. Thoracoscopy—state of the art. Eur Respir J. 1998;11:213–21.
57. Metintas M, Ak G, Dundar E, et al. Medical thoracoscopy vs CT scan-guided Abrams pleural needle biopsy for diagnosis of patients with pleural effusions. Chest. 2010;137(6):1362–8.
58. Adams RF, Gray W, Davies RJ, Gleeson FV. Percutaneous image-guided cutting needle biopsy of the pleura in the diagnosis of malignant mesothelioma. Chest. 2001;120(6):1798–802.
59. American Thoracic Society. Diagnosis and initial management of nonmalignant diseases related to asbestos. Am J Respir Crit Care Med. 2004;170:691–715.
60. Cugell DW, Kamp DW. Asbestos and the pleura. A review. Chest. 2004;125:1103–17.
61. Hosoda Y, Hiraga Y, Sasagawa S. Railways and asbestos in Japan (1928-1987)-epidemiology of pleural plaques, malignancies and pneumoconioses. J Occup Health. 2008;50(4):297–307.
62. Lichtenstein D, Mézière G, Biderman P, et al. The comet-tail artifact an ultrasound sign of alveolar-interstitial syndrome. Am J Respir Crit Care Med. 1997;156:1640–6.
63. Smargiassi A, Pasciuto G, Pedicelli I, et al. Chest ultrasonography in health surveillance of asbestos-related lung diseases. Toxicol Ind Health. 2017;33(6):537–46. 748233716686916.
64. Yang PC, Luh KT, Chang DB, et al. Value of sonography in determining the nature of pleural effusion: analysis of 320 cases. Am J Roentgenol. 1992;159(1):29–33.
65. Reuss J. Sonographic imaging of the pleura: nearly 30 years experience. Eur J Ultrasound. 1996;3:25–39.
66. Steinberg HV, Erwin BC. Metastases to the pleura: sonographic detection. J Clin Ultrasound. 1987;15:276–9.
67. Goerg C, Schwerk WB, Goerg K, et al. Pleural effusion: an "acoustic window" for sonography of pleural metastases. J Clin Ultrasound. 1991;19:93–7.

7 Chest Wall Disorders

Francesco Feletti, Bruna Malta,
and Andrea Aliverti

7.1 Introduction

7.1.1 Study Techniques

The use of thoracic ultrasound (TUS) is becoming increasingly popular in the study of the chest wall and its alterations to both the soft tissue and skeletal components [1].

With an average thickness of 27 (±5) mm [2], the chest wall must be studied sonographically with medium-high (5–10 MHz) to high (>10 MHz) frequency transducers [1].

However, to cope with the limited penetration capacity and the restricted field of view of linear probes, it may be helpful to use convex transducers with frequencies between 3.5 and 5 MHz [3], especially in the case of extensive lesions or when the fat layer is particularly represented.

In certain cases, to ensure more reliable results, comparative evaluations of the same scans on both sides of the thorax can be useful.

7.1.2 Normal Finds

To locate pathological findings, it is imperative to recognize the natural appearance of the different chest wall components.

In an intercostal scanning, along the direction of the costal arches, underneath the thin echogenic layer of the skin, there is a subcutaneous connective tissue that shows highly variable echogenicity depending on the fat content and the degree of hydration.

Deep to the skin, the superficial fascia appears as a subtle echogenic line that delimits the muscular planes above.

The chest wall muscles, which present a streaked structure (echogenicity typical of skeletal muscle), have a variable thickness in different regions of the chest.

Electronic Supplementary Material The online version of this chapter (https://doi.org/10.1007/978-3-319-93055-8_7) contains supplementary material, which is available to authorized users.

F. Feletti (✉)
Dipartimento di Diagnostica per Immagini, Ausl della Romagna, Ospedale S. Maria delle Croci, Ravenna, Italy

Dipartimento di Elettronica, Informazione e Bioingegneria, Politecnico di Milano, Milan, Italy
e-mail: francesco.feletti@auslromagna.it

B. Malta
Dipartimento di Diagnostica per Immagini, Ausl di Ferrara, Ospedale Universitario di Ferrara, Ferrara, Italy
e-mail: mltbrn@unife.it

A. Aliverti
Dipartimento di Elettronica, Informazione e Bioingegneria, Politecnico di Milano, Milan, Italy
e-mail: andrea.aliverti@polimi.it

F. Feletti et al. (eds.), *Thoracic Ultrasound and Integrated Imaging*,
https://doi.org/10.1007/978-3-319-93055-8_7

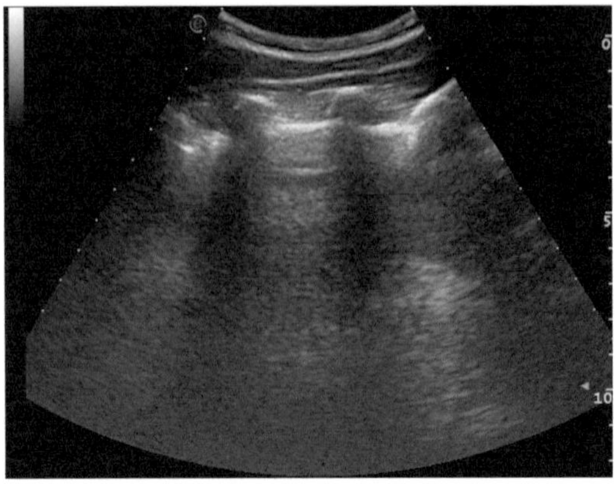

Fig. 7.1 Bat sign. *Bat sign* is the eponym used to describe the intercostal space transversally sounded, because the upper margin of the ribs resembles the wings of a bat seen in front, while the interposed pleural line represents the body

Deep to the chest wall muscles, in lean subjects, it is possible to identify the endothoracic fascia. It looks like an echogenic line, separated from the pleura only by a thin echogenic layer of fat tissue.

By rotating the probe perpendicularly to the ribs, the intercostal soft tissues are seen between two transversally scanned ribs (Fig. 7.1).

Typically, the bone structure of the thoracic cage partially reflects and partially absorbs ultrasounds, generating coarse rear shadow cones.

Costal acoustic shadows should be considered as standard criteria to be referred to; they are not present in subcutaneous emphysema because the air trapped in soft tissues masks the costal plane.

Instead, less intense and crisp costal shadows mean an increase in bone permeability to ultrasounds, and this may be due to an osteolytic lesion.

Therefore, every time costal shadows are less evident or abnormal, an X-ray examination is required.

7.2 Main Indications of Method

Thoracic ultrasound allows detailed and straightforward visualization of chest wall soft tissue alterations which, unlike in chest X-rays, may not be visible at all or may only result in minimal signs that are difficult to identify and interpret.

TUS is also sensitive enough to detect changes in the skeletal component, including costal fractures.

For these reasons, apart from diagnostic possibilities, the nonuse of ionizing radiation, rapidity of execution, availability, and low cost, TUS can be used alongside clinical examination and traditional radiology, especially in chest pain and in the study of any palpable swelling of the thoracic wall.

7.2.1 Chest Pain

While the visceral pleura and the lungs are insensitive to painful stimuli, thoracic pain is mediated by nerve fibres of the chest wall and the parietal pleura. Both the chest wall and the pleura are easily evaluated by TUS.

Therefore, TUS, along with clinical examination, can quickly exclude some of the most common causes of chest pain (Table 7.1), allowing for more rational use of traditional radiology and CT, with consequent benefits in diagnostic, radioprotection, and economic terms.

7.2.2 Studying Palpable Thoracic Wall Alterations

Thoracic ultrasound is often used as an initial examination when studying thoracic wall swelling.

Depending on the case, TUS may be the starting point or an intermediate step of the diagnostic process, which is useful for indicating other examinations or confirming a diagnosis that is already hypothesized based on anamnesis and the overall clinical picture.

Many of the conditions discussed below appear clinically as palpable masses.

7.2.3 Limitations

The main limitations of the chest wall ultrasound study are preexisting conditions which inhibit penetration of the ultrasound waves or hinder

Table 7.1 Most common causes of chest pain (underlined the causes that may give signs to TUS) [4] ECG: electrocardiogram; CTPA: computed tomography pulmonary angiography; CT: computed tomography.

Chest wall disorders	Possible ultrasound signs
Costal fractures	Lighthouse phenomenon (Fig. 7.2) Cortical interruption Bone fragments
Hematoma	<24 h isoechogenic or hyperechogenic collection with fine and dense echoes >24/<72 h hypo-anechogenic collection >72 h complex structure training
Neoplastic invasion of the chest wall	Echopermeability of bone components Infiltrating hypoechoic mass Local tissue softening
Chest wall abscesses	Complex structures, sometimes with gas bubbles
Pleurisy	Pleural line interruption Subpleural infiltrates Possible pleural effusion
Pleural empyema	Sometimes corpuscular pleural effusion
Pneumothorax	No gliding sign Presence of A lines
Lung diseases	
Pneumonia	Liver hepatitis, aerial bronchogram, hypervascularization, pleural effusion, B lines
Pulmonary embolism	Possible subpleural hypoecogens Pleural effusion. Diagnosis requires laboratory examinations and possibly angiopneumo CT
Mediastinal pathologies	
Acute aortic dissection	Expanded aorta with interspaced flaps in suprasternal or parasternal scans
Myocardial infarction	Normal TUS; diagnosis requires ECG and laboratory tests; possible role of echocardiography
Pericarditis	There may be a small pericardial effusion Diagnosis requires ECG
Esophageal breakage	TUS is not informative Diagnosis by X-ray or CT

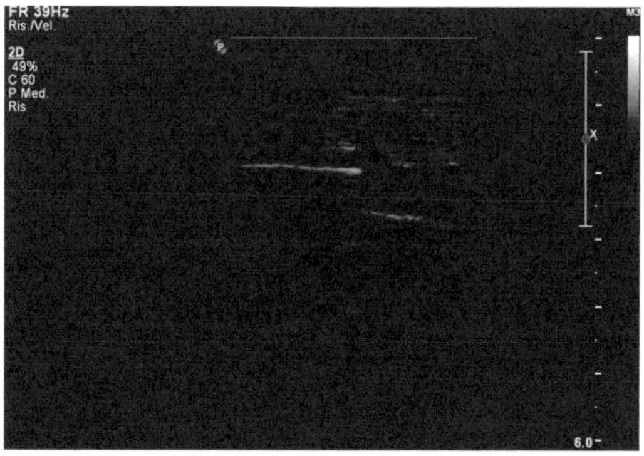

Fig. 7.2 Lighthouse phenomenon. The *lighthouse phenomenon* is a reverberation artifact that is generated between bone fragments in costal fractures

proper positioning of the probe such as subcutaneous emphysema, scarring or skin lesions, and external devices applied to the chest as electrodes or surgical dressings [5].

7.3 Soft Tissue Pathology

7.3.1 Hematomas

The sonographic appearance of hematomas changes over time.

In the acute phase (within 12–24 h of trauma), chest wall hematomas generate small, intense,

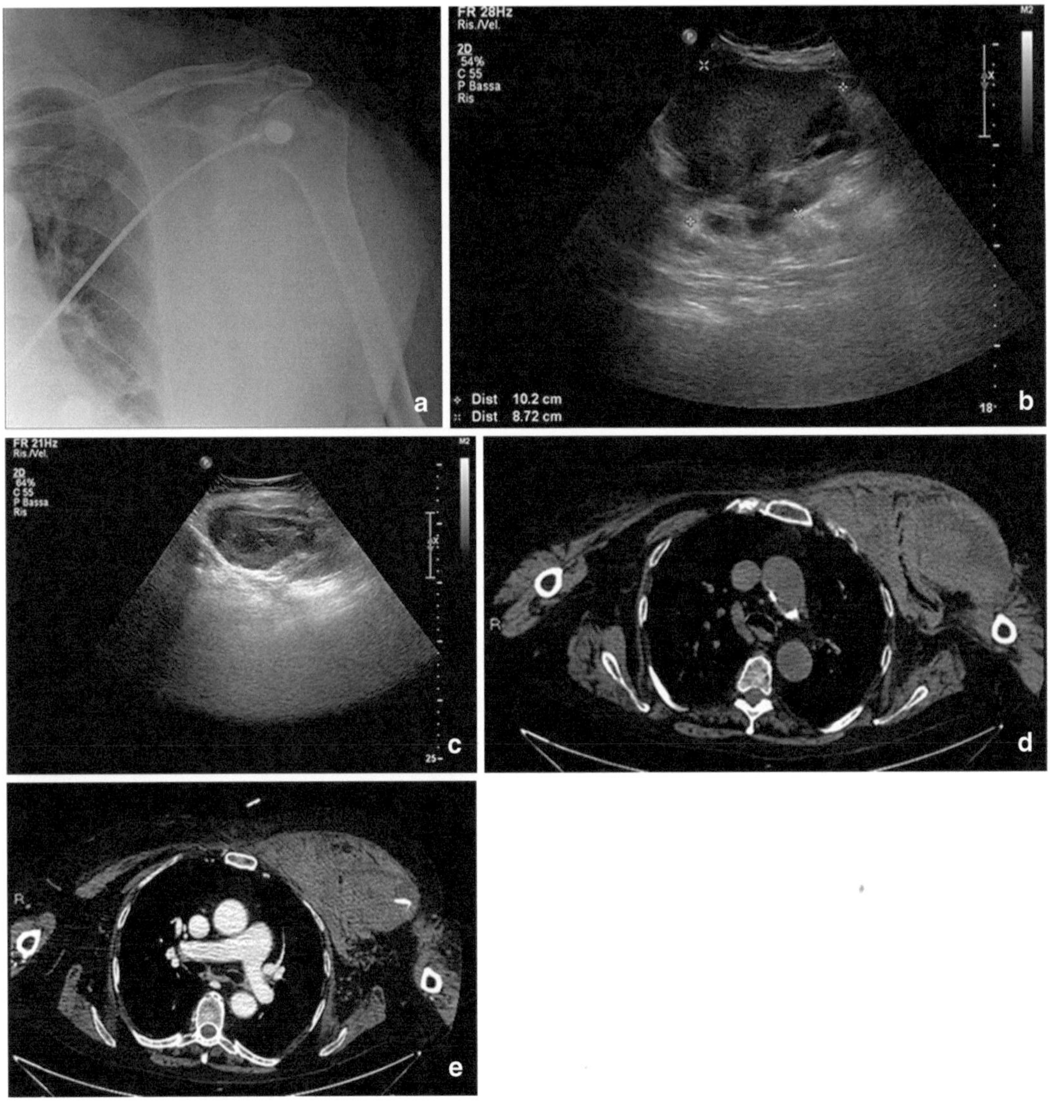

Fig. 7.3 Pectoral hematoma. The X-ray showed a soft tissue thickening (**a**). TUS (**b**, **c**) showed a complex echostructure formation that, together with the case history, allowed the diagnosis of a hematoma. The CT (**d**, **e**), on the other hand, made it possible to determine the anatomical relationships with the surrounding structures and to identify an active blood spill

Fig. 7.4 Hemorrhagic effusion in the presence of a costal fracture (arrow). The hematoma appeared as shaded hyperechogenicity which made the interfaces between the muscular planes of the thoracic wall less evident

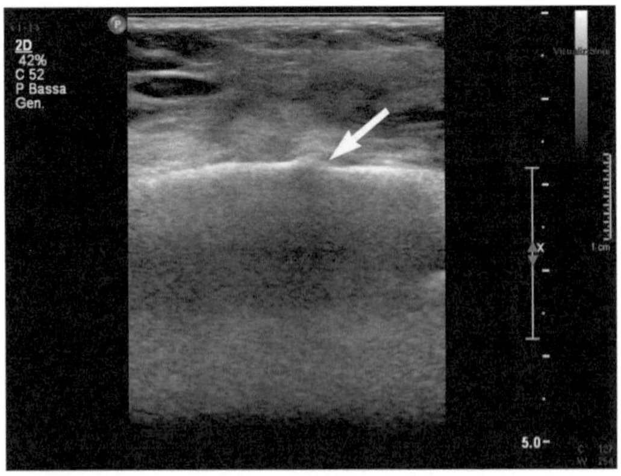

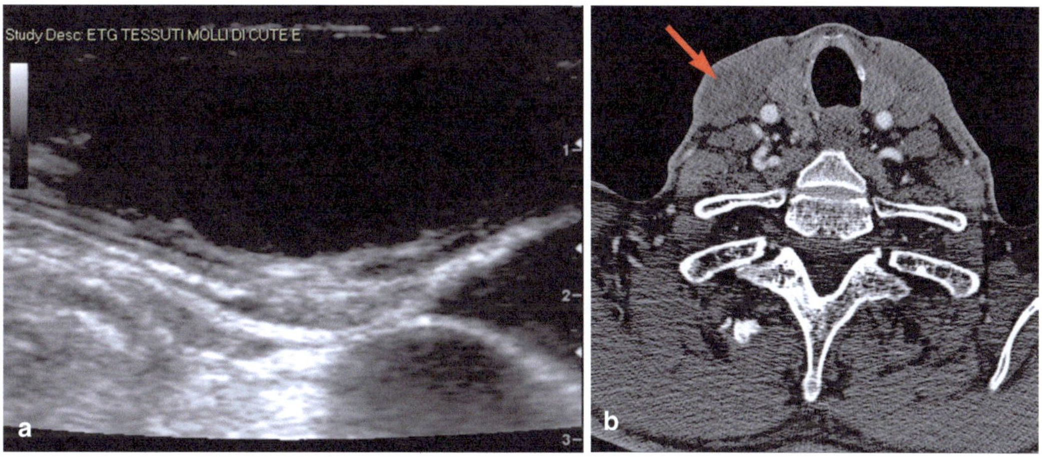

Fig. 7.5 Hematoma of the sternocleidomastoid muscle. The swelling at the base of the neck was evident in the ultrasound and showed an uneven appearance (**a**). A CT-angiography was then conducted to exclude active bleeding; the lesion was visible with the CT (**b**), although it was poorly delimited (arrow) due to the limited resolution of tissue contrast offered by this method, decidedly lower than the TUS, and there were no visible contrast spillages

uniform, and dense echo signals (Figs. 7.3a–e; and 7.4, Video 7.1).

Subsequently, following the lysis of red blood cells, they assume the appearance of hypo-anechoic collections, sometimes uneven, due to the persistence of clots in the context (Fig. 7.5a, b).

Subsequently, smaller hematomas are reabsorbed.

Instead, larger ones are organized and have a complex structure with predominantly liquid contents.

At this stage, hematomas have an oval or melted shape with rounded edges and the echogenic wall may be thinner or thicker.

7.3.2 Cellulitis and Abscesses

Typically, cellulitis has a cobblestone appearance, while abscesses are complex structures with inhomogeneous intensity, size, and distribution of echoes [7] (Fig. 7.6a–c).

Usually, the echo layout within a lesion does not change with decubitus changes; this aspect, however, is not always easy to evaluate.

The abscess enters differential diagnosis with hematoma. However, a hematoma may become infected and become secondary into an abscess. As a result, the ultrasound data must always be complemented by anamnesis, objective examination, and laboratory findings (Fig. 7.7a–c).

7.3.3 Seroma

Seromas are free or partially organized posttraumatic or postsurgical lymphatic groups, while lymph cysts are congested, lymphatic vessels dilated upstream from an obstruction.

Both seroma and lymphatic cysts appear as anechoic, more or less elongated structures, with lateral acoustic shadows and back reinforcement (Fig. 7.8).

When studying a seroma group of the chest wall, it is essential to measure it and locate it with respect to the pleura, both to understand its origin and to address any ultrasound-guided interventional or surgical procedures.

7.3.4 Primary Expansion Processes

Tumours that originate from the chest wall are most often of mesenchymal origin. There are also several tumorlike masses which originate from the soft tissues of the chest wall.

Along with TUS, it is useful to evaluate the anatomical relationships of these expansive

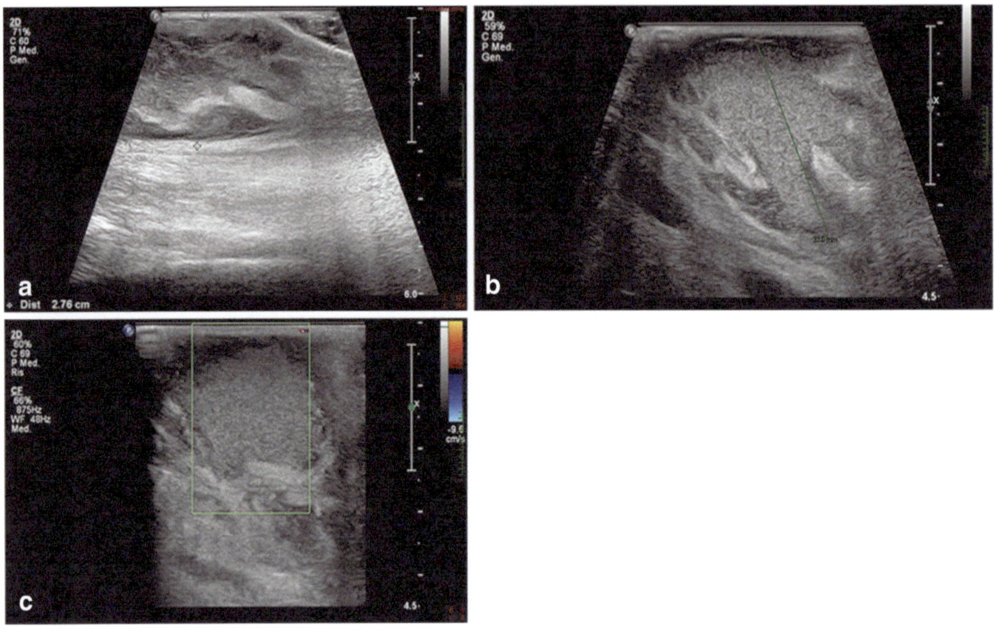

Fig. 7.6 Right subcutaneous dorsal abscess in a 38-year-old diabetic male patient. Ultrasound examination (**a**, **b**, **c**) revealed a complex mass of about 3 cm in the axillary region. The formation was hyperechogenic and characterized by thin, thickly crammed echoes

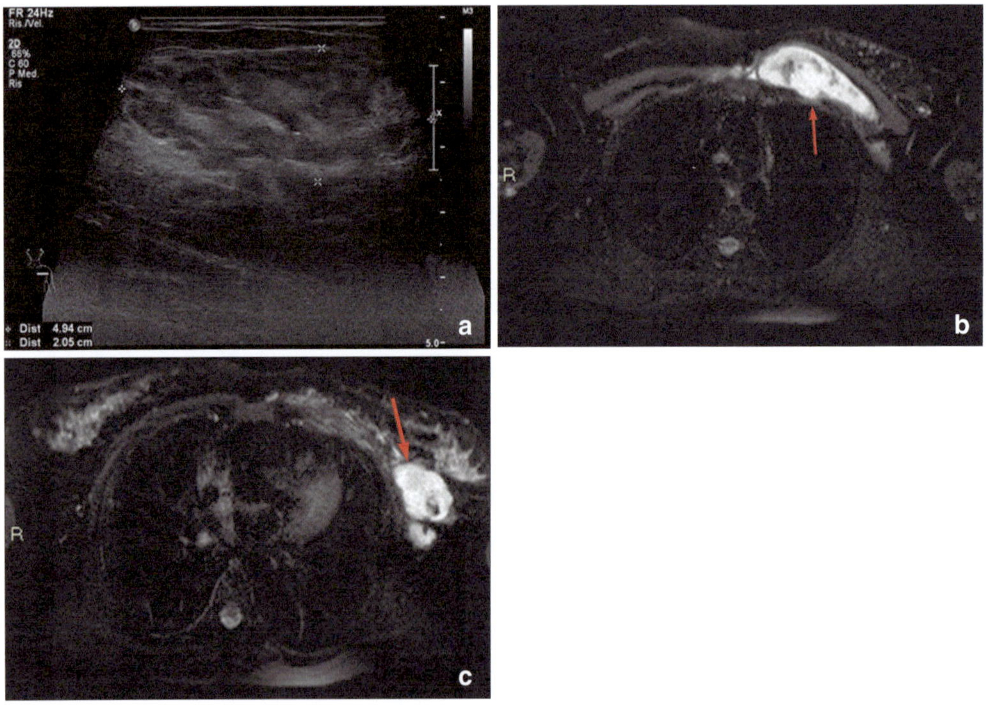

Fig. 7.7 Abscess of the chest wall. The ultrasound examination (**a**) showed the presence of a complex mass of about 5 cm in the left subclavian space. Echostructural characteristics alone did not allow for differential diagnosis from a hematoma. The MRI (**b**, **c**) showed the subfascial seat and extension to the axilla. The hyperintense aspect on T2w sequences and hypointense on T1w sequences were characterized by minute hypointense elements more evident in T1w sequences, which were attributed to a gas component. Contrast impregnation was poor and peripheral. The findings have been referred to as confluent abscessual collections

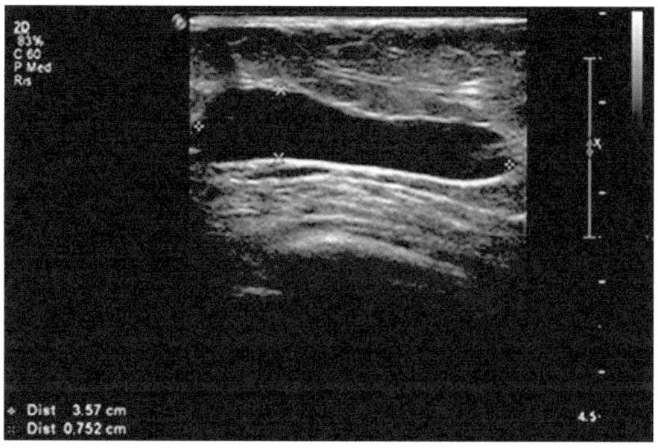

Fig. 7.8 Dysontogenetic lymphatic cyst. Soft tissue subcutaneous cyst in the left mammary site in a 5-year-old child. This formation was present from birth

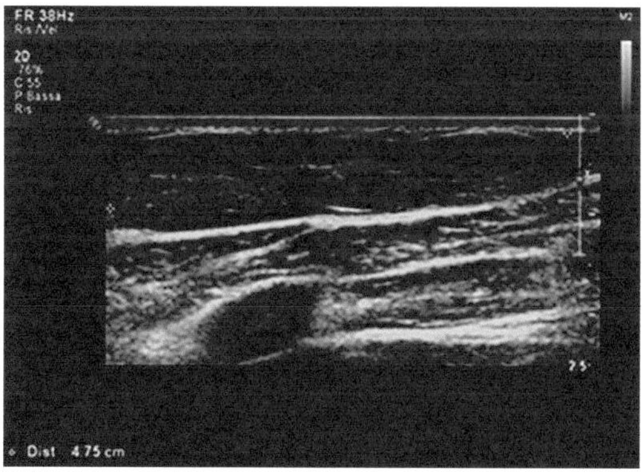

Fig. 7.9 Suprafascial lipoma of the right lateral thoracic wall. TUS showed the hyperechoic mass with regular margins and homogeneous echostructure of about 5 cm

processes with the pleura to confirm the extrathoracic origin of the lesion.

The pleura creates a cleavage plane and a natural barrier to the extension of the tumours and can be compressed and dislocated while the lung is not generally involved.

Therefore, even when they protrude in the chest cavity, these lesions retain obtuse joints with the chest wall.

7.3.5 Lipoma and fibrolipoma

Lipomas are the most common benign tumours in the chest wall, found both on the surface and at greater depths; deep lipomas are less frequent and generally larger.

Surface lipomas (Fig. 7.9) are found in the subcutaneous and are palpable. They are disk-shaped with a greater diameter parallel to the skin surface, compressible, and partially movable on the underlying planes.

Deep forms are intramuscular or intrafascial (Fig. 7.10a–e) and have varied, sometimes bizarre, shapes [7].

Sometimes large lipomas can widen an intercostal space or cause costal erosions through compression.

Finally, lipomatosis of the thoracic wall is a relatively rare condition characterized by multiple lipomas spread along the thoracic wall.

Regardless of location, lipomas have smooth, well-defined margins, poor internal structure, and uniform echogenicity, without signals at colour Doppler imaging (Fig. 7.11a–c).

Often lipomas contain intralesional fibrotic lines along the major axis of the lesion, that give them a streaked appearance.

As a result of traumas or inflammation, adiponecrosis may render the interior architecture less orderly, with hypo-anechoic areas and sometimes with small calcifications.

Fibroma and fibrolipoma have been frequently reported as benign tumours originating from the fibrous connective tissue of the chest wall [8]: they can be intrafascial, intramuscular, and, less frequently, subcutaneous.

They generally have regular contours, with a molten form and intermediate echogenicity (Fig. 7.12).

7.3.6 Desmoids

Deep, extra-abdominal fibromatosis (desmoids) generally affect the dorsal chest wall, shoulder, or thigh.

They are lesions which originate from muscular aponeurosis with intrafascial growth, oval or fusiform in general, with well-defined contours and hypoechoic and inhomogeneous ultrasound structures (Fig. 7.13a–c).

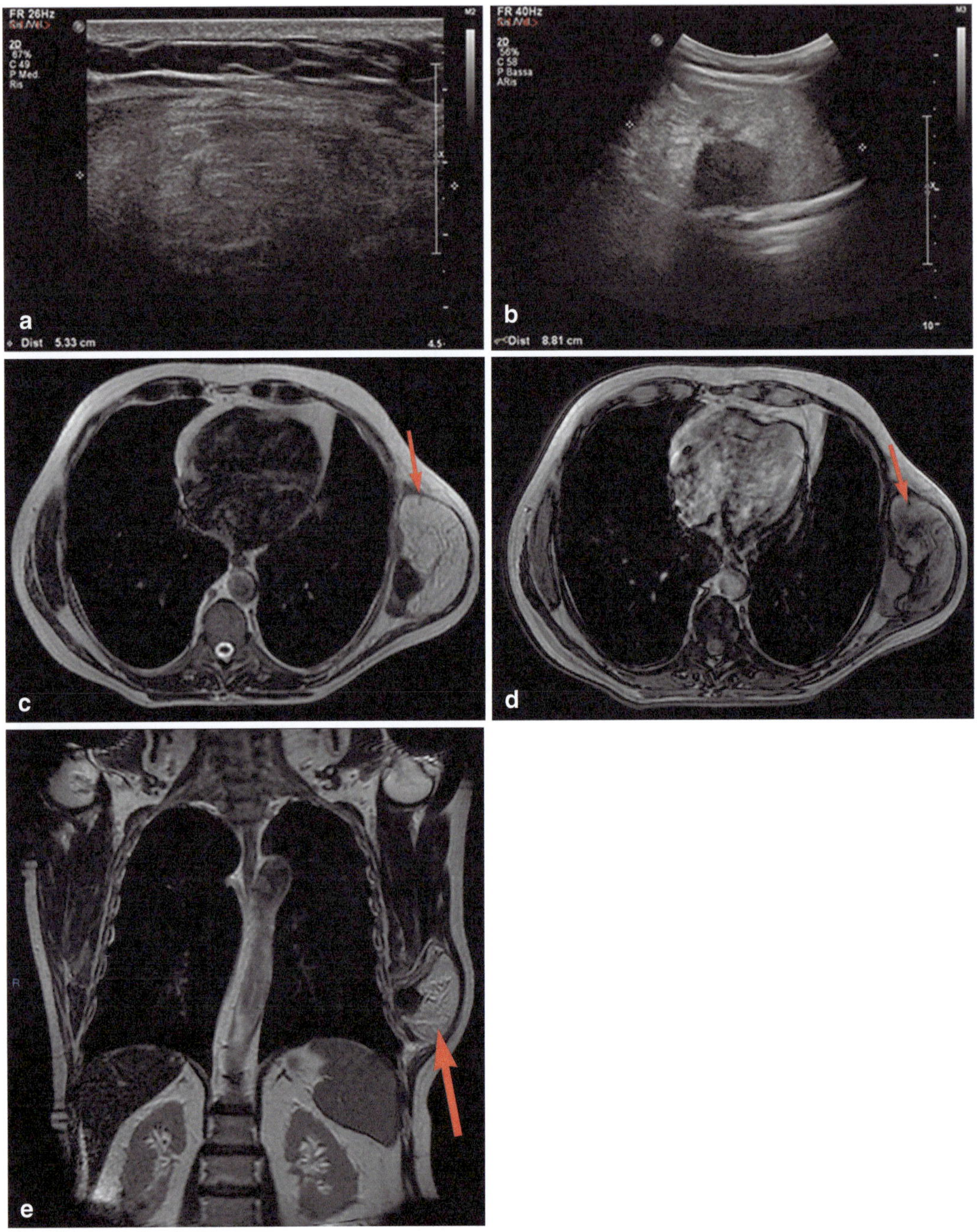

Fig. 7.10 Fibrolipoma of the left serratus anterior muscle. The TUS (**a**, **b**) focused on the voluminous palpable tumefaction and documented the presence of a coarse solid subfascial formation, of about 10 cm, with a nonhomogeneous echostructure, mainly hyperechogenic, with a central hypoechogenic area. MRI (**c**–**e**) confirmed the predominantly adipose nature of the lesion. Histological diagnosis of the atypical fibrolipomatous tumour was posed

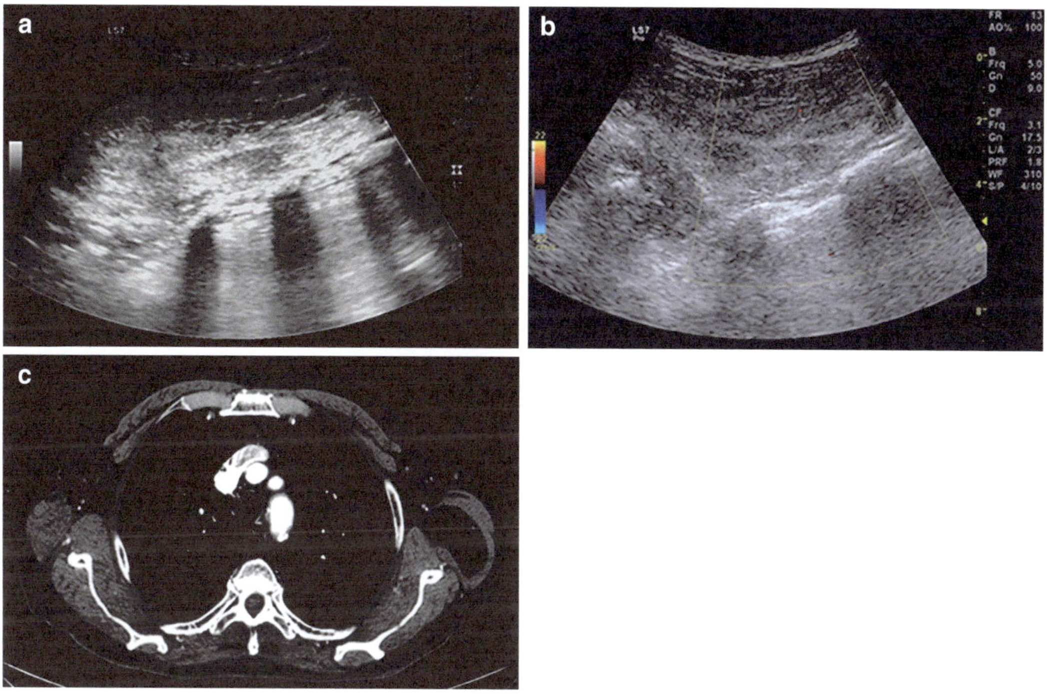

Fig. 7.11 Ultrasound (**a**, **b**) and CT (**c**) of coarse lipoma in the context of the left latissimus dorsi muscle. The colour-Doppler (**b**) showed no vascular signals. The CT confirmed uniform adipose density of the lesion

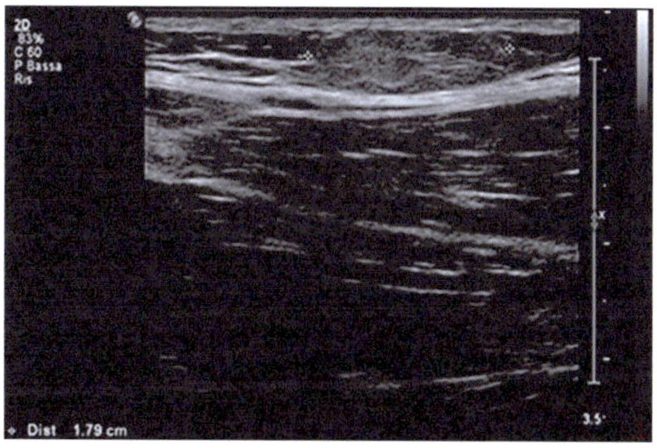

Fig. 7.12 Fibrolipoma. Typical appearance with regular contours and slightly hyperechogenic compared to muscle tissues

These lesions have a variable clinical course; they are generally locally aggressive and often reoccur if they are not removed with wide surgical margins.

7.3.7 Lymphangioma

Lymphangiomas are malformations of the lymphatic vessels, preferentially localized in the head and neck but also found in the mediastinum and axilla.

They can either be directly located or extend to the chest wall.

Under ultrasound examination, they appear as smooth (Fig. 7.14), micro- or macrocyst (i.e., hygroma, cystic) formations, uni- or multilocular.

7.3.8 Epidermal Inclusion Cyst

Epidermal inclusion cysts are localized in the thickness of the skin and the subcutaneous tissue.

They depend on the accumulation of secretive products within the sebaceous glands, for example, as a result of the occlusion of their excretory ducts.

They appear as round cysts with homogeneous hypoechoic content, although sometimes they may exhibit some hyperechogenic spots in the context, caused by the crystallization of sebaceous material.

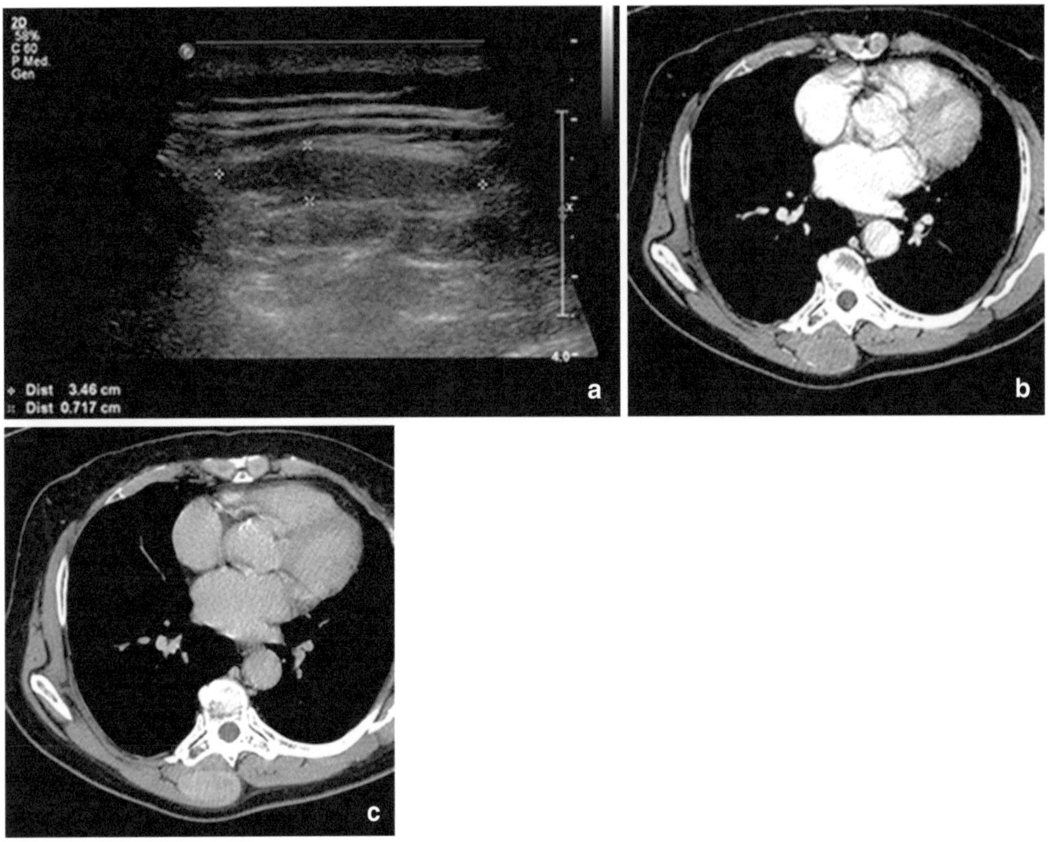

Fig. 7.13 Desmoid thoracic wall. Tumefaction of the back, in the paramedian area, with an ultrasound appearance (**a**) of an elongated subfascial lesion, hypoechogenic with regular contours, with scarce signals at colour Doppler imaging. With a CT (**b**, **c**), the lesion showed a peripheral neoformed vessel in the arterial phase and a homogeneous densitometric increase in the venous phase

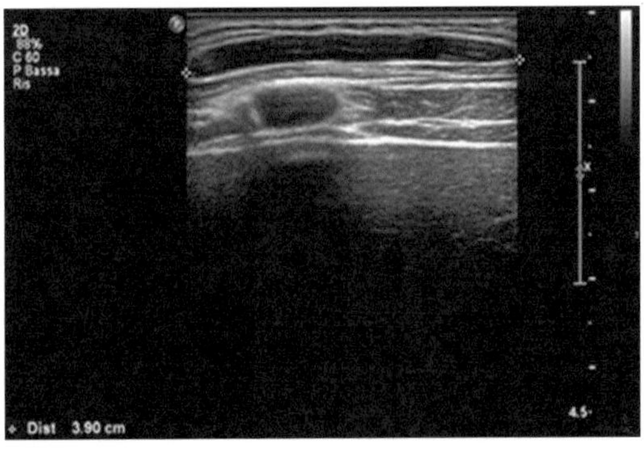

Fig. 7.14 Lymphangioma. An 8-year-old patient. Soft tumefaction. Elongated anechogenic formation with a smooth and thin wall, easily compressible above the costal muscular plane

7.3.9 Elastofibroma

Elastofibroma dorsi is a pseudotumoral lesion, often bilateral, which affects the posterolateral portion of the chest wall, between the apex of the scapula the latissimus dorsi and rhomboid.

It is composed of adipose and fibroelastic tissue, and it is common in subjects engaged in manual occupations, leading to the assumption of a possible reactive genesis as an expression of repeated rubbing movements of the lower angle of the scapula on the adjacent structures.

It is common in older people and females.

Generally, it has semilunar morphology, is located below the muscle plane, and has variable echogenicity depending on the percentage of fatty components (Fig. 7.15a–c).

It features typical hypoechoic or circular internal bands, arranged obliquely in relation to the skin surface and related to the fibroelastic component.

Its typical location, its appearance in TUS, and its possible bilaterality orient the diagnosis [9].

7.3.10 Hemangioma

Hemangiomas are benign vascular tumours and can, although rarely, affect the chest wall [10, 11].

TUS most often reveals them as complex, spongy masses characterized by multiple convoluted vascular spaces [10] (Fig. 7.16a, b).

Angiomas may sometimes simulate a cyst presenting itself as a single cavity with anechoic

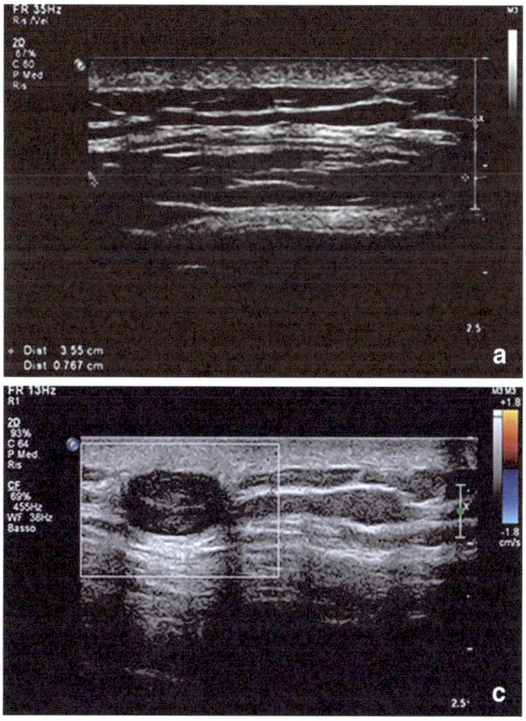

Fig. 7.15 Elastofibroma dorsi. The patient was a young man dedicated to manual activities. The TUS (**a**–**c**) revealed an elongated, semilunar formation, with a diameter of 3.5 cm in the subcutaneous tissue of the right dorsal thoracic wall, below the scapular apex. The almost isoechogenic formation of the muscle showed a typical longitudinal striation, regular contours, and the absence of vascular signals at colour Doppler imaging

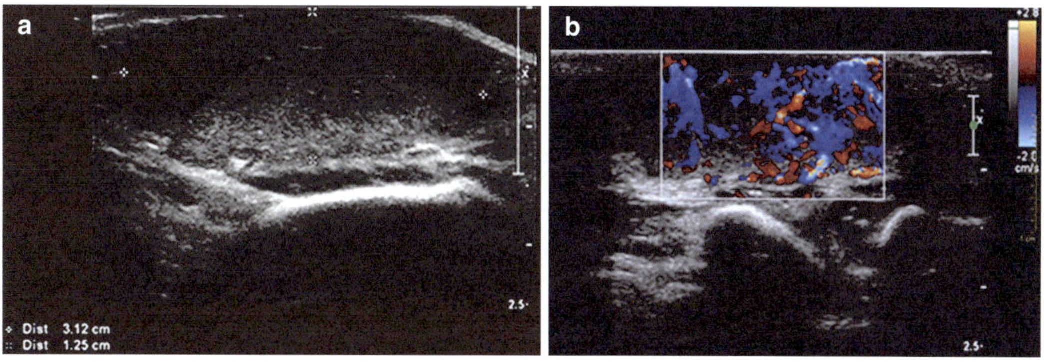

Fig. 7.16 Semilunar angioma in newborn. Formation in the subcutaneous, resting on the underlying muscular fascia with a diameter of about 3 cm, hyperechogenic (**a**) and intensely vascularized with afferent and efferent vessels (**b**)

content. Sometimes, however, multiple septa give the lesion a hyperechogenic appearance similar to that of a solid lesion.

The colour-Doppler shows the vascular signal in dilated vessels, and the flow may be arterial or venous (Fig. 7.17a–c).

7.3.11 Myositis Ossificans

Although rare in this anatomical region, myositis ossificans should be considered in the differential diagnosis of the thoracic wall and thoracic pain masses [12].

It is a metaplastic bone proliferation that develops in the context of the skeletal muscle and sometimes in subcutaneous layers (Fig. 7.18).

Generally, it follows a traumatic event, although there are non-traumatic forms, and the affected area, in the beginning, appears tumulus and sore.

Ossification occurs within a few weeks on the periphery of a fibroblast-like lesion [13], and in TUS, it produces typical acoustic absorption and is therefore easily recognizable.

Therefore, TUS is essential for early diagnosis of the disease when calcifications may not yet be visible on a plain chest X-ray [12].

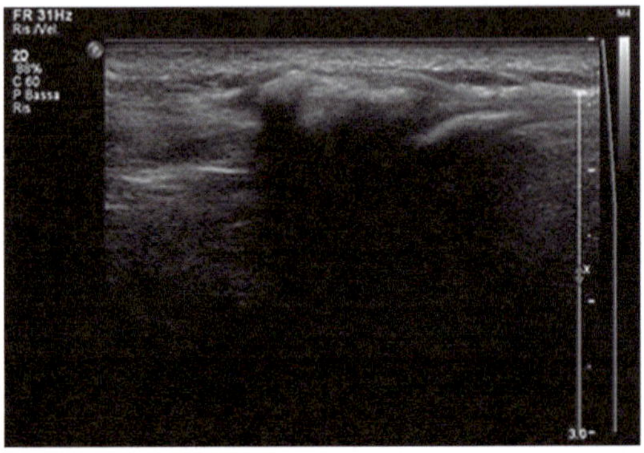

Fig. 7.18 Myositis ossificans. Typical hyper-reflective appearance with rear acoustic barrier due to previous trauma

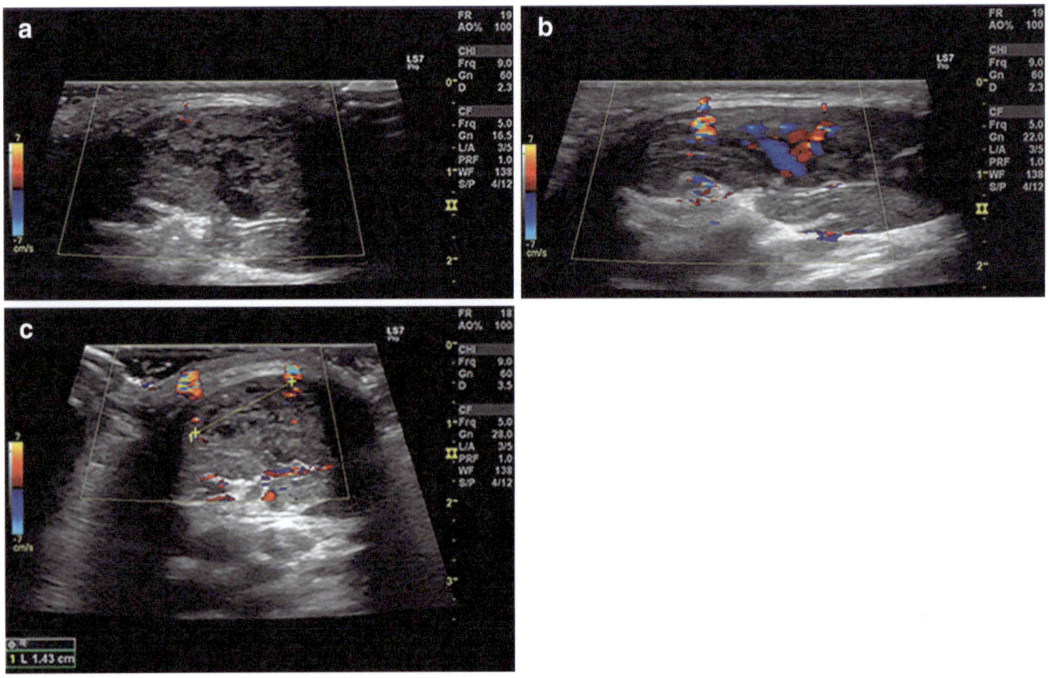

Fig. 7.17 Muscular angiomyolipoma. Ultrasound aspects (**a**–**c**). Dishomogeneous echostructure formation (vascular, adipose, and muscular components) showing marked vascularization in Doppler colour

7.3.12 Neurogenic Tumours

The neurogenic tumours originate from the spinal nerve roots or the intercostal nerves.

Neurogenic tumours generally appear as regular, hypoechoic, and often with back wall reinforcement formations.

In some cases, TUS can document the continuity of the lesion with the source nerve: the tumour tissue subverts the typical fascicular collated nerve structure.

7.3.13 Primary Malignant Tumours

Primary malignant tumours of the chest wall are mainly sarcomas (chondrosarcomas, osteosarcomas, and Ewing sarcoma family of tumours), plasma cell neoplasms (multiple myeloma and plasmacytoma), and malignant peripheral nerve sheath tumours [14].

Sarcomas of the chest are rare and generally originate from the chest wall tissues, while the primary sarcomas of the pleura are rare.

Generally, sarcomas are bulky lesions with uneven edges and are markedly inhomogeneous due to the coexistence of prominent sects and nodules, an expression of the aberrant proliferation of mesenchymal tissues, fibrous hyperechogenic tissue, and hypo- or anechogenic necrotic regions.

In colour-Doppler, they often appear hyper vascularized with neoformed vessels.

Dynamic TUS can show tumour fixity to deeper structures [8] before and after muscle contraction.

Moreover, ultrasound study allows the evaluation of possible infiltration of bone tissue, which appears with irregularities and cortical interruption.

Ultrasound can ultimately guide biopsy maneuvers for histological characterization. The rib cage is often involved in *multiple myeloma* [15] (Fig. 7.19a–g).

Malignant peripheral nerve sheath tumour is associated with neurofibromatosis type 1, and the transformation of a benign neurofibroma (Fig. 7.20a–c) should be suspected when a patient with neurofibromatosis type 1 is experiencing pain [14].

7.3.14 Lymph Nodes

Ultrasound examination of pectoral, axillary, and laterocervical lymph node assessments exceeds the accuracy of clinical examination [16].

High-frequency linear probes (7.5–12 MHz) are used for the study of surface lymph nodes.

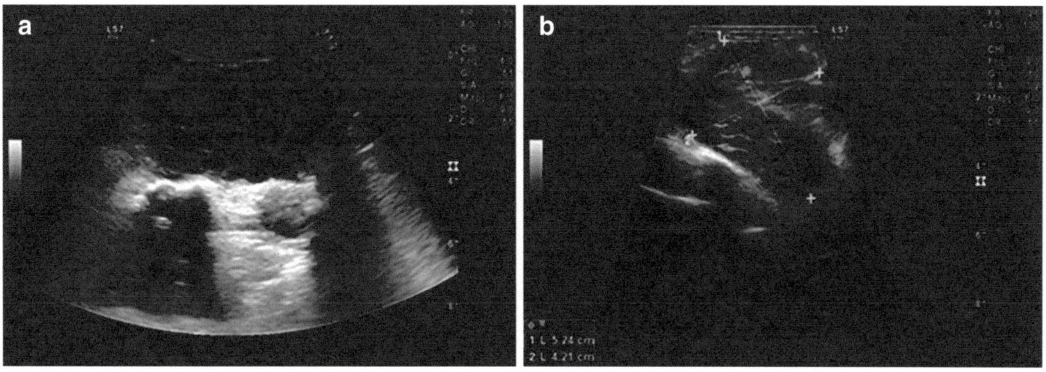

Fig. 7.19 Infiltrating heteroplasia of the thoracic wall in an 82-year-old male patient. The TUS showed a coarse, parasternal lesion of about 5 cm in the chest wall with uneven echostructure, hypo-anechogenic areas (**a**, **b**), and vascular signals in Doppler colour (**c**). Note the irregularity of the underlying bone surface. An X-ray, in LL projection, showed osteolysis of the sternum body (**d**, arrow). This aspect was confirmed by CT (**e**, **f**), which also highlighted the infiltration of surrounding muscular structures. An echo-guided biopsy (**g**) allowed the identification of the expansive lesion, resulting in the diagnosis of multiple myeloma

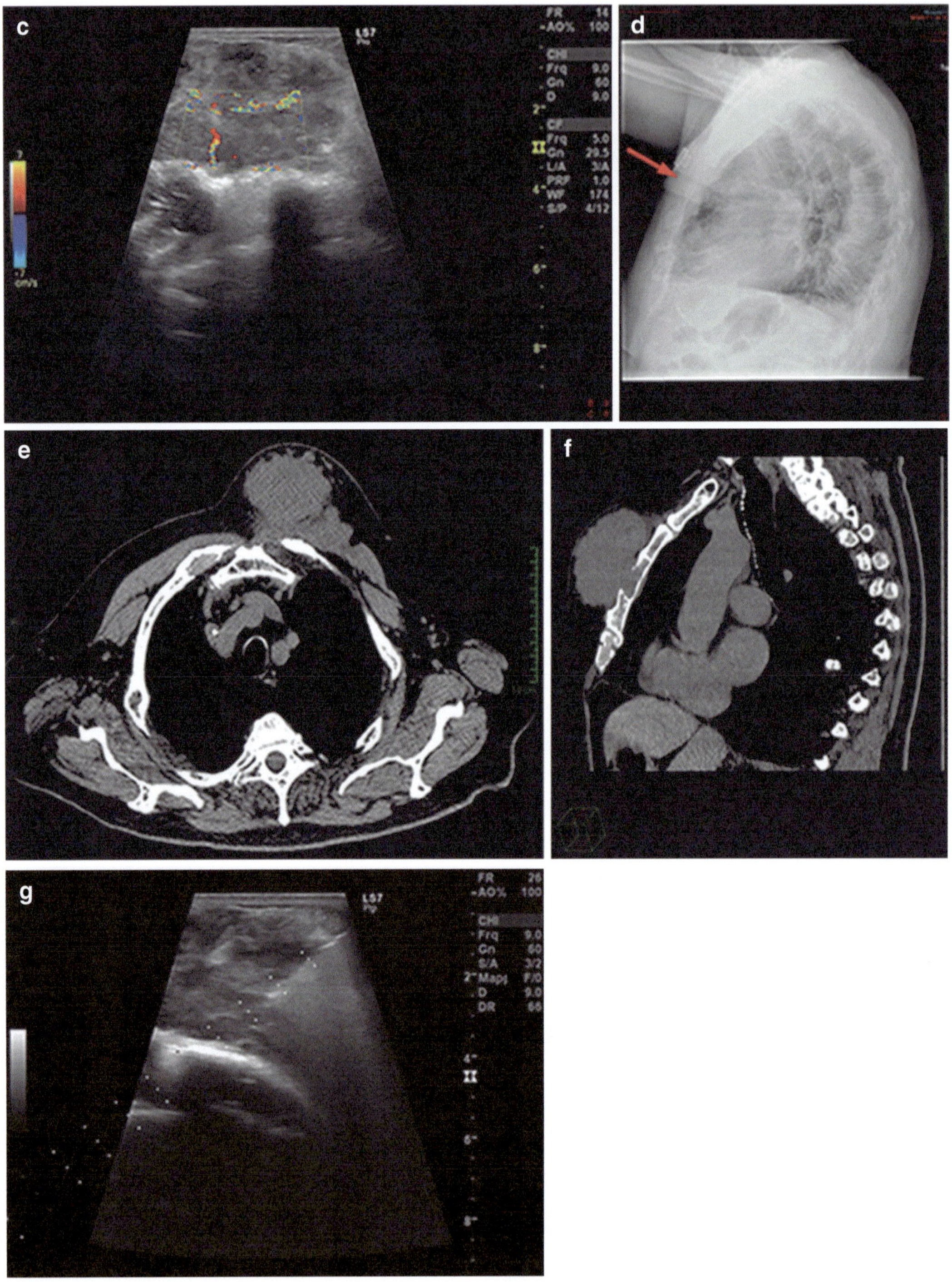

Fig. 7.19 (continued)

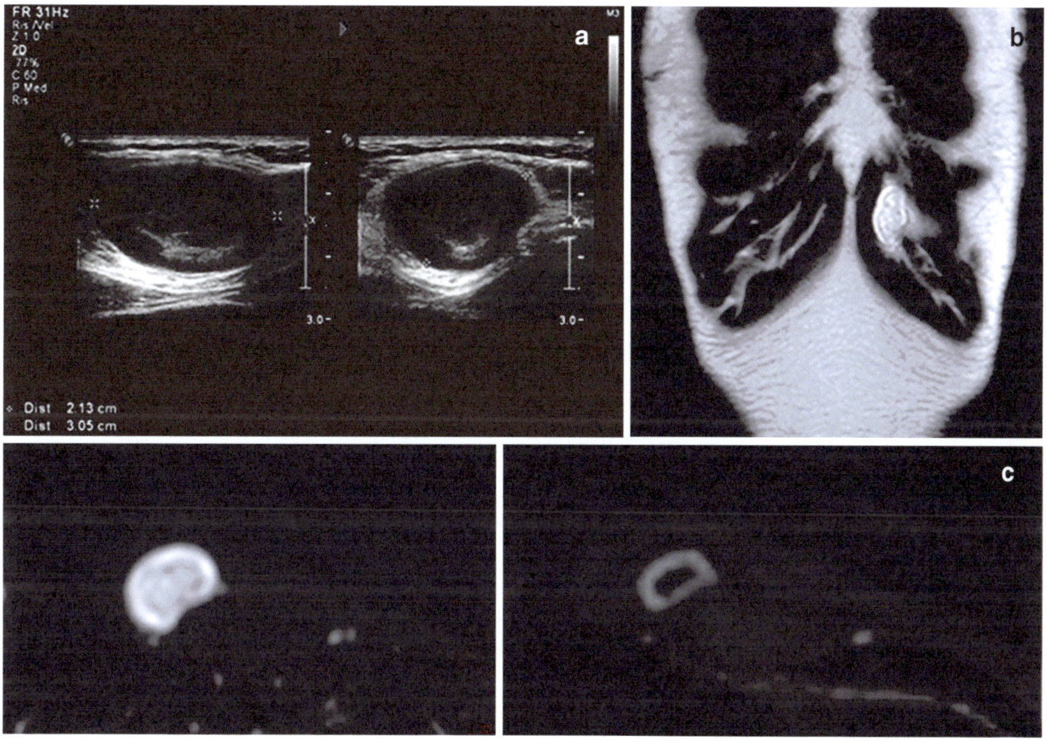

Fig. 7.20 Parasternal neurofibroma in neurofibromatosis. With an ultrasound, the palpable swelling of the thoracic wall showed an oval, unevenly hypoechogenic lesion with regular contours of 2.2 × 3.4 cm (**a**). MRI: Coronal acquisition T2w (**b**); axial acquisition T2w SPAIR(**c**); axial after administration of gadolinium (**d**). With an MRI, the lesion showed low signal in T1w sequences and was hyper intensive in T2w (**b, c**). After administration of contrast medium, enhancement was mainly peripheral (**d**)

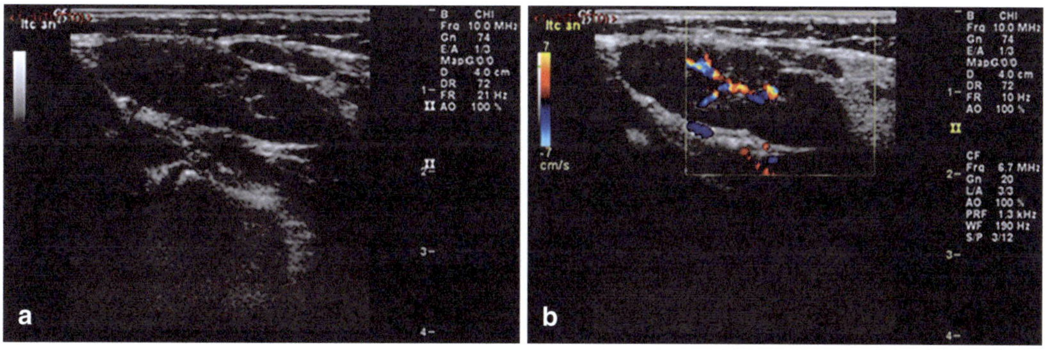

Fig. 7.21 Ultrasound of reactive normal lymph node (**a**), oval-shaped, with hyperechogenic hilum and regular Doppler vascular pattern (**b**)

The normal lymph node has a homogeneously hypoechogenic cortical area [17] and a central or eccentric, hyperechogenic, oval, or linear component.

This second echostructural element depends on the lymphatic sinus interfaces that converge toward the bone marrow and represents an essential sign of normality [17].

In the normal lymph node, with colour- and power-Doppler, only tiny, predominantly central components are seen; they generally have a radial distribution around the central hyperechogenic component [18, 19] (Fig. 7.21a, b).

The *roundness index* (RI) is the ratio between the longitudinal diameter and the transverse lymph node diameter; an oval shape (RI > 1)

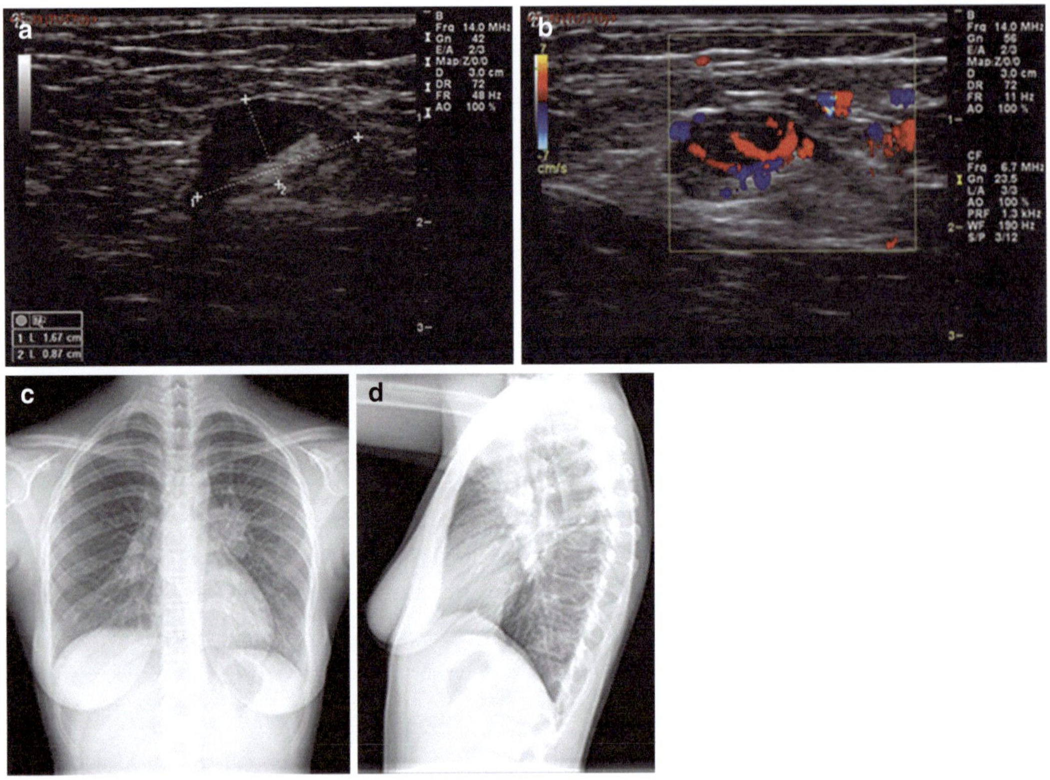

Fig. 7.22 Ultrasound of axillary lymph node in a young patient with non-Hodgkin's lymphoma (**a**, **b**). Evident roundish morphology and vascularization accentuated and altered in Doppler colour. In X-ray examination (**c**, **d**), the enlargement of the pulmonary hila linked to the lymphadenopathic padding is highlighted

orientates toward a reactive nature; vice versa a rounded morphology is indicative of neoplastic involvement (Fig. 7.22a–d).

The roundness index and the central hyperechogenic component [20] represent the most reliable ultrasound parameters to distinguish reactive lymphoma from neoplastic ones.

Focal hypoechoic necrosis areas are typically present in non-Hodgkin's centrocytic or centroblastic type lymphomas and metastases but may also be present in tuberculous lymphadenitis [17, 21].

The ultrasound appearance of neoplastic lymph nodes is unspecific (Fig. 7.23a–d); however, those involved in lymphoproliferative and secondary malignant diseases are often hypoechoic, while metastatic lymph nodes in epithelial neoplasms tend to be more echogenic and inhomogeneous. Nonetheless, the absence of the central echogenic zone is not always synonymous with neoplastic lymph node because it may also depend on the widespread infiltration of fat present in infectious outcomes [22]; in these cases, sometimes fibrotic or macrocalcifications that appear echographically as streaks or hyperechogenic spots are present.

Lymph node microcalcifications are common (65–70% of cases) in the lymph node metastases of medullary and papillary thyroid cancer that mainly affect the cervical, pre-tracheal, and paratracheal lymph nodes [23].

The typical vascular pattern of lymph nodes remains unaltered in hyperplastic-reactive lymph nodes, while it is disrupted in malignant lymphadenopathies, both in the displacement and incarceration of vessels by neoplastic infiltration and neoangiogenic processes [19].

In malignant or tuberculous lymphadenopathies, the colour-Doppler can show eccentric and asymmetric hilar vascularization, and peripheral linear or multifocal flow signals with loss of normal radial distribution or even the absence of vascularization [18, 19].

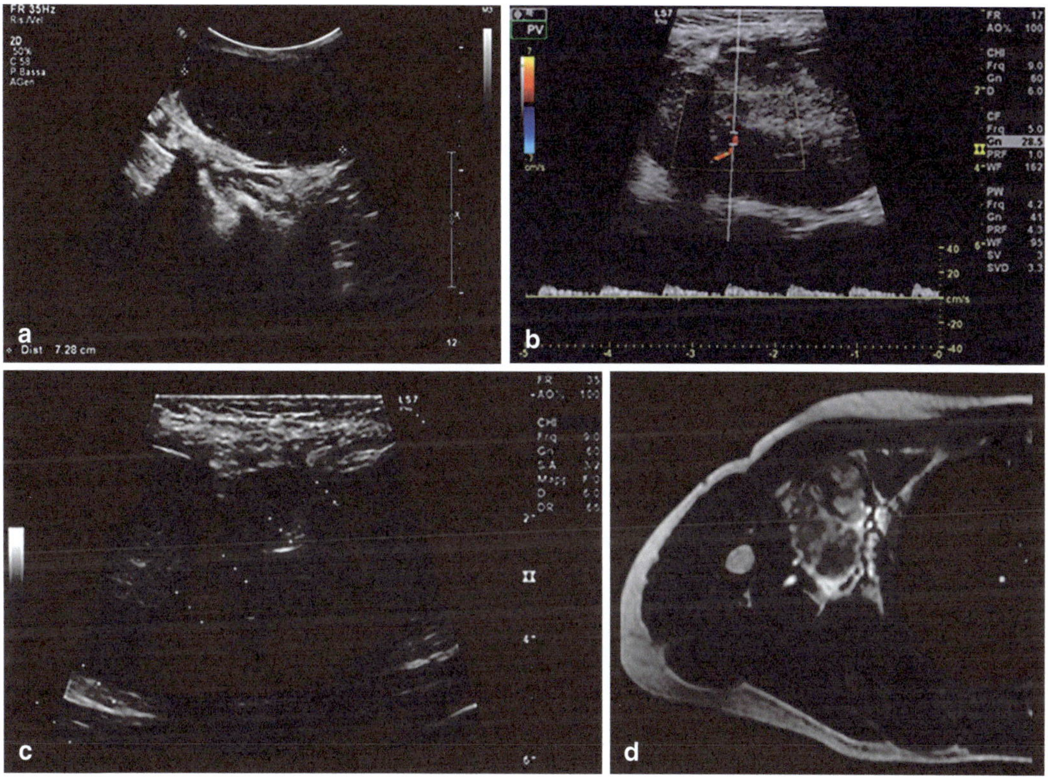

Fig. 7.23 Metastases of the chest wall. TUS with convex probe (**a**), linear probe with Doppler colour (**b**), echo-guided biopsy (**c**), and MRI (**d**): T1W axial image after administration of contrast medium. Solid oval formation of soft tissues (max. diameter 8 cm) with an uneven echostructure, fairly regular contours, and some arterial vessels visible with Doppler. Diagnosis of axillary lymph node metastases from melanoma with unknown origins in a 40-year-old patient

However, any result of a peripheral or mixed vascular pattern—i.e., both central and peripheral—suggests the neoplastic nature of lymphadenopathy [24].

7.3.15 Axillary Lymphadenopathies in Breast Cancer

The ultrasound study of the breast is beyond the scope of this discussion. However, it is advisable to recall the classification of axillary lymph nodes and the role of TUS in patients with breast cancer.

Axillary lymph nodes are classified in three levels based on anatomic relationships with small pectoral muscle.

Lymph nodes placed below the inferior margin of the said muscle belong to level I; those posterior or between the lateral and medial muscle margins are classified as level II; and those medially placed at the upper edge of the muscle, including intravascular lymph nodes, belong to level III.

The ultrasonic probe study is useful in the study of non-palpable lymph nodes at the lower level and the study of palpable lymph nodes of all levels [25].

7.3.16 Supraclavicular Lymphadenopathies

Over the last 20 years, the superiority of noninvasive imaging methods such as TUS and CT compared to palpation evaluation in the detection of overlapping lymph node metastases has been established [26].

To study overlapping lymph nodes with TUS, starting from the base of the neck, one must move sideways with both transverse and longitudinal scans, extending the study by about 4 cm above the clavicle head [27].

In patients with lung cancer, there are often (41–51% of cases) non-palpable metastatic lymph nodes [28] visible ultrasonically, and TUS has higher accuracy, sensitivity, and specificity than contrast-enhanced CT for primary supraclavicular lymph node metastases in lung cancer [29].

Supraclavicular occult metastases are present in 30% of patients with uterine cervical cancer involving abdominal para-aortic lymph nodes and in 15% of patients with oesophagus carcinoma but may also be present in breast cancer, gastric cancer, pancreas adenocarcinoma, and prostate cancer [30].

Finally, the US-guided FNA of supraclavicular adenopathy is a safe and straightforward tool for diagnosing and staging metastatic lymph nodes in the lung [16] and oesophagal cancer [31] and can also confirm the diagnosis in patients suspected of sarcoidosis [31].

7.3.17 Metastases and Neoplastic Invasion

In lung cancer, TUS with colour-Doppler can evaluate thoracic wall invasion with sensitivity and specificity superior to CT, complementing CT or MRI for preoperative staging [32] and being useful in operational planning [33] (Fig. 7.24a–g).

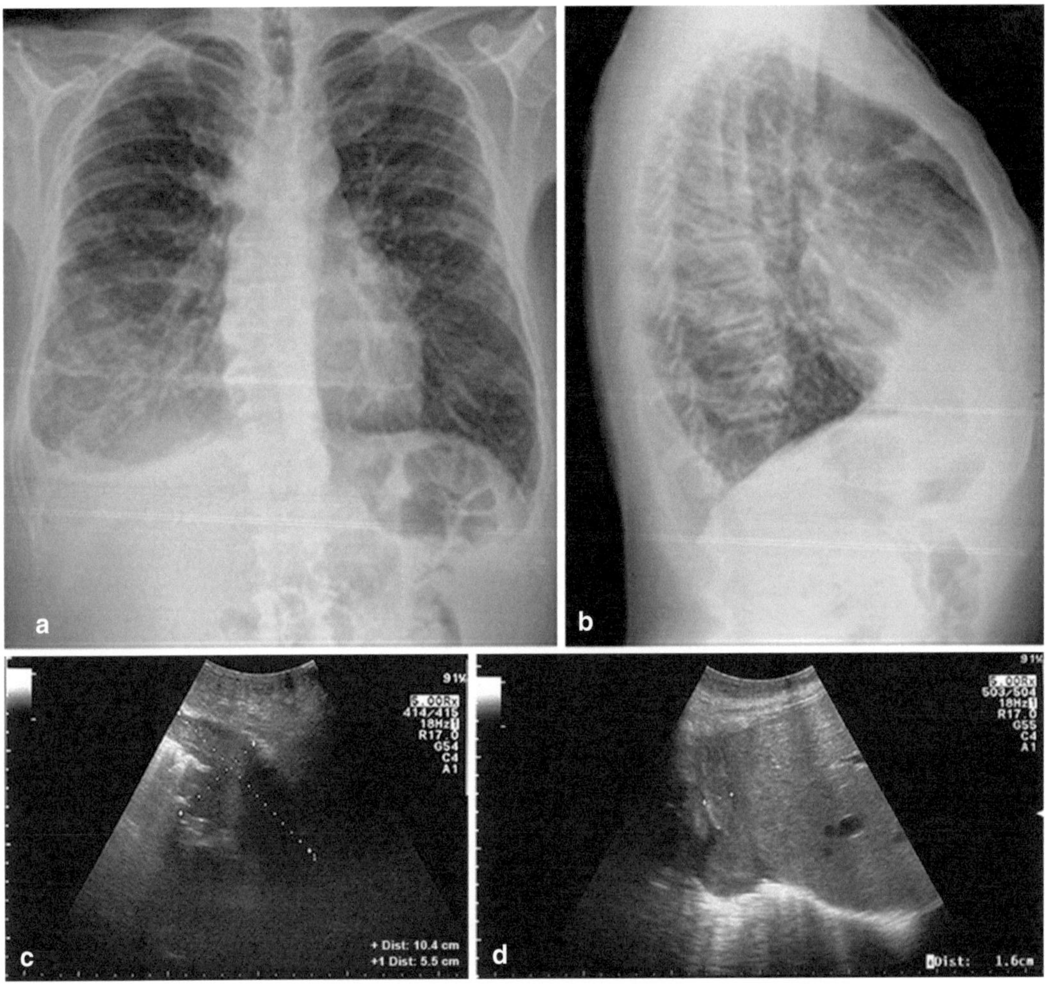

Fig. 7.24 Pulmonary neoplasia infiltrating the chest wall and the diaphragm. X-rays (**a**, **b**); TUS with convex probe (**c**, **d**) and detail of the chest wall with linear probe (**e**); CT (**f**, **g**). The infiltration of the thoracic wall and diaphragm was evident at the TUS, while the CT was more effective in determining the extension of the pathology

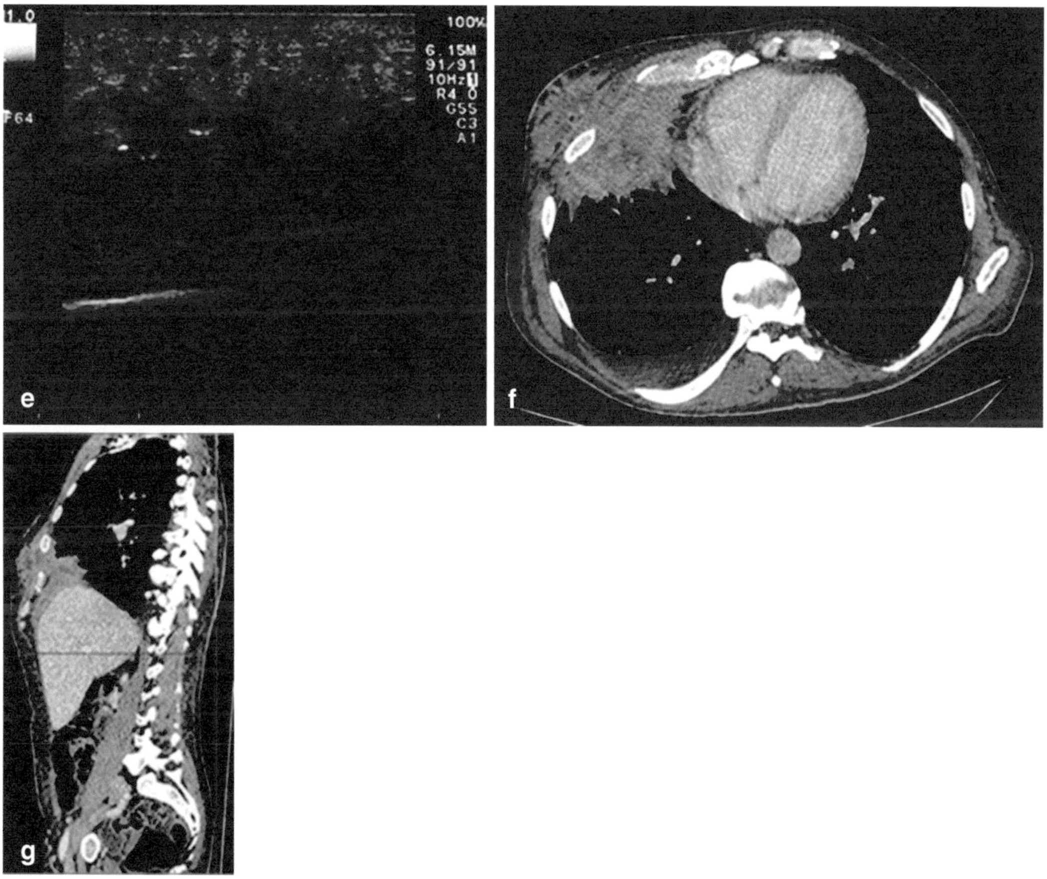

Fig. 7.24 (continued)

Hodgkin's lymphoma sometimes (6.4% of cases) involves the chest wall as the initial or secondary location [34].

The thoracic wall is most often reached by contiguity from an early mediastinal localization in advanced stages of the disease [35] frequently involving the chest skeleton. Instead, recurrences are frequent in the internal lymphatic chain because it is usually excluded from the fields of radiotherapy [36].

On the contrary, non-Hodgkin lymphomas in the chest appear as isolated chest masses, usually in locations that are difficult for ultrasound examination: mediastinal, paratracheal, hernia, and pericardial sites [34, 36].

Finally, soft tissues of the chest wall may sometimes be affected by hematogenic metastases of various malignant neoplasms.

7.3.18 Parietal Emphysema

Overall, parietal emphysema creates an acoustic barrier with the consequent formation of *dirty* acoustic shadows, making it impossible to study the underlying structures and often limiting the visibility of the ribs.

In particular, air causes reverberation artefacts that are classified as E lines and W lines [37] depending on the depth they originate from (Fig. 7.25a, b).

Specifically, E lines are generated at the same depth as the air trapped in a single tissue plane, while W lines are produced at various depths by aerial bubbles scattered between different tissue planes.

Sonographers must learn to recognize tissue emphysema in order to avoid gross interpretative errors.

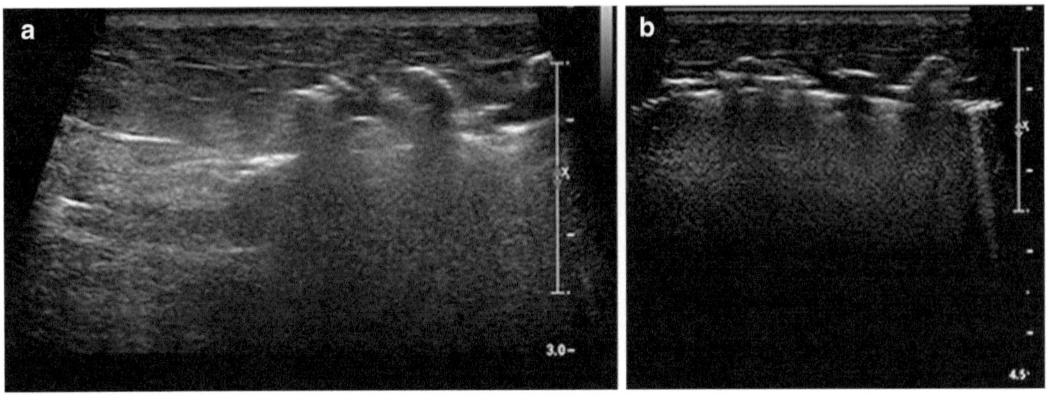

Fig. 7.25 Parietal emphysema (**a, b**). Partial posterior acoustic damming, caused by the presence of air bubbles in the soft tissues of the chest wall

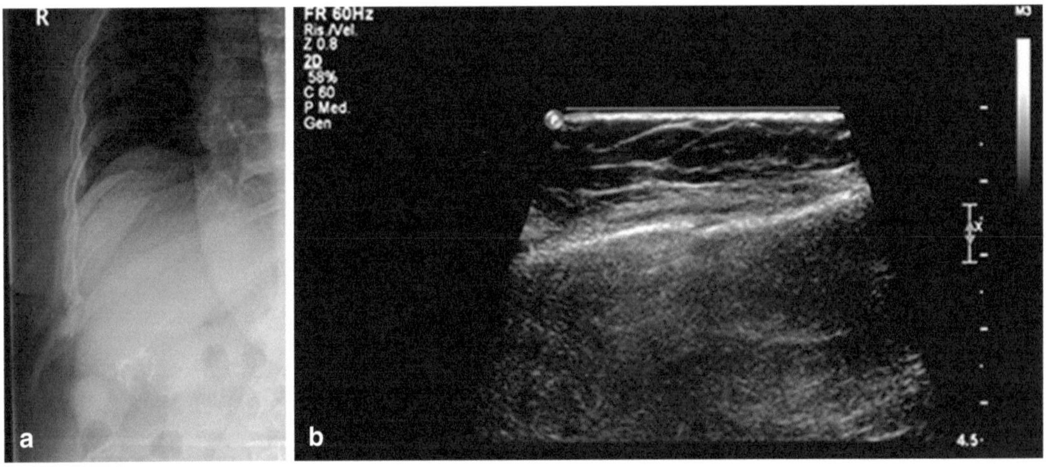

Fig. 7.26 Uncertain cortical irregularity in X-ray examination (**a**) of the eighth right rib at middle axillary, promptly confirmed by the visualization of the cortical bone interrupted in ultrasound examination (**b**)

In particular, E lines and W lines must be distinguished from B lines for their different diagnostic meaning; both E and W lines are formed in soft chest wall tissues, are fixed, and prevent the ribs from appearing, while B lines are generated at the pleural line level and are modified with respiratory acts.

The presence of B lines excludes pneumothorax. Instead, E and W lines indicate the presence of subcutaneous emphysema, a condition often associated with pneumothorax [38].

If the parietal emphysema is not too widespread, one can attempt to create acoustic access to the underlying structures by applying moderate pressure to the transducer, using ribs as fixed points to squeeze and shift the air bubbles.

7.4 Pathology of Scheletric Components

7.4.1 Fractures

The radiological diagnosis of bone fractures in the chest is not always easy, particularly if the radiogram is performed immediately after trauma and in the case of undisplaced fractures.

TUS allows for the identification of twice the amount of rib fractures compared to the standard chest radiogram performed with specific projections [39] (Fig. 7.26a, b).

It can also detect associated conditions such as pleural effusion, pneumothorax, pulmonary contusions, and chest wall haemorrhages [40].

In costal, cranial, and scapular fractures, TUS allows direct visualization of the interruption of the bone cortical, any fragments, and, if the fracture is disintegrated, the uneven levels of the fracture stumps (Fig. 7.27a–c).

The *lighthouse phenomenon*, also called *chimney phenomenon*, consists of reverberation echoes extending from the margin of the fracture to the bottom [40, 41].

This sign can be summoned by exerting minimal pressure at the point where the patient reports pain [42] and can be the only visible echographic sign in composite fractures.

To precisely locate sternal fractures, it is useful to refer to the joints between the manubrium, the sternal body, and the xiphoid process.

Fractures of the chest cage can form hematomas of variable size.

In the beginning, hematoma appears hypoanechoic, while about two weeks after the trauma, an increasing number of echoes and small acoustic shadows appear. They are signs of the repairing processes, and the first calcifications [40].

After consolidation, a more or less evident hump can remain in the bone profile [40, 43] (Fig. 7.28a, b).

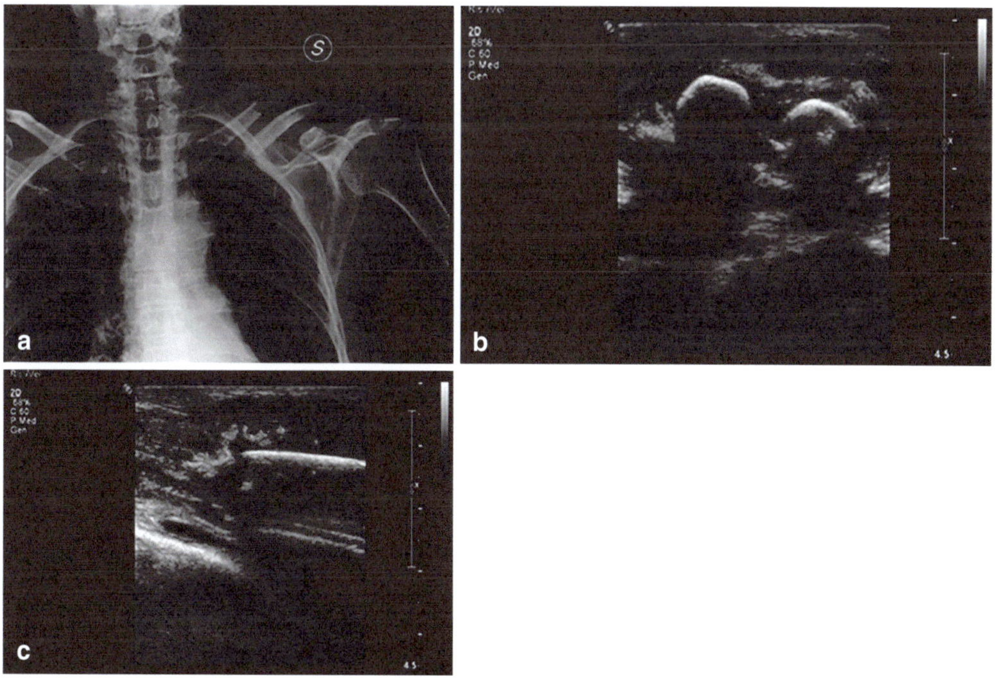

Fig. 7.27 Fracture at the middle third of the left collarbone. X-ray (**a**) and ultrasound (**b**, **c**)

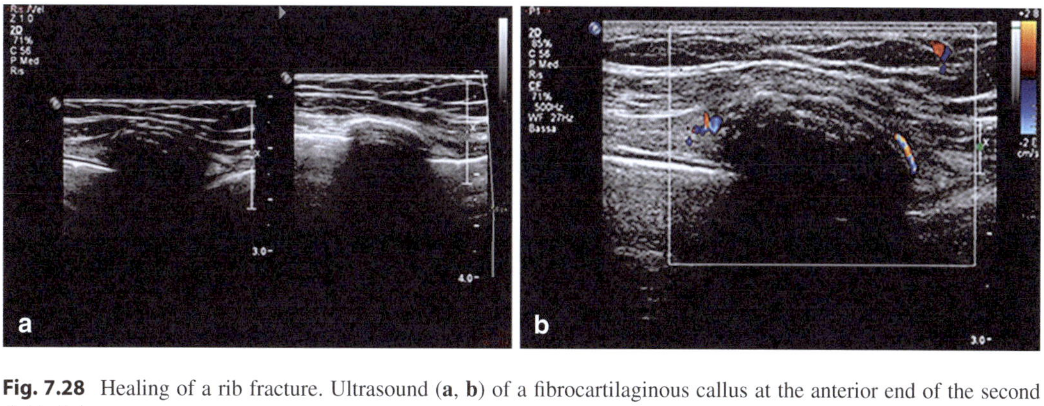

Fig. 7.28 Healing of a rib fracture. Ultrasound (**a**, **b**) of a fibrocartilaginous callus at the anterior end of the second right rib in a young woman

7.4.2 Osteomyelitis

Clinical diagnosis of osteomyelitis, cellulite, and abscess of soft chest wall tissues is challenging.

In osteomyelitis, inflammation related to bone necrosis and ischemic phenomena in the microcirculation produces an exudate that emerges from the cortical bone, forming fluid collections [44], which may sometimes contain a gaseous component or, in tuberculous forms, minute calcifications [45].

Fluid collections caused by osteomyelitis are located directly on the bone surface, while fluids originating from soft tissues (i.e., cellulite, lymphedema, abscess, or hematoma) remain separate from the cortical bone because the soft tissues remain attached to the bone.

Therefore, a fluid collection in direct contact with the bone is a sensitive sign of osteomyelitis and, when associated with the clinical data, allows for diagnosis [44].

However, this is a non-specific sign since fluid collections in direct contact with cortical bone can also be small hemorrhagic outbreaks in the presence of costal metastases [45].

7.4.3 Neoplastic Osteolytic Lesions

The thoracic cage may be home to metastases of several cancers (Fig. 7.29a–f) and in particular bronchogenic cancer, plasmacytoma, and breast, prostate, and kidney tumours.

While osteoblastic injuries do not show up in TUS, most osteolytic metastases can be detected because they reduce bone calcium content and increase ultrasound permeability.

In some cases, a well-conducted ultrasound can even allow the pleura to be seen behind a costal lesion [46].

More commonly, these lesions result in the reduction in sharpness or the disappearance of the back acoustic shadow [46, 47].

Upon examination, the neoplastic tissue component generally looks like a hypoechoic mass, while periosteal edema appears to be a localized thickening of soft tissues.

Ultrasound ultimately provides the guide to bioptic sampling for the characterization of osteolytic lesions of the chest cage [48] (Fig. 7.30a–d).

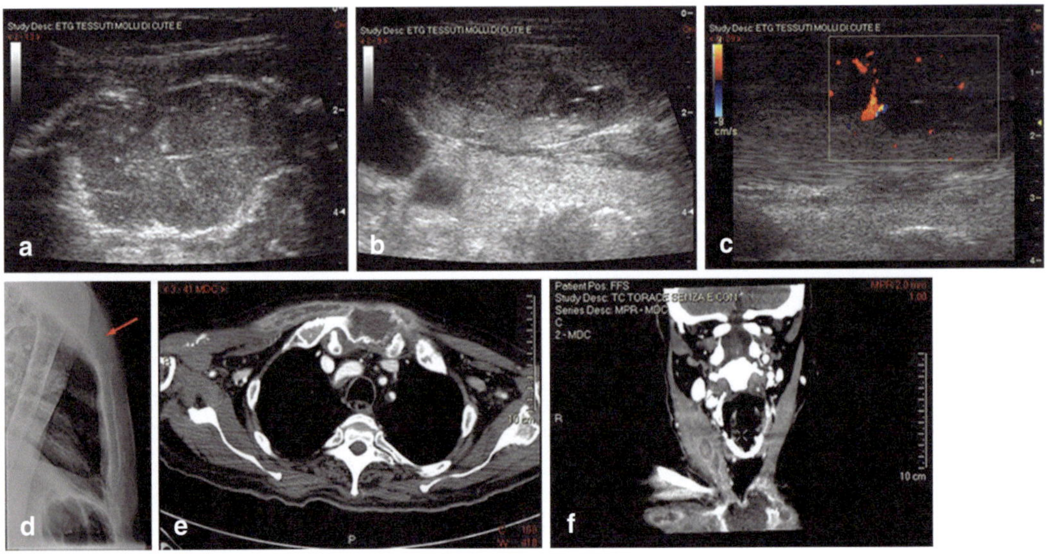

Fig. 7.29 Metastasis within the sternocleidomastoid muscle from colon neoplasm. In correspondence with painful swelling, the TUS showed a solid lesion that interrupted the cortical bone of the sternal manubrium (**a**). Hypoechogenic lesions were present in the sternocleidomastoid muscle, (**b**) with signs of lesion neovascularization in Doppler colour (**c**). An X-ray, in LL projection, confirmed sternal osteolysis (**d**, arrow). The axial scan CT showed the lithic area of the sternal manubrium (**e**). Injuries in the sternocleidomastoid muscle were also visible, better demonstrated in coronal reconstruction (**f**)

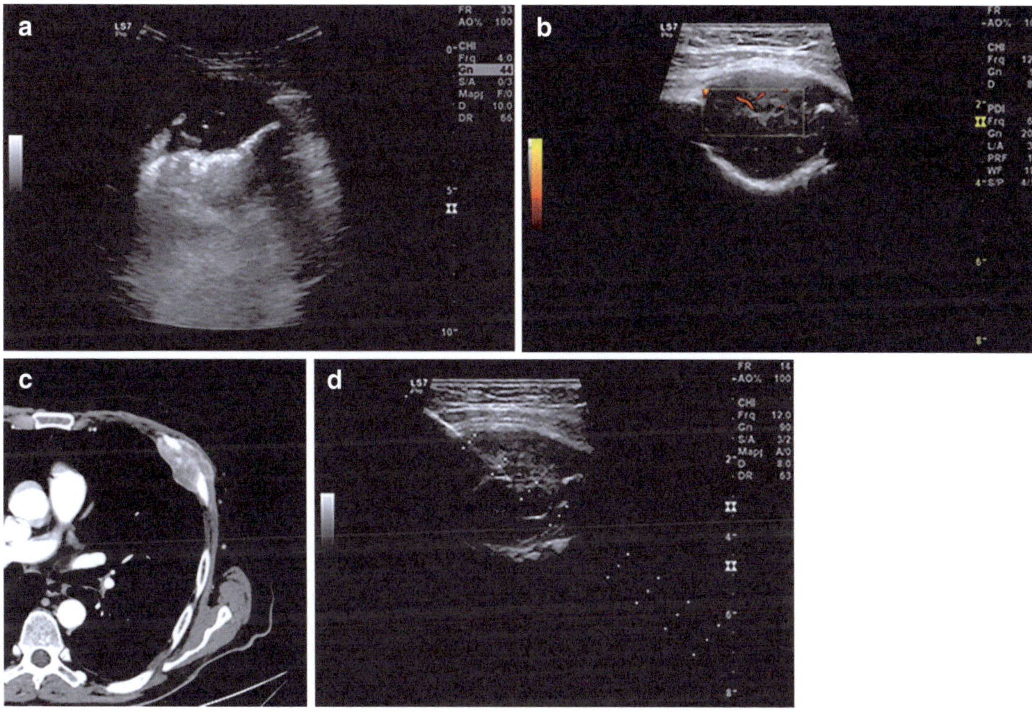

Fig. 7.30 Costal metastases from bladder cancer. The TUS was performed to assess a painful swelling of the anterior-lateral chest wall in the lower third of the left hemithorax. A solid lesion (**a**) interrupted the cortical bone of the mid-anterior arc of cost, with uneven echostructure and signs of lesion neovascularization in Doppler colour (**b**). Axial CT scan (**c**) confirmed the finding. An echo-guided biopsy (**d**) allowed the identification of the expansive lesion, resulting in the diagnosis of bladder cancer metastases

7.5 Conclusions

Ultrasound study is useful in supporting clinical evaluation and other imaging methods in different diagnostic pathways, both in conditions affecting soft tissues and chest wall skeletal components.

TUS also has purely specialist applications, including an essential role in staging certain cancers, biopsy procedures, and operational planning.

The method is easily available, economical, radiation-free, and easy to execute. There are some limitations however, mainly related to conditions which hinder the correct positioning of the probe or that limit the penetration of the ultrasound beam, as in the case of parietal emphysema.

References

1. Lee RKL, Griffith JF, Ng AWH, Sitt JCM. Sonography of the chest wall: a pictorial essay. J Clin Ultrasound. 2015;43:525–37.
2. Broggio D, Lechaftois X, Abline O, Fleury B, Vial A, Corrèze P, Franck D, Merzoug V. Energy dependent chest wall thickness equations for male lung monitoring with germanium detectors. Health Phys. 2014;106(3):405–14.
3. Aliotta A, Ferraioli G, Livraghi T. Standard per una corretta esecuzione dell'esame ecografico. In: Journal of ultrasound, speciale 2009. XXI Congresso Nazionale SIUMB. Milano: Elsevier; 2009. p. 33–5.
4. Mathis G. Chest sonography. Berlin: Springer; 2008. p. 229.
5. Gardelli G, Feletti F, Nanni A, Mughetti M, Piraccini A, Zompatori M. Chest ultrasonography in the ICU. Respir Care. 2012 May;57(5):773–81.
6. Feletti F, Mucci V, Aliverti A. Chest Ultrasonography in Modern Day Extreme Settings: From Military Setting and Natural Disasters to Space Flights and Extreme Sports. Can Respir J. 2018: 8739704.
7. Cammarota T, et al. Ecografia in dermatologia. Milano: Poletto Editore; 1998. p. 79–93.
8. Athanassiadi K, Kalavrouziotis G, Rondogianni D, Loutsidis A, Hatzimichalis A, Bellenis I. Primary chest wall tumors: early and long-term results of surgical treatment. Eur J Cardiothorac Surg. 2001 May;19(5):589–93.
9. Falidas E, Arvanitis D, Anyfantakis G, et al. Painful elastofibroma dorsi: a report of a case and

a brief review of the literature. Case Rep Orthop. 2013;2013:794247.
10. Tarantino CC, Vercelli A, Canepari E. Angioma of the chest wall: a report of 2 cases. J Ultrasound. 2011;14(1):18–21.
11. Dzian A, Hamzík J. Intercostal hemangioma of the chest wall. Kardiochir Torakochirurgia Pol. 2016;13(1):58–60.
12. Ergun T, Lakadamyali H, Lakadamyali H, Gokay E. Myositis ossificans in the right inferior thoracic wall as an unusual cause of lower thoracic-upper abdominal pain: report of a case. Surg Today. 2008;38(10):962–4.
13. Saussez S, Blaivie C, Lemort M, Chantrain G. Non-traumatic myositis ossificans in the paraspinal muscles. Eur Arch Otorhinolaryngol. 2006;263(4):331–5.
14. Bueno J, Lichtenberger JP 3rd, Rauch G, Carter BW. MR imaging of primary chest wall neoplasms. Top Magn Reson Imaging. 2018;27(2):83–93.
15. Oymak FS, Karaman A, Soyuer I, et al. Pulmonary and chest wall involvement in multiple myeloma. Tuberk Toraks. 2003;51(1):27–32.
16. Tian HY, Xu D, Liu JP, Mao WM, Chen LY, Yang C, Wang LP, Shi KY. Contribution of ultrasound-guided fine-needle aspiration cell blocks of metastatic supraclavicular lymph nodes to the diagnosis of lung cancer. J Cancer Res Ther. 2015;11(Suppl):C234–8.
17. Vassallo P, Wernecke K, Roos N, Peters PE. Differentiation of benign from malignant superficial lymphadenopathy: the role of high-resolution US. Radiology. 1992;183(1):215–20.
18. Na DG, Lim HK, Byun HS, et al. Differential diagnosis of cervical lymphadenopathy: usefulness of color Doppler sonography. AJR Am J Roentgenol. 1997;168(5):1311–6.
19. Wu CH, Chang YL, Hsu WC, et al. Usefulness of Doppler spectral analysis and power Doppler sonography in the differentiation of cervical lymphadenopathies. AJR Am J Roentgenol. 1998;171(2):503–9.
20. Stiglich F, Barbonetti C, Di Lorenzo E, et al. Diagnostic reliability of ultrasonography in the preoperative staging of the N parameter in head and neck neoplasms. Radiol Med. 1991;81(6):838–43.
21. Som PM. Lymph nodes of the neck. Radiology. 1987;165:593–600.
22. Rubaltelli L, Proto E, Salmaso R, et al. Sonography of abnormal lymph nodes in vitro: correlation of sonographic and histologic findings. AJR Am J Roentgenol. 1990;155(6):1241–4.
23. Gorman B, Charboneau JW, James EM, et al. Medullary thyroid carcinoma: role of high resolution US. Radiology. 1987;162:147–50.
24. Dragoni F, Cartoni C, Pescarmona E, et al. The role of high resolution pulsed and color Doppler ultrasound in the differential diagnosis of benign and malignant lymphadenopathy: results of multivariate analysis. Cancer. 1999;85(11):2485–90.
25. Lee SC, Jain PA, Jethwa SC, Tripathy D, Yamashita MW. Radiologist's role in breast cancer staging: providing key information for clinicians. Radiographics. 2014;34(2):330–42.
26. Kendirlinan R, Özkan G, Bayram M, et al. Ultrasound guided fine-needle aspiration biopsy of metastases in nonpalpable supraclavicular lymph nodes in lung cancer patients. Multidiscip Respir Med. 2011;6(4):220–5.
27. van Overhagen H, Brakel K, Mark W, et al. Metastases in supraclavicular lymph nodes in lung cancer: assessment with palpation, US, and CT. Radiology. 2004;232:75–80.
28. Lee DH, Yoon TM, Lee JK, Lim SC. Supraclavicular lymph node excision biopsy in patients with suspected supraclavicular lymph node metastasis of lung cancer: experience in a Tertiary Hospital. Chonnam Med J. 2017;53(1):69–72.
29. Liu Z, Cheng W, Li P, Sun Y, Wang Q. Clinical value of ultrasound in the diagnosis of supraclavicular lymph node metastasis of primary lung cancer. Zhongguo Fei Ai Za Zhi. 2014;17(9):663–8.
30. Fultz PJ, Feins RH, Strang JG. Detection and diagnosis of nonpalpable supraclavicular lymph nodes in lung cancer at CT and US. Radiology. 2002;222(1):245–51.
31. Patrick J, Fultz L, Amy R, et al. Sonographically guided biopsy of supraclavicular lymph nodes: a simple alternative to lung biopsy and other more invasive procedures. AJR. 2003;180:1403–9.
32. Sripathi S, Mahajan A. Comparative study evaluating the role of color Doppler sonography and computed tomography in predicting chest wall invasion by lung tumors. J Ultrasound Med. 2013;32(9):1539–46.
33. Tahiri M, Khereba M, Thiffault V, Ferraro P, Duranceau A, Martin J, Liberman M. Preoperative assessment of chest wall invasion in non-small cell lung cancer using surgeon-performed ultrasound. Ann Thorac Surg. 2014;98(3):984–9.
34. Bae YA, Lee KS. Cross-sectional evaluation of thoracic lymphoma. Radiol Clin N Am. 2008;46:253–64.
35. Guermazi A, Brice P, De Kerviler EE, et al. Extranodal Hodgkin disease: spectrum of disease. Radiographics. 2001;21:161–79.
36. Sharma A, Fidias P, Hayman A, et al. Pattern of lymphoadenopathy in thoracic malignancies. Radiographics. 2004;24:419–39.
37. Lichtenstein D. Lung ultrasound in the critically ill. Berlin: Springer; 2015. p. 105.
38. Lichtenstein D. General ultrasound in the critically ill. Berlin: Springer; 2005. p. 107–13.
39. Bitschnau R, Gehmacher O, Kopf A. Ultrasound diagnosis of rib and sternal fracture. Ultraschall Med. 1997;18:158–61.
40. Paik SH, Chung MJ, Park JS, et al. High-resolution sonography of the rib: can fracture and metastasis be differentiated? AJR. 2005;184:969–74.
41. Beckh S, Bölcskei PL, Lessnau KD. Real-time chest ultrasonography. A comprehensive review for the pulmonologist. Chest. 2002;122:1759–73.

42. Mathis G, Blank W. The chest wall in chest sonography. 2nd ed. Berlin: Springer; 2008. p. 12–22.
43. Dubs-Kunz B. Sonography of chest wall. Eur J Ultrasound. 1996;3:103–11.
44. Abiri MM, Kirpekar R, Ablow RC. Osteomyelitis: detection with US. Radiology. 1997;172:509–11.
45. Park CM, Chung KB, Suh WH. Osteomyelitis: detection with US. Radiology. 1991;178:890a.
46. Sugama Y, Tamaki S, Kitamura S, et al. Ultrasonographic evaluation of pleural and chest wall invasion of lung cancer. Chest. 1998;93:275–9.
47. Vogel B. Ultrasonographic detection and guided biopsy of thoracic osteolysis. Chest. 1993;104(4):1003–5.
48. Targhetta R, Balmes P, Marty-Double C. Ultrasonically guided aspiration biopsy in osteolytic bone lesions of the chest wall. Chest. 1993;103:1403–8.

Mediastinal Pathologies

8

Christoph F. Dietrich, Nathan Atkinson,
and Christian Jenssen

8.1 Introduction

Lymphadenopathy is the most common pathology in the mediastinum. Thorough mediastinal lymph nodal evaluation, including tissue sampling, can be performed with a variety of imaging techniques: conventional ultrasound, endoscopic techniques (e.g., bronchoscopy), radiological methods (e.g., computed tomography, fluoroscopy, and magnetic resonance imaging), nuclear medicine techniques (e.g., positron emission tomography, PET), and surgical procedures (e.g., mediastinoscopy and video-assisted thoracoscopy) [1, 2].

Chest imaging by computed tomography (CT) with intravenous contrast enhancement provides detailed anatomical information of the mediastinum, hilum, lung parenchyma, and chest wall. Fluorodeoxyglucose (FDG)-PET scanning, preferably in combination with CT, provides physiological information and lesion metabolic activity; however due to the limitations of imaging techniques, enlarged or FDG avid nodes should be sampled to prevent over- or under-staging [1].

Minimally invasive surgical methods of mediastinal staging of non-small cell cancer (NSCLC) and sampling of mediastinal lymph nodes include standard cervical mediastinoscopy, video-assisted mediastinoscopy (VAM) and lymphadenectomy (VAMLA), and video-assisted thoracoscopic surgery (VATS). VAM facilitates better visualization and has an improved lymph node yield (including the opportunity of performing lymph node dissection) than standard mediastinoscopy [3, 4]. The major limitation of cervical mediastinoscopy is its inability to access lymph node stations 5 and 6. Therefore, several methods are used to supplement cervical mediastinoscopy, such as the transcervical extended mediastinoscopy (TEMLA) [1].

Endobronchial ultrasound-guided transbronchial needle aspiration (EBUS-TBNA) and endoscopic ultrasound-guided fine-needle aspiration (EUS-FNA) have replaced surgical staging as the initial investigation of choice for mediastinal tissue evaluation [3, 5–18]. Regardless of the numerous advantages, ultrasound-derived techniques are not yet utilized to their full potential in respiratory medicine [1]. Complications may be encountered. Mediastinitis with abscess formation has been

C. F. Dietrich (✉)
Medical Department 2, Caritas-Krankenhaus Bad Mergentheim, Academic Teaching Hospital of the University of Würzburg, Würzburg, Germany
e-mail: christoph.dietrich@ckbm.de

N. Atkinson
John Radcliffe Hospital, Oxford University Hospitals NHS Trust, Oxford, UK

C. Jenssen
Department of Internal Medicine, Krankenhaus Märkisch Oderland Strausberg/Wriezen, Academic Teaching Hospital of the Medical University of Brandenburg "Theodor Fontane", Neuruppin, Strausberg, Germany

F. Feletti et al. (eds.), *Thoracic Ultrasound and Integrated Imaging*,
https://doi.org/10.1007/978-3-319-93055-8_8

observed after transesophageal biopsy of mediastinal lymph nodes [19]. Therefore, prophylactically administered antibiotics may be considered for EUS-guided biopsies, but studies on this topic are lacking. Similar complications have not been observed in EBUS-TBNA; therefore, no antibiotic prophylaxis is recommended [1].

The aim of this book chapter is to discuss mediastinal pathology. Lung pathologies are discussed elsewhere, and we recommend published papers on anatomy [20–30], mediastinal imaging [1, 2], lung ultrasound [31–33], and mediastinal ultrasound imaging of sarcoidosis [34], cystic fibrosis [35, 36], chronic virus hepatitis C [37], and other diseases.

8.2 Transcutaneous Mediastinal Ultrasound (TMUS)

Transcutaneous ultrasound has excellent resolution in the head and neck regions, including cervical and supraclavicular nodes. In addition, mediastinal ultrasound detects and guides sampling of pathological lymph nodes [20, 24] and masses [38] in the supra-aortic, prevascular, pericardial, and upper- and lower-located paratracheal regions, as far as the aortopulmonary window. Studies on mediastinal ultrasound published 20 years ago demonstrated the suprasternal and parasternal approach, when compared with CT, had a sensitivity of 69–100% for the detection of pathological lymph nodes in the mediastinal regions mentioned above [20, 21, 24, 38]. Detection of abnormal lymph nodes in the supra-aortic, supraclavicular, and head and neck regions, respectively, by TMUS and TMUS-guided biopsy is highly specific for N3 or M1 stage (Fig. 8.1) [1, 39].

As mediastinal ultrasound is infrequently applied, and in most centers not utilized routinely, the value of TMUS is still discussed with some controversy. The specifics of examination technique have previously been detailed and summarized in review articles [22, 30, 33, 40] and in textbooks [1, 41–43] and so are not repeated here.

8.2.1 Definition of Mediastinal Regions Using TMUS

The definitions used in lymph node evaluation are similar to CT, EUS, and EBUS criteria. The criterion for adequate visualization of the different regions is listed in Table 8.1 [1].

8.2.2 Detection of Normal Lymph Nodes

The diagnostic evaluation by ultrasound of mediastinal regions depends upon differences in echogenicity between pathological lymph nodes and

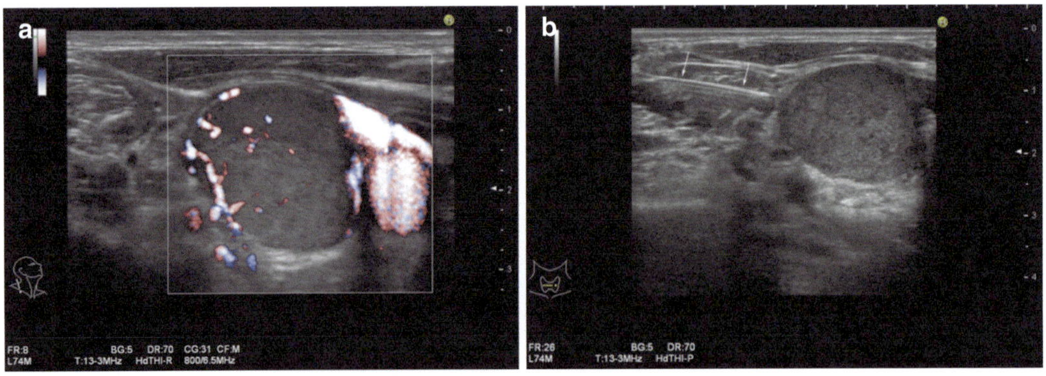

Fig. 8.1 In a patient with radiological suspicion of lung cancer, a highly suspicious supraclavicular lymph node was detected by transcutaneous ultrasound (N3 disease). The lymph node is round and hypoechoic. Color-coded Doppler ultrasound exhibits peripheral neovascularization as a typical feature of lymph node metastasis (**a**). US-guided core biopsy (**b**; 18 Gauge core needle, arrows) confirmed metastatic lymph node infiltration by non-small cell lung cancer

Table 8.1 Anatomic structures within each mediastinal region, necessary to positively visualize for an adequate transcutaneous ultrasound (TMUS) examination

Region	Key anatomic structures to identify
Supra-aortic	Whole aortic arch with all branches and both brachiocephalic veins (suprasternal approach)
Paratracheal	Right brachiocephalic vein, brachiocephalic trunk and ascending aorta, right pulmonary artery (suprasternal approach)
Aortopulmonary	Whole aortic arch, pulmonary trunk (suprasternal approach)
Prevascular	Ascending aorta and pulmonary artery (right and left parasternal approach)
Subcarinal	Ascending aorta, right pulmonary artery, left atrium in two planes (right and left parasternal approach)
Pericardial	Right atrium, right and left ventricles, pericardial fat pads bilaterally (right and left parasternal approach)

the adjacent tissue. This led to the belief that, unlike CT, TMUS was unable to differentiate normal lymph nodes from surrounding tissue. However, using high-resolution ultrasound and color Doppler imaging, lymph nodes are detectable in healthy subjects. Normal lymph nodes can be regularly detected in the right paratracheal region, aortopulmonary window [28, 29], and occasionally subcarinal region. The lower detection rate in the subcarinal region may be a consequence of the deep location of this region within the mediastinum and of artifacts caused by cardiac movement [1].

8.2.3 Mediastinal Ultrasound in Cadaveric Studies

Cadavaric correlation of mediastinal ultrasound confirms normal lymph nodes can be detected; 20 human cadavers (11 male, 9 female, 66.4 ± 10.9 years, range, 45–76 years), all without known diseases affecting mediastinal lymph nodes, were examined before and after autopsy to validate sonographic findings with histological examination [29]. Ultrasound detected lymph nodes in the paratracheal region in 85% of cadavers and in the aortopulmonary window in 90%. The longitudinal diameter of detected paratracheal nodes was 8–22 mm and 8–17 mm in the aortopulmonary window. Sonographic lymph node measurements correlated well with morphometric measurements of macro-pathological specimens. Ultrasound had a sensitivity for lymph node detection of 75% in the paratracheal region and 91% in the aortopulmonary window. In this study all normal lymph nodes were oval in shape and no round lymph nodes were found. In only one-fifth (21%) could a lymph node sinus be identified. Histologic examination revealed lymphatic tissue in all sonographically detected lymph nodes suggesting a high specificity (Table 8.2) [1, 28, 29]. Furthermore, normal lymph nodes were detectable more frequently in the paratracheal region and aortopulmonary window of cadavers compared to the respective mediastinal regions of healthy volunteers. A possible explanation of this finding lies in the better image resolution obtained by application of the transducer to the region of interest in cadavers. A difference in age may also have an impact [1].

8.2.4 Mediastinal Ultrasound in Healthy Subjects

Ultrasound detected lymph nodes in 35% of healthy subjects in the paratracheal region, 45% in the aortopulmonary window, and 12.5% in the subcarinal region. All detected lymph nodes had a hypoechogenic appearance. In healthy subjects the longitudinal diameter of lymph nodes detected ranged between 10 and 19 mm in paratracheal chains and 12–19 mm in the aortopulmonary window. Lymph nodes >6 mm were not detected in the supra-aortic, prevascular, and the pericardial regions by mediastinal ultrasound [29] which is in accordance to the literature [25]. The superior pericardial recessus were reliably differentiated from lymph nodes in the aortopulmonary window, due to the typical location and shape [1, 29, 44].

Table 8.2 Lymph nodes detected by ultrasound in the mediastinum of 20 human cadavers [1, 28, 29]

Mediastinal region	Proportion of cadavers with detectable lymph nodes	Number of lymph nodes (detected by ultrasound)	Lymph node size (determined by ultrasound) (mm)	Lymph node size (morphometric measurement) (mm)
Paratracheal	17/20	1.9 ± 1.0	11 × 6	11 × 6
Aortopulmonary window	18/20	1.7 ± 0.7	11 × 5	11 × 4

The number of lymph nodes is given as mean ± standard deviation. The lymph node size is given as the mean longitudinal diameter × mean transverse diameter

8.3 Mediastinal Imaging

8.3.1 Comparative Measurements of Mediastinal Lymph Node Size by Imaging Technique

Computed tomography (CT) is the anatomical standard for the description of intrapulmonary lesions and mediastinal abnormalities. When evaluating mediastinal lymph nodes, the clinical significance of computed tomography is less certain since CT mainly relies on size criteria. Cutoff values for the short-axis diameter of between 10 and 15 mm have defined abnormal lymph nodes for decades [26, 27] with false-positive and false-negative findings in about 25% of cases indicating a low accuracy [45–47]. In two systematic analyses, the cumulative sensitivity of CT in mediastinal staging of non-small cell lung cancer (NSCLC) was estimated to be 55% and 61%, with a specificity of 81% and 79%, respectively [3, 48]. The lower the cutoff value, the higher the sensitivity, at the cost of specificity [49]. PET-CT has not been able to resolve the problem of nodal size [1].

Directly comparing measurements of mediastinal lymph node size obtained by computed tomography with those obtained by ultrasound techniques is difficult, because lymph nodes orientate longitudinally in the mediastinum while CT images section transversally. In contrast, ultrasound allows measurement of lymph node size in any plane. Therefore, lymph node size measured sonographically correlates better with morphometric assessment than to measurements obtained by axial computed tomography [50]. Two recent comparative cohort studies found only a weak agreement between thoracic CT and EBUS for size estimation of mediastinal and hilar lymph nodes [51, 52]. Using EBUS-TBNA, malignant cells were obtained from 24% of lymph nodes initially interpreted as normal in size by CT criteria [1, 52]. Therefore, selection of lymph nodes for EUS-FNA or EBUS-TBNA should not be guided by CT size alone.

8.3.2 Mediastinal Lymph Node Anatomy and Diagnostic Reach of Ultrasound Techniques

To ensure efficient performance of all mediastinal ultrasound techniques, it is important to have a thorough knowledge of mediastinal anatomy and insight into how ultrasound images relate to nodal stations. According to the International Association for the Study of Lung Cancer (IASLC) classification, mediastinal lymph nodes (MLN) are divided into different lymph node regions [53, 54]. In the following paragraphs and Table 8.1, lymph node anatomy and the evaluation criteria are summarized [1].

8.3.2.1 Mediastinal Lymph Node Evaluation by Transcutaneous Mediastinal Ultrasound (TMUS)

TMUS allows standardized examination of the supra-aortic region, prevascular region, right-sided upper and lower paratracheal regions (regions 2R, 4R), aortopulmonary window (region 5), and subcarinal region (region 7) under most circumstances [20, 21, 23, 24, 30, 40, 55]. In addition, the precardial region can be easily evaluated [1].

8.3.2.2 EBUS and EUS: A Complimentary Approach

EBUS and EUS are complimentary methods for the evaluation of mediastinal lesions, as each can reach differing mediastinal and hilar nodal stations [56]. The added value of EUS to EBUS includes additional diagnostic access to the lower mediastinum and aortopulmonary window in selected cases and evaluation of the left adrenal gland and other infradiaphragmatic metastatic sites (Table 8.3, Fig. 8.2). Patients tolerate EUS far easier than EBUS (with less cough and dyspnea), which is particularly relevant for the nodal regions accessible to either technique; the left paratracheal region (station 4L) and the often involved subcarinal region (station 7). The implementation of endosonographic techniques in lung cancer staging algorithms has also reduced the need for surgical staging modalities (e.g., mediastinoscopy, thoracoscopy, thoracotomies), though they remain valuable in staging nodes suspicious in CT/PET imaging but with negative features at EBUS/EUS [57] as well as in clinical N1 NSCLC [58]. This approach has been emphasized in recent guidelines [1, 3, 8, 59–61].

Both EUS and EBUS have been successfully used in the assessment of mediastinal tumor spread of patients with extrathoracic neoplastic diseases [62–65], for the evaluation of mediastinal lymphadenopathy of unknown origin, and have been particularly useful in the diagnosis and differentiation of mediastinal granulomatous disease and malignant lymphoma [64, 66–78]. The examination technique using longitudinal probes is described in current textbooks and articles [1, 79–81].

Table 8.3 Modified lymph node classification according to the International Association for the Study of Lung Cancer (IASLC) and diagnostic reach of EUS, EBUS, and TMUS (modified from [2])

No	Region	EUS	EBUS	TMUS
1	Low cervical, supraclavicular, and sternal notch node regions	–	–	+++
2	Upper paratracheal region (left (2L), right (2R))	++	+++	++
3a	Prevascular region	+	+++	++
3p	Retrotracheal region	+++	+++	–
4	Lower paratracheal region (left (4L), right (4R))			
	4L	++	+++	(+)
	4R	(+)	+++	++
5	Aortopulmonary window	+	(+)	(+)
6	Paraaortal region	(+)	–	–
7	Subcarinal region	+++	+++	–
8	Lower paraesophageal region	+++	–	–
9	Pulmonary ligament	+++	–	–
10	Hilar lymph nodes (left (10L), right (10R))			
	10L	++	+++	–
	10R	+	+++	–
11	Interlobar lymph nodes	–	++	–
12	Lobar lymph nodes	–	+[a]	–
13	Segmental lymph nodes	–	+[a]	–
14	Subsegmental lymph nodes	–	+[a]	–

+++ ultrasound evaluation is always possible and FNA is easy to perform, ++ ultrasound evaluation and FNA are often but not always possible, + ultrasound evaluation and FNA are sometimes possible, (+) ultrasound evaluation is partially possible, but FNA is (often) not feasible, – ultrasound evaluation and FNA are restricted and only possible if LNs are grossly enlarged. In the case of lung cancer, ipsilateral pulmonary LNs (hilar, lobar, segmental, and subsegmental) are defined as N_1-LNs, mediastinal and subcarinal as N_2-LNs and supraclavicular and scalenus LNs as well as contralateral pulmonary LNs as N_3-LNs

[a]Only radial EBUS using miniprobes

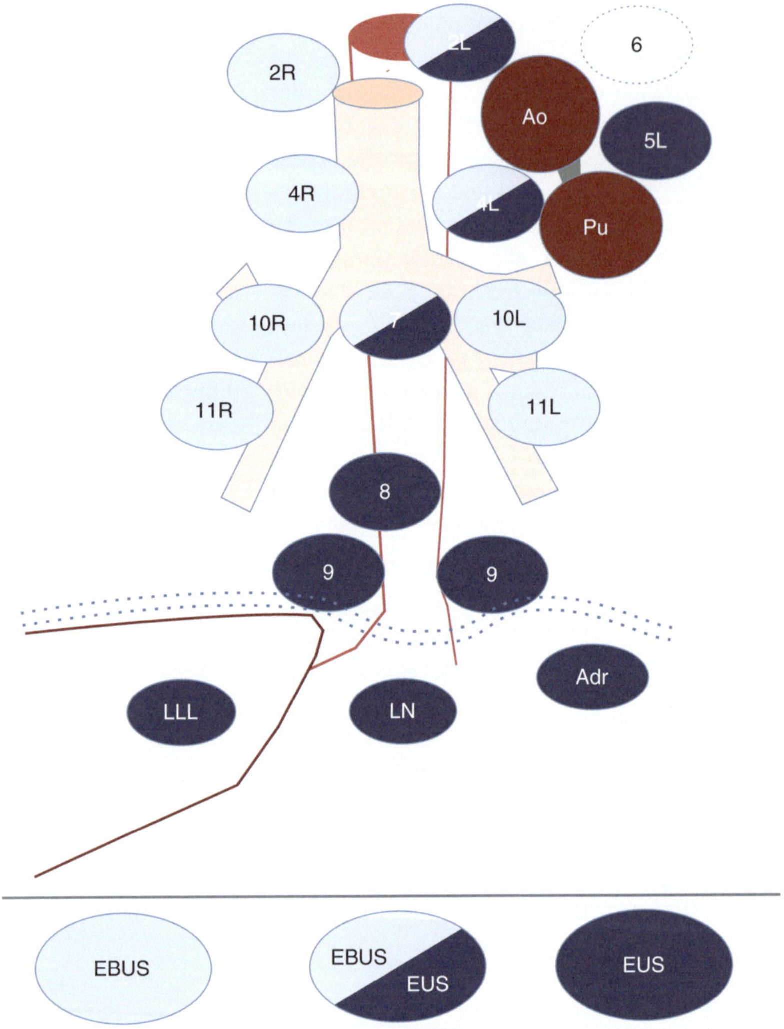

Fig. 8.2 Complimentary diagnostic reach of endobronchial and endoscopic ultrasound: Mediastinal lymph node stations accessible by EBUS only are marked light blue. Mediastinal lymph node stations accessible by EUS only are marked dark blue. Mediastinal lymph node stations within the reach of both EUS and EBUS are marked light and dark blue. Station 6 is visible with EUS; however EUS-FNA is possible only from a high esophageal position or by traversing the aorta (*Adr* left adrenal, *Ao* aorta, *EBUS* endobronchial ultrasound, *EUS* endoscopic ultrasound, *LLL* left liver lobe, *LN* infradiaphragmatic lymph nodes, *Pu* pulmonal artery)

8.3.3 Clinical Work-Up of Mediastinal Lymphadenopathy Using Ultrasound Techniques

Enlargement of mediastinal lymph nodes is a frequent finding in inflammatory and neoplastic diseases. Conventional chest radiography and thoracic CT are first-line diagnostic methods to evaluate suspected mediastinal lymphadenopathy [3, 59]. In addition, ultrasound modalities offer guidance for biopsy and intervention, and deliver higher spatial resolution. Ultrasound methods allow not only size-related criteria as shown for CT and magnetic resonance imaging (MRI) but also evaluation of the lymph node architecture [82, 83], lymph node vascularity and perfusion [84–87], resistance index [88], lymph node elasticity [89–92], and changes of perfusion during anti-angiogenetic treatment [1, 84]. This multiparametric sonographic evaluation may be helpful to differentiate very hypoechoic lymph nodes from cystic masses (Fig. 8.3) and to direct EUS-FNA or EBUS-TBNA (Figs. 8.4 and 8.5).

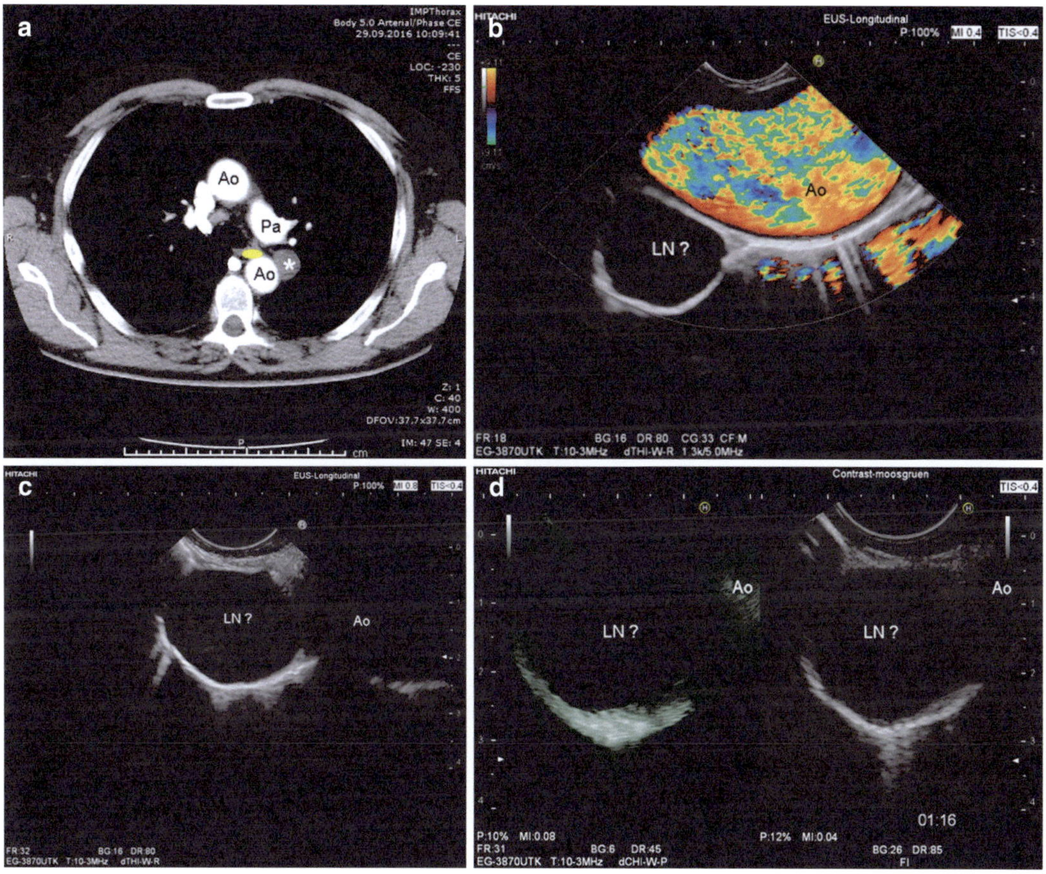

Fig. 8.3 A well-circumscribed para-aortic lesion (station 6) was identified on CT in a 72-year-old male patient and suspected to be an enlarged lymph node (**a**). With EUS the lesion appears to be anechoic (**b**). After optimizing scope position, the lesion reveals a slightly inhomogeneous hypoechoic echopattern. EUS-FNA would be technically feasible (**c**). However, contrast-enhanced EUS reveals complete lack of vascularization (**d**). Therefore, the lesion was diagnosed a bronchogenic cyst, and due to the high risk of mediastinitis, EUS-FNA was avoided (*asterisk*, *Ln?* lesion suspected to be a lymph node, *Ao* aorta, *Pa* pulmonal artery, *yellow oval* position of the longitudinal echoendoscope within the esophageal lumen)

8.3.3.1 Cytological/Histological Diagnosis of Mediastinal Lymphadenopathy

Tissue diagnosis of mediastinal lymphadenopathy using ultrasound-guided techniques (TMUS, EUS, EBUS) is highly accurate [2, 93, 94], has a low interobserver variability [95], and is safe with a serious adverse event rate of 0.05–0.11% (EBUS-TBNA) and 0.16–0.30% (EUS-FNA) [96, 97]. The use of ancillary studies facilitates diagnosis of granulomatous lymphadenopathy and mediastinal lymph node metastasis as well as subtyping and genotyping of NSCLC and malignant lymphoma [2, 93].

8.3.3.2 Cytological/Histological Confirmation of Lung Cancer

Conventional bronchoscopy fails to establish the diagnosis in up to one-third of patients with suspected lung cancer. In patients with suspected lung carcinoma adjacent to the trachea or bronchi without mucosal (endobronchial) abnormalities, EBUS is superior to CT for biopsy guidance. This is due to improved diagnostic yield and a much lower rate of complications including pneumothorax and bleeding when the tumor is perivascularly located [98, 99]. In addition, EUS can be used to biopsy centrally located intrapulmonary periesophageal tumors if conventional

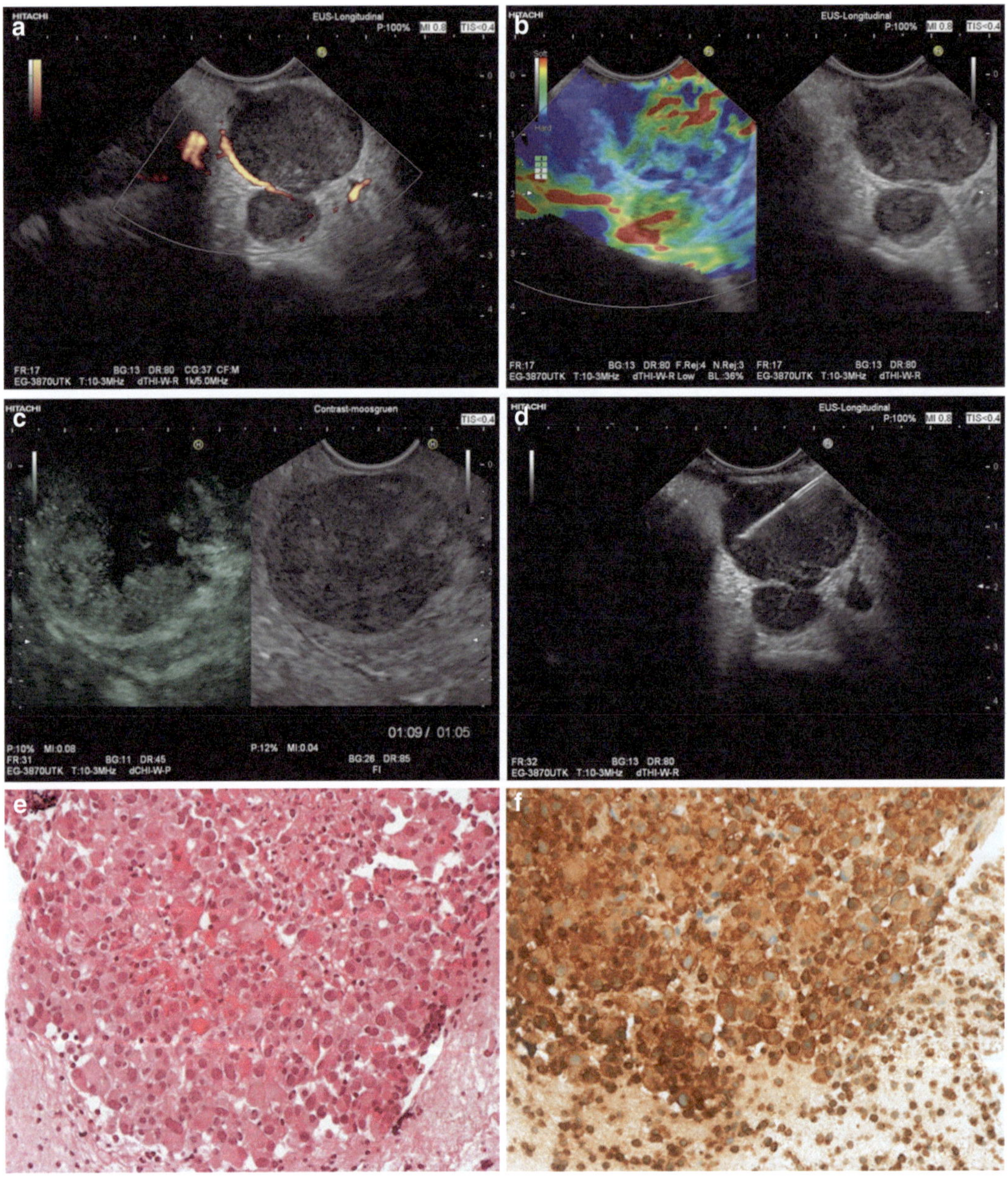

Fig. 8.4 Large suspicious mediastinal lymph nodes (Station 7/8) in a 58-year-old female patient who had undergone a nephrectomy for renal cell cancer 2 years prior (**a**). EUS-elastography shows heterogeneous elasticity with soft central parts and harder peripheral parts (**b**). Contrast-enhanced endoscopic ultrasound reveals central necrosis (**c**). To avoid a false-negative finding and infection, only the peripheral parts of the lesion were targeted by EUS-FNA (22-gauge aspiration needle) (**d**). Histology revealed clear cell carcinoma with focal necrosis (**e**; hematoxylin-eosin, ×200). Immunohistochemistry (**f**; vimentin staining strongly positive; not shown, CD10 and RCC stains positive; CK7, CK20, and TTF-1 stains negative) was highly suggestive for metastasis of renal cell cancer. Histological images were kindly provided by Dr. Krisztina Zels, Institute of Pathology Königs Wusterhausen, Germany

methods fail [100]. In a group of 123 patients with an undiagnosed but suspected malignant lung lesion (paratracheal, parabronchial, para-esophageal) or with a peripheral lung nodule and PET-positive mediastinal lymph nodes who had undergone at least one diagnostic flexible bronchoscopy or CT-guided transthoracic needle aspiration attempt, EBUS-TBNA and/or EUS-FNA had a high diagnostic efficacy; an endosonographic approach to the diagnosis of lung cancer avoided expensive surgical procedures in 106 cases, leading to significant cost savings [101]. In the case of subpleural localization of a suspected advanced lung cancer, transcutaneous ultrasound-guided biopsy is feasible and safe (Fig. 8.6).

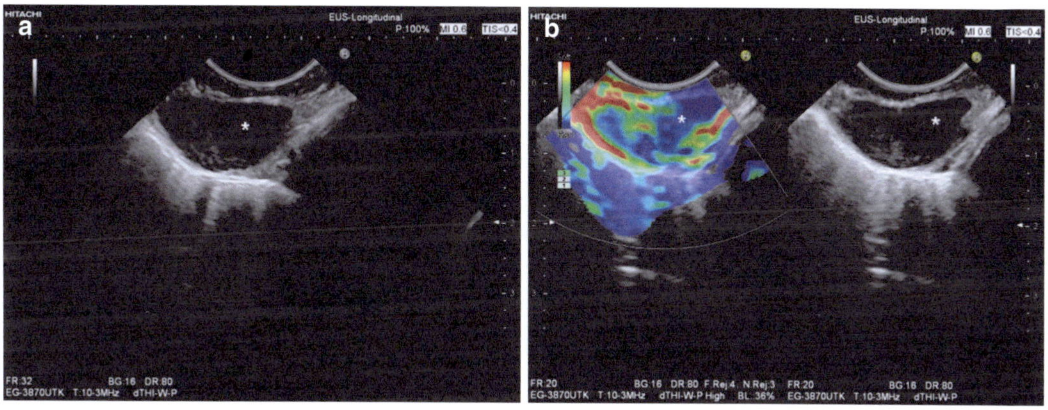

Fig. 8.5 Enlarged oval mediastinal lymph node (station 7) with an intranodal hypoechoic area (asterisk) in a 62-year-old male patient with gastric cancer (**a**). EUS-elastography reveals that the hypoechoic intranodal area (asterisk) is definitely harder than the other parts of the node. EUS-FNA was directed to the hypoechoic, harder nodal area suspected to be a focal malignant infiltration (**b**). For cytology and histology, see Fig. 8.9

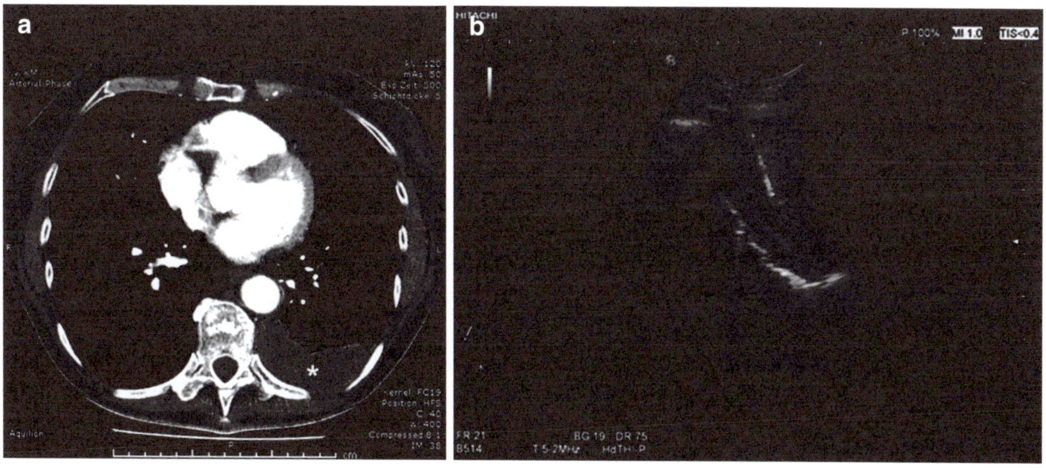

Fig. 8.6 In a 61-year-old female patient with a large subpleural mass (asterisk) of the left lower lobe on CT (**a**), transcutaneous ultrasound-guided biopsy was performed using an 18-gauge core needle (**b**). Histology revealed squamous cell carcinoma (**c**, hematoxylin-eosin, ×100; **d**, p63 staining, ×200). EBUS-TBNA of a large hypoechoic ipsilateral interlobar node (11L) with heterogeneous elasticity (**e**) revealed reactive lymphadenopathy; no metastatic infiltration was found (not shown). Histological images kindly provided by Dr. Uta Kerlikowski, Institute of Pathology Königs Wusterhausen, Germany

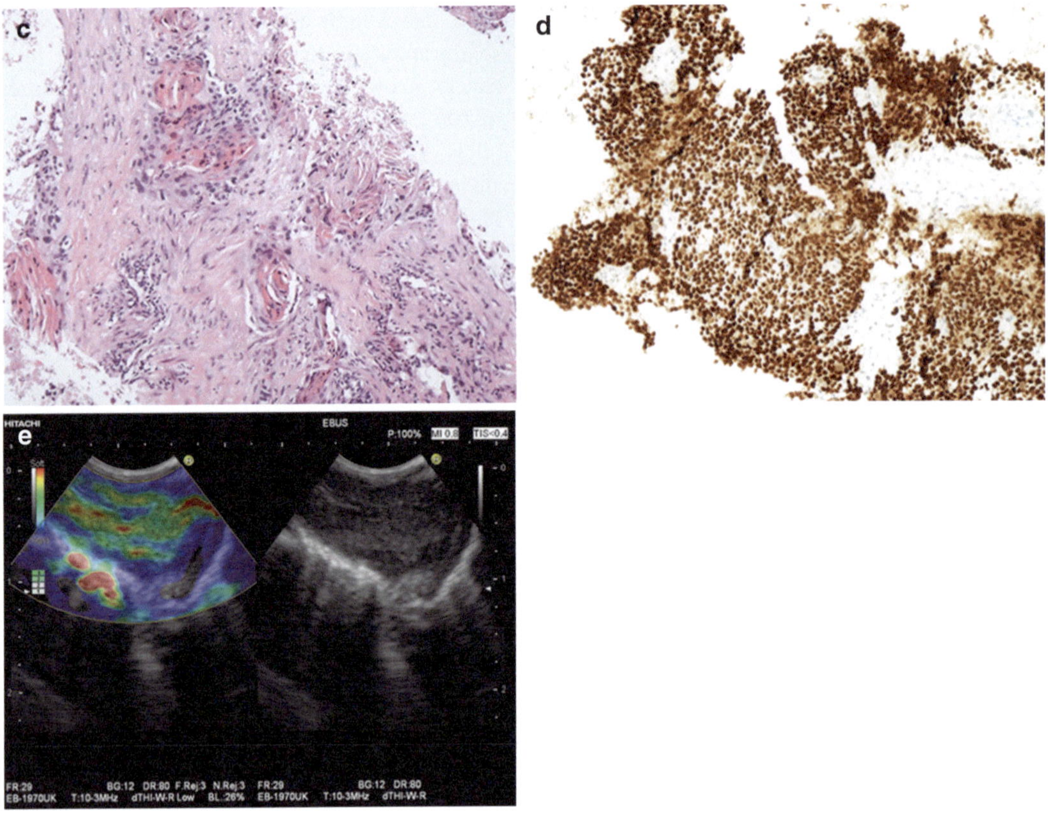

Fig. 8.6 (continued)

8.4 Mediastinal Pathology

8.4.1 Introduction

Ultrasound of the head and neck regions is well established in evaluating cervical and supraclavicular lymphadenopathies [102, 103]. In addition, transcutaneous mediastinal ultrasound (TMUS) is able to detect normal and pathological lymph nodes in the deeper mediastinal region, though this is not widely recognized and requires particular expertise [1]. Nonetheless, ultrasound-derived techniques changed the pathway of mediastinal disease evaluation. Conventional transcutaneous ultrasound imaging of the chest wall and pleural effusions has gained importance [31, 104, 105]. Nowadays, thoracentesis and chest tube placement are preferably performed only after sonographic evaluation of the chest [1].

8.4.2 Malignant Mediastinal Lymphadenopathy in Non-small Cell Lung Cancer Patients

Malignant mediastinal lymph node infiltration has a major impact on treatment of patients with non-small cell lung cancer; patients without malignant nodal involvement or N1 disease are commonly offered immediate surgical resection or radiotherapy with curative intent, whereas those with more advanced nodal involvement (N2, N3) are treated with chemoradiation or palliative chemotherapy [1, 3, 5, 6, 59, 60, 106]. According to recent meta-analyses, the pooled sensitivity of EBUS-TBNA (88–93%) and EUS-FNA (83–89%) in nodal staging of NSCLC [2, 8, 93] can be further improved by combining EBUS-TBNA and EUS-FNA (or transesophageal FNA using an EBUS-bronchoscope, EUS-B-

FNA) by an average of 21% (compared with the esophageal approach alone) and 13% compared with EBUS-TBNA alone [8]. Moreover, the combined endosonographic approach is significantly more accurate than PET-CT alone [15] and may prevent >50% of scheduled surgical staging procedures by providing tissue proof of advanced disease in patients with suspected lung cancer and enlarged or PET-positive lymph nodes [2, 8, 93]. However, negative endosonography findings should be verified by surgical staging before initiating treatment with curative intent [8].

Ultrasound-guided sampling should be performed under the premise that distant metastases (M1, e.g., adrenal or left liver lobe) are excluded first, followed by lymph node staging in the order N3 (contralateral, cervical) → N2 (ipsilateral mediastinal and subcarinal lymph nodes) → N1 (ipsilateral hilar lymph nodes). In suspected N2 disease, infiltration of only single N2 lymph nodes (N2a, stage IIIA3) has to be differentiated from infiltration of more than one N2 lymph node region, bulky N2 lymph node involvement, or large N2 lymph nodes with extracapsular invasion (N2b, stage IIIA4) (Figs. 8.7 and 8.8) [2, 8, 93].

8.4.3 Mediastinal Staging of Extrathoracic Malignancies

As has been shown for pancreatobiliary cancer, up to 10% of extrathoracic malignancies metastasize to mediastinal lymph nodes [107]. Both EUS and EBUS have been successfully used to assess tumor spread to mediastinal lymph nodes (M1 disease) in patient cohorts of various extrathoracic malignant diseases [62–64, 66, 108–111]. In particular, the utility of EUS-guided sampling of mediastinal lymph nodes has been reported in the staging of patients with gastric, pancreatic [107, 112], breast [113], upper GI [114, 115], head and neck [116], and colorectal [117] cancers and lymphoma [118–125]. A recent meta-analysis (five studies, n = 533 patients) demonstrated the value of EBUS-TBNA for the diagnosis of mediastinal and hilar lymph node metastases from extrathoracic malignancy; pooled sensitivity was 85%, and specificity was 99% [126]. Acquisition of specimens eligible for immunohistochemistry is important for reliable differentiation between mediastinal nodal metastases of extrathoracic cancer vs. non-small cell lung cancer (Fig. 8.9) [1, 2, 93], which sonographic techniques facilitate.

8.4.4 Lymphoma

In a retrospective study (40 consecutive patients with Hodgkin's (n = 29) and non-Hodgkin's (n = 11)), TMUS was clearly superior to chest radiography and comparable to CT for monitoring mediastinal lymphomas [127]. Thymic enlargement due to involvement by Hodgkin disease is more frequently observed than previously reported. Thymic gland involvement is sonographically visible due the hypoechoic structure. In contrast TMUS was not helpful for differentiating the normal-sized typically tongue-shaped thymus from surrounding fatty tissue after treatment, due to equivalent echogenicity of the gland and surrounding fat [38]. Elastography and contrast-enhanced techniques might overcome this problem, but data are lacking [82]. Lymphoma and other tumors in the anterior mediastinum can also be biopsied under ultrasound guidance via a suprasternal and strict parasternal approach. Using the parasternal approach, non-visible lymphoma might be made visible by mediastinal shift when a patient is positioned from a decubitus to a strict left or right lateral position [1, 55, 81]. With a pooled diagnostic accuracy of approximately 69% (EBUS-TBNA), endosonography-guided tissue sampling is an useful initial, minimally invasive diagnostic test to establish a diagnosis and subtype mediastinal involvement of malignant lymphoma, particularly if flow cytometry, immunohistochemistry, and cytogenetic examinations are used [2, 93, 128–130]. The diagnostic yield of EBUS-TBNA for diagnosing lymphoma relapse is higher than for de novo diagnosis of malignant lymphoma [128–130].

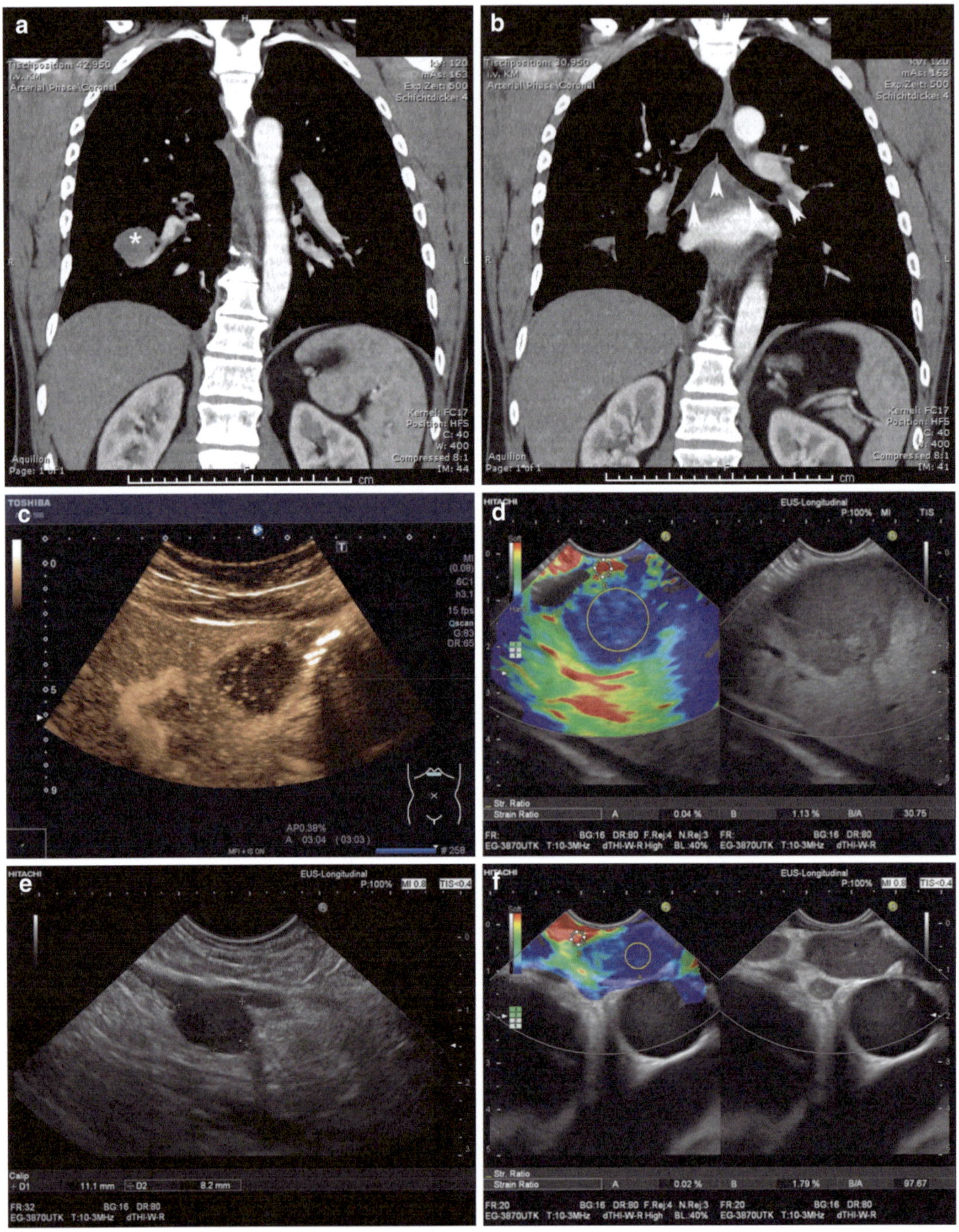

Fig. 8.7 Forty-five-year-old male patient with a suspicious mass lesion of the apical right lower lobe (**a**; asterisk) and mediastinal lymphadenopathy (**b**; subcarinal, ipsilateral, and contralateral hilum, marked with arrowheads) on CT. A solitary mass lesion of the left liver lobe showed typical features of malignancy with contrast-enhanced ultrasound (**c**; late phase hypoenhancement, between markers) and EUS-elastography (**d**; very high strain ratio of 30.75). Sequential EUS-FNA using a 20-gauge core needle was performed of the liver lesion (**e**; potentially $M1_{hep}$), a small nodule of the left adrenal gland (potentially $M1_{adr}$, between markers), suspicious lymph nodes at mediastinal stations 10L (**f**; very high strain ratio of 97.7, potentially N3) and 7 (potentially N2). Histology revealed poorly differentiated pulmonary adenocarcinoma in all sampling locations with the exception of the adrenal gland (shown is only the liver biopsy; (**g**) hematoxylin-eosin, ×100; (**h**) CK7 staining ×100; (**i**) TTF-1 staining ×100; synaptophysin and p63 negative, not shown). Final endosonographic diagnosis was poorly differentiated pulmonary adenocarcinoma, cT1 cN3 $M1_{hep}$. Histological images were kindly provided by Dr. Uta Kerlikowski, Institute of Pathology Königs Wusterhausen, Germany

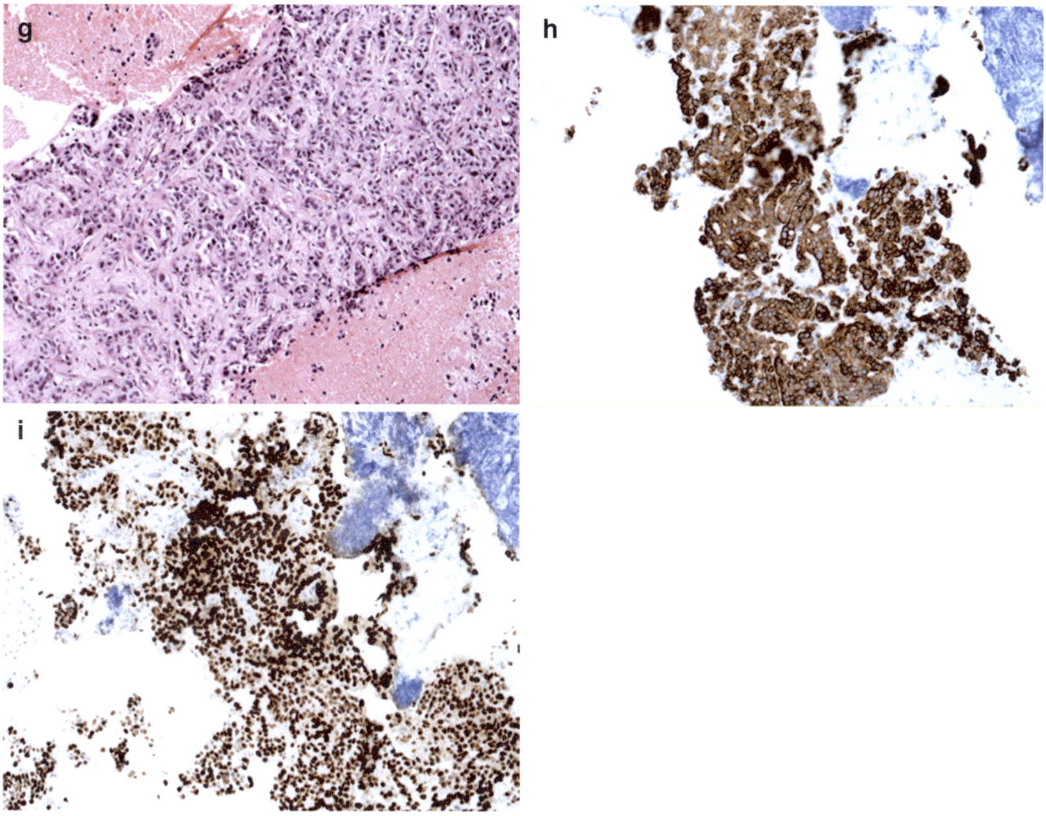

Fig. 8.7 (continued)

8.4.5 Benign Mediastinal Lymphadenopathy

8.4.5.1 Sarcoidosis and Tuberculosis

Depending on the geographic distribution, sarcoidosis and tuberculosis are the two most important inflammatory causes of mediastinal lymphadenopathy [1, 2, 34, 66, 68, 69, 74, 131].

Sarcoidosis

Sarcoidosis-related lymphadenopathy is typically visualized as symmetrically distributed clusters of mediastinal lymph nodes around large vessels. The typically oval-shaped lymph nodes may reach a size of up to 60 mm with mixed echogenicity depending on disease stage [34]. Color Doppler imaging, contrast-enhanced ultrasound techniques, and elastography have shown that typically the lymph node architecture is preserved and a hilum can be displayed [102, 132, 133]. Both EUS-FNA and EBUS-TBNA are suitable for gaining a definitive tissue diagnosis of sarcoidosis (Fig. 8.10), whereas pure transbronchial biopsy fails in about one-third of cases. Published data indicate that the sensitivity (80–90%) and accuracy of EUS-FNA and EBUS-TBNA are superior to simple mucosal biopsies either with or without "blind" transbronchial puncture [70, 71, 73, 74, 134]. Special techniques (cytology and cell block analysis) might further improve the diagnostic yield of ultrasound-guided biopsies [73]. Meta-analysis (14 studies including 2097 patients) found a diagnostic yield of 79% in the diagnosis of sarcoidosis by EBUS-TBNA; pooled sensitivity and specificity were 84% and 100%, respectively [135].

In conclusion, for the diagnosis of sarcoidosis, endosonographic techniques are superior to the combination of endobronchial mucosa and transbronchial lymph node biopsies. Besides conventional cytological smears, cell blocks are recommended to increase diagnostic yield [1, 2, 93, 130].

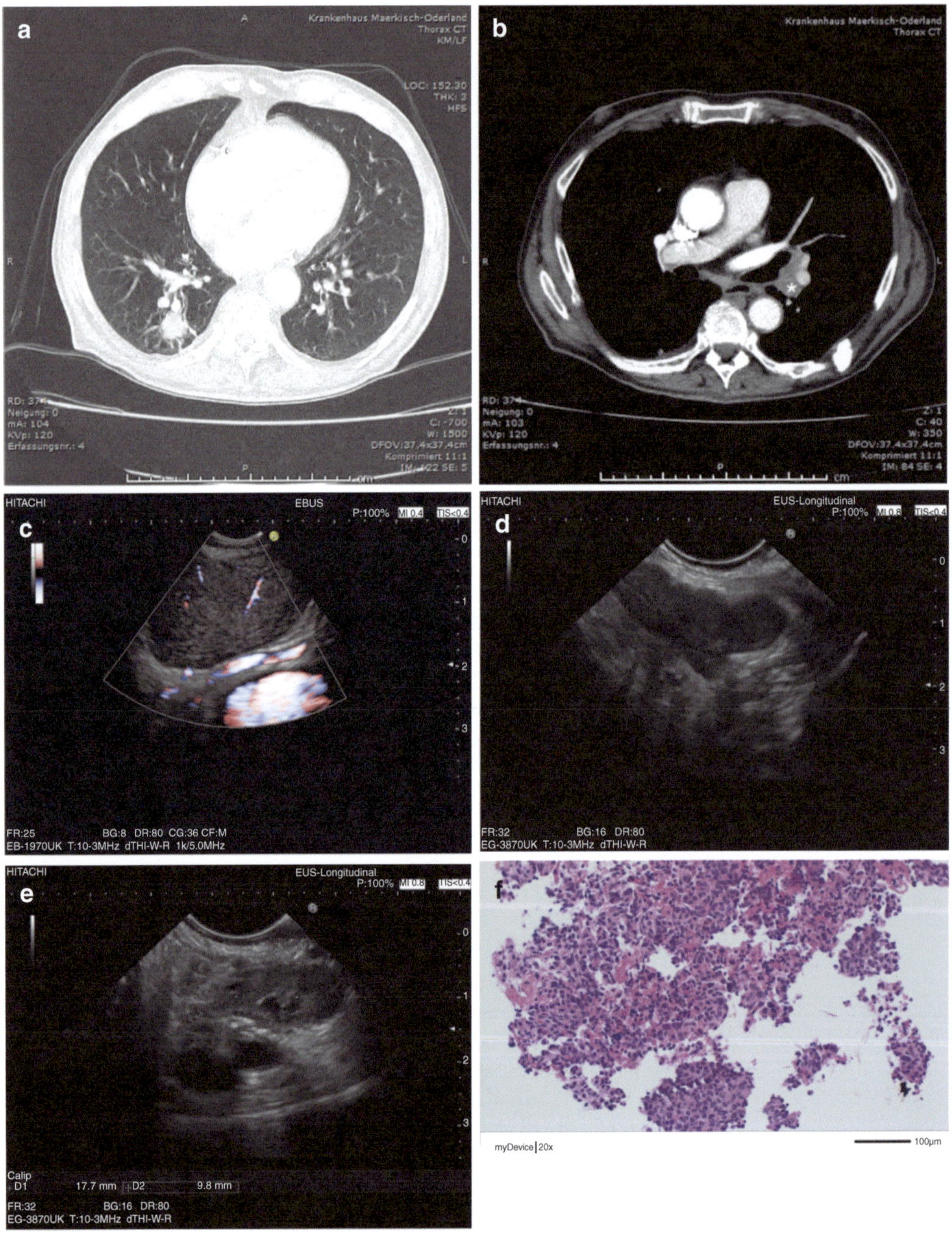

Fig. 8.8 Sixty-two-year-old patient with suspicion of peripheral lung cancer of the right lower lobe (**a**) and enlarged mediastinal and hilar lymph nodes (**b**, shown is station 11L, asterisk) as shown by thoracic CT. Bronchoscopy was negative. EBUS revealed a well-defined large hypoechoic lymph node at station 11L (**c**), whereas EUS showed a lumpy left adrenal without any clear defined mass lesion (**d**) and a well-demarcated mass lesion of 18 x 10 mm with small cystic changes in the pancreatic body (**e**, between markers). EUS-FNA (22-gauge aspiration needle) of the left adrenal (presumable M1adr), the pancreatic mass lesion (assumed to also be a metastasis), and EBUS-TBNA (22-gauge aspiration needle) of the 11L lymph nodes (presumable N3) were performed. Sampling of the left adrenal and of the 11L-lymph nodes proved metastatic infiltration by a poorly differentiated adenocarcinoma (**f**, core histology of the left adrenal, hematoxylin-eosin, x20) of pulmonary origin (**g**, TTF-1 strongly positive, x20). Surprisingly, EUS-FNA of the pancreatic mass lesion showed a neuroendocrine tumor (**h**, hematoxylin-eosin; (**i**) synaptophysin x20: strongly positive) with a Ki67 proliferation index of 3% (**j**). Final endosonographic diagnoses were poorly differentiated pulmonary adenocarcinoma, cT1 cN3 $M1_{adr}$ and pancreatic neuroendocrine tumor G2. Histological images were kindly provided by Dr. Gunnar Schröder, Institute of Pathology Königs Wusterhausen, Germany

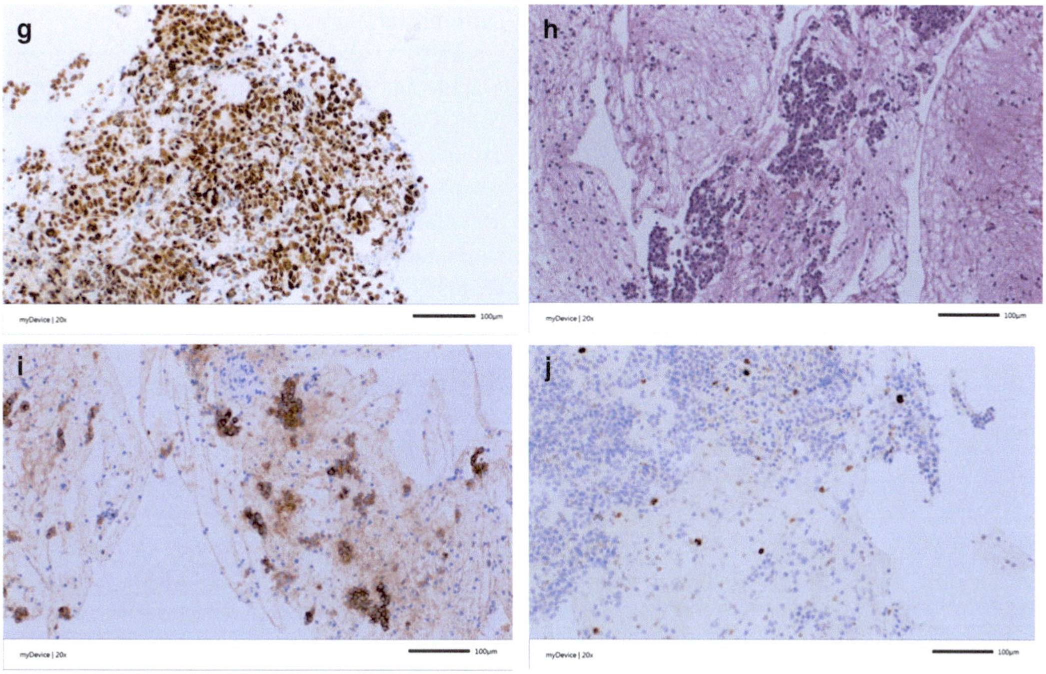

Fig. 8.8 (continued)

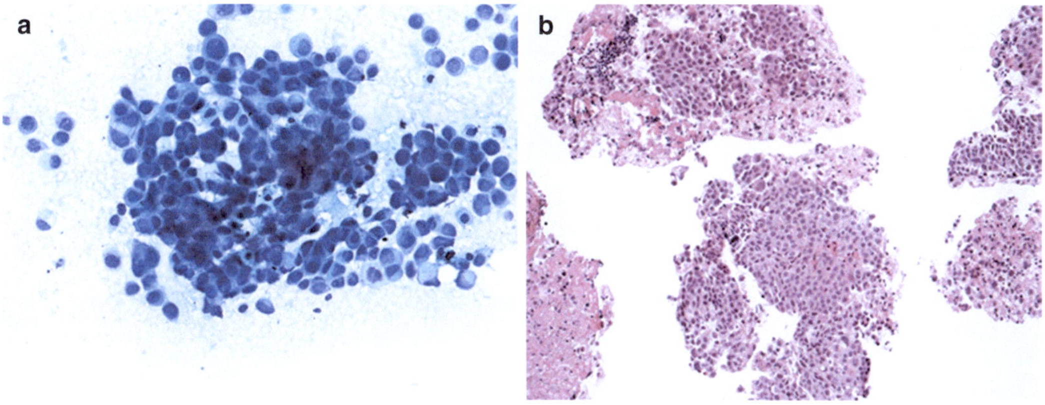

Fig. 8.9 EUS-FNA (22-gauge aspiration needle) of a mediastinal lymph node suspected of focal metastatic infiltration in a 62-year-old male patient with histologically proven adenocarcinoma of the stomach (see Fig. 8.5); positive cytological and histological findings implying M1 stage was established: smear cytology (**a**, Papanicolaou stain, ×200) and core histology (**b**, hematoxylin-eosin, ×100) show poorly differentiated carcinoma. The immunohistochemical phenotype (**c**, CK 7 strongly positive; not shown, negative staining with p63, TTF-1, and p16) is consistent with lymphatic metastasis of poorly differentiated gastric adenocarcinoma and argues against adenocarcinoma or squamous cell carcinoma of pulmonary origin. Palliative treatment was initiated. Cytological and histological images were kindly provided by Dr. Uta Kerlikowski, Institute of Pathology Königs Wusterhausen, Germany

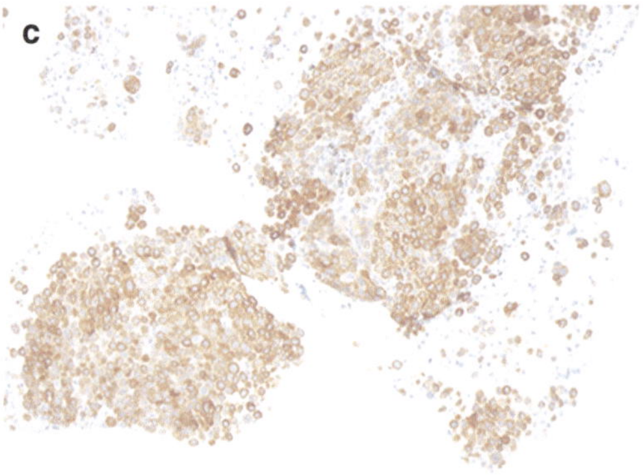

Fig. 8.9 (continued)

Differential Diagnoses

Under particular circumstances, including geographic and other epidemiologic criteria, tuberculosis and atypical mycobacteriosis must be excluded as causes of unexplained mediastinal lymphadenopathy. Several studies have shown acceptable diagnostic accuracy for the diagnosis of mediastinal lymph node tuberculosis by EUS-FNA and EBUS-TBNA. Cytopathological criteria, identification of acid-fast bacilli using Ziehl-Neelsen technique or acridin-orange staining, culture, and polymerase chain reac-

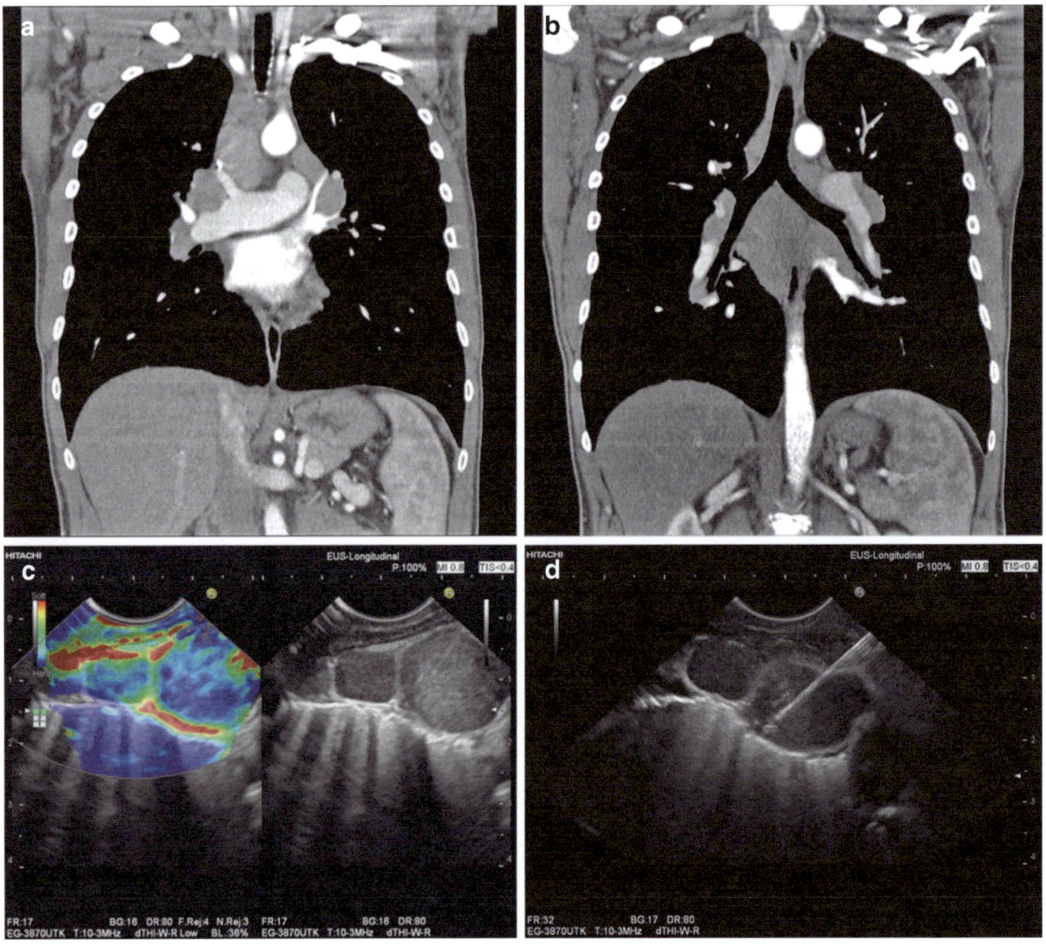

Fig. 8.10 In a 44-year-old male patient with bilateral hilar and mediastinal lymphadenopathies on CT (**a, b**), malignant lymphoma was suspected. EUS revealed multiple large hypoechoic and elastographically heterogeneous lymph nodes with a diameter of up to 50 × 30 mm at all accessible mediastinal lymph node stations (**c**; lymph node station 8 is shown). EUS-FNA was performed using a 22-gauge core needle (**d**). Cytology (**e;** Papanicolaou stain, ×200) and histology (**f**; hematoxylin-eosin, ×100) showed epitheloid cell granuloma with giant cells and perifocal fibrosclerosis without necrosis. Ziehl-Neelsen stain for acid-resistant bacilli (**g**) and polymerase chain reaction for mycobacteria were negative. A diagnosis of sarcoidosis was established. Cytological and histological images were kindly provided by Dr. Uta Kerlikowski, Institute of Pathology Königs Wusterhausen, Germany

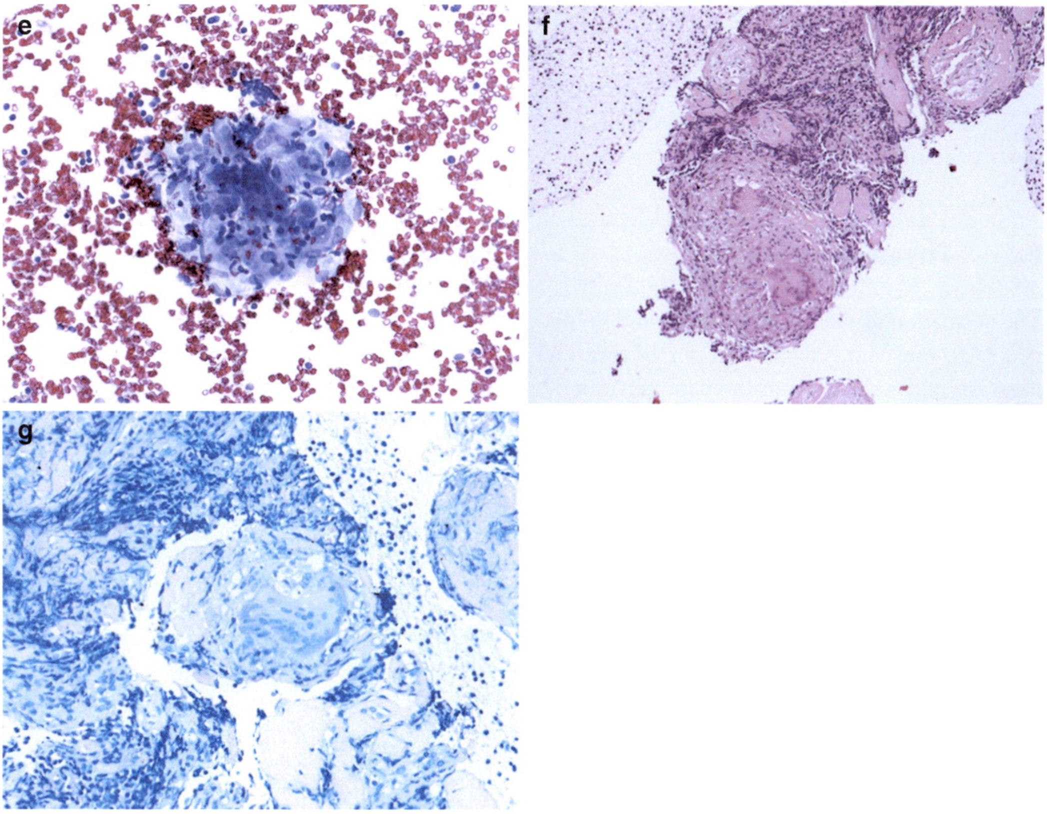

Fig. 8.10 (continued)

tion (PCR) are used as complimentary tools to establish the final diagnosis [2, 67–69, 75, 93, 130, 136]. Concurrent systemic symptoms may be encountered [137]. Besides tuberculosis, atypical mycobacteriosis, sarcoidosis, and other granulomatous diseases, paraneoplastic "sarcoid-like reactions" (SLR) must be included in the differential diagnosis of granulomatous lymphadenopathy. SLR have been observed in association with malignancies and as a sequelae of chemotherapy or radiation. PET studies may misinterpret positive uptake in patients with SLR [1, 138–140].

8.4.5.2 Mediastinal Ultrasound in Patients with Cystic Fibrosis

The respiratory tract is involved in almost all patients with cystic fibrosis, and respiratory failure accounts for about 90% of their morbidity and mortality. Extrapulmonary manifestations are also often encountered [36]. TMUS evaluation of healthy subjects and patients with cystic fibrosis demonstrated a significantly higher lymph node detection rate in the paratracheal region and aortopulmonary window in patients with cystic fibrosis, and the total lymph node volume was larger. Mediastinal ultrasound was helpful for the detection of inflammatory activity in patients with cystic fibrosis [35]. Similar studies using EUS and EBUS have not been published [1].

8.4.5.3 Mediastinal Ultrasound in Chronic Hepatitis C Virus Infection

Mediastinal lymphadenopathy can be considered an extrahepatic manifestation of chronic hepatitis C (HCV). TMUS was able to detect slightly enlarged mediastinal lymph nodes in patients with HCV. Patients with larger perihepatic lymph nodes were also found to have larger mediastinal lymph nodes, a trend suggesting a systemic pathomechanism. However the mechanism of lymphadenopathy in either the liver hilum [141–143] or mediastinum in HCV and other viral or autoimmune liver diseases remains unknown [37]. Similar studies using EUS and EBUS have not been published.

8.5 Thymus

The evaluation of the normal thymus and thymic neoplasia presenting as an anterior mediastinal mass should include transthoracic ultrasound, especially in pediatric patients, computed tomography, and/or magnetic resonance imaging for staging and to determine tumor resectablity. Staging is based on the margins and extent of the tumor, the presence of invasion into adjacent structures, and metastases. The World Health Organization (WHO) classification is used for definite diagnosis of thymic neoplasms, and the Masaoka staging system is also used for prognostic reasons including overall survival. The differential diagnosis includes age-dependent thymus hyperplasia, thymoma, thymic carcinoma, lymphoma, mediastinal germ cell tumor (→ beta-HCG and alpha fetoprotein), metastases, and retrosternal thyroid. The clinical assessment of resectability is the major diagnostic feature. The definitive diagnosis requires surgery in curative intention or biopsy and histological evaluation of the specimen.

8.6 Mediastinal Vessels

The description of the anatomy and topography of the mediastinal vessels and their pathological findings is not elaborated in this chapter. We refer to the currently published guidelines of the European Federation of Societies for Ultrasound in Medicine and Biology (EFSUMB) [144–146].

8.7 Conclusion

TMUS, EUS, and EBUS are powerful and safe complimentary minimally invasive techniques for the evaluation of mediastinal lymphadenopathy, diagnosis of mediastinal masses including centrally located lung cancers, and staging of NSCLC. The introduction and large-scale implementation of state-of-the art multiparametric ultrasound techniques and ultrasound-guided sampling (in particular EBUS-TBNA and EUS-FNA) for the assessment of mediastinal disease have improved the accuracy of mediastinal imaging and of lung cancer staging and reduced the need for more invasive and surgical diagnostic techniques, therefore, representing a paradigm shift in thoracic medicine.

Acknowledgment The authors wish to express their gratitude to Mrs. Eileen Mühsig, Dr. Uta Kerlikowski, Dr. Krisztina Zels, and Dr. Gunnar Schröder (Institute of Pathology Königs Wusterhausen, Germany) for excellent collaboration and for providing the cytological and histological images of this chapter.

References

1. Dietrich CF, Annema JT, Clementsen P, Cui XW, Borst MM, Jenssen C. Ultrasound techniques in the evaluation of the mediastinum, part I: endoscopic ultrasound (EUS), endobronchial ultrasound (EBUS) and transcutaneous mediastinal ultrasound (TMUS), introduction into ultrasound techniques. J Thorac Dis. 2015;7:E311–25.
2. Jenssen C, Annema JT, Clementsen P, Cui XW, Borst MM, Dietrich CF. Ultrasound techniques in the evaluation of the mediastinum, part 2: mediastinal lymph node anatomy and diagnostic reach of ultrasound techniques, clinical work up of neoplastic and inflammatory mediastinal lymphadenopathy using ultrasound techniques and how to learn mediastinal endosonography. J Thorac Dis. 2015;7:E439–58.
3. Silvestri GA, Gonzalez AV, Jantz MA, Margolis ML, Gould MK, Tanoue LT, Harris LJ, et al. Methods for staging non-small cell lung cancer: diagnosis and management of lung cancer, 3rd ed: American College of Chest Physicians evidence-based clinical practice guidelines. Chest. 2013;143:e211S–50S.
4. Adebibe M, Jarral OA, Shipolini AR, McCormack DJ. Does video-assisted mediastinoscopy have a better lymph node yield and safety profile than conventional mediastinoscopy? Interact Cardiovasc Thorac Surg. 2012;14:316–9.
5. Detterbeck FC, Postmus PE, Tanoue LT. The stage classification of lung cancer: diagnosis and management of lung cancer, 3rd ed: American College of Chest Physicians evidence-based clinical practice guidelines. Chest. 2013;143:e191S–210S.

6. De Leyn P, Dooms C, Kuzdzal J, Lardinois D, Passlick B, Rami-Porta R, Turna A, et al. Revised ESTS guidelines for preoperative mediastinal lymph node staging for non-small-cell lung cancer. Eur J Cardiothorac Surg. 2014;45:787–98.
7. Vansteenkiste J, De Ruysscher D, Eberhardt WE, Lim E, Senan S, Felip E, Peters S. Early and locally advanced non-small-cell lung cancer (NSCLC): ESMO Clinical Practice Guidelines for diagnosis, treatment and follow-up. Ann Oncol. 2013;24(Suppl 6):vi89–98.
8. Vilmann P, Clementsen PF, Colella S, Siemsen M, De Leyn P, Dumonceau JM, Herth FJ, et al. Combined endobronchial and esophageal endosonography for the diagnosis and staging of lung cancer: European Society of Gastrointestinal Endoscopy (ESGE) guideline, in cooperation with the European Respiratory Society (ERS) and the European Society of Thoracic Surgeons (ESTS). Endoscopy. 2015;47:545–59.
9. Liberman M, Sampalis J, Duranceau A, Thiffault V, Hadjeres R, Ferraro P. Endosonographic mediastinal lymph node staging of lung cancer. Chest. 2014;146:389–97.
10. Wallace MB, Pascual JM, Raimondo M, Woodward TA, McComb BL, Crook JE, Johnson MM, et al. Minimally invasive endoscopic staging of suspected lung cancer. JAMA. 2008;299:540–6.
11. Annema JT, van Meerbeeck JP, Rintoul RC, Dooms C, Deschepper E, Dekkers OM, De Leyn P, et al. Mediastinoscopy vs endosonography for mediastinal nodal staging of lung cancer: a randomized trial. JAMA. 2010;304:2245–52.
12. Herth FJ, Krasnik M, Kahn N, Eberhardt R, Ernst A. Combined endoesophageal-endobronchial ultrasound-guided, fine-needle aspiration of mediastinal lymph nodes through a single bronchoscope in 150 patients with suspected lung cancer. Chest. 2010;138(4):790–4.
13. Hwangbo B, Lee GK, Lee HS, Lim KY, Lee SH, Kim HY, Lee HS, et al. Transbronchial and transesophageal fine-needle aspiration using an ultrasound bronchoscope in mediastinal staging of potentially operable lung cancer. Chest. 2010;138:795–802.
14. Szlubowski A, Zielinski M, Soja J, Annema JT, Sosnicki W, Jakubiak M, Pankowski J, et al. A combined approach of endobronchial and endoscopic ultrasound-guided needle aspiration in the radiologically normal mediastinum in non-small-cell lung cancer staging–a prospective trial. Eur J Cardiothorac Surg. 2010;37:1175–9.
15. Ohnishi R, Yasuda I, Kato T, Tanaka T, Kaneko Y, Suzuki T, Yasuda S, et al. Combined endobronchial and endoscopic ultrasound-guided fine needle aspiration for mediastinal nodal staging of lung cancer. Endoscopy. 2011;43:1082–9.
16. Kang HJ, Hwangbo B, Lee GK, Nam BH, Lee HS, Kim MS, Lee JM, et al. EBUS-centred versus EUS-centred mediastinal staging in lung cancer: a randomised controlled trial. Thorax. 2014;69:261–8.
17. Lee KJ, Suh GY, Chung MP, Kim H, Kwon OJ, Han J, Um SW. Combined endobronchial and transesophageal approach of an ultrasound bronchoscope for mediastinal staging of lung cancer. PLoS One. 2014;9:e91893.
18. Oki M, Saka H, Ando M, Kitagawa C, Kogure Y, Seki Y. Endoscopic ultrasound-guided fine needle aspiration and endobronchial ultrasound-guided transbronchial needle aspiration: are two better than one in mediastinal staging of non-small cell lung cancer? J Thorac Cardiovasc Surg. 2014;148:1169–77.
19. von Bartheld M, van der Heijden E, Annema J. Mediastinal abscess formation after EUS-guided FNA: are patients with sarcoidosis at increased risk? Gastrointest Endosc. 2012;75:1104–7.
20. Wernecke K, Peters PE, Galanski M. Mediastinal tumors: evaluation with suprasternal sonography. Radiology. 1986;159:405–9.
21. Wernecke K, Potter R, Peters PE, Koch P. Parasternal mediastinal sonography: sensitivity in the detection of anterior mediastinal and subcarinal tumors. AJR Am J Roentgenol. 1988;150:1021–6.
22. Wernecke K. The examination technic and indications for mediastinal sonography. Rofo. 1989;150:501–8.
23. Wernecke K, Vassallo P, Peters PE, Potter R, Luckener HG. [Diagnostic imaging of mediastinal tumors. Sensitivity and specificity of sonography in comparison with computed tomography and conventional x-ray diagnosis]. Radiologe. 1990;30:532–40.
24. Wernecke K, Vassallo P, Potter R, Luckener HG, Peters PE. Mediastinal tumors: sensitivity of detection with sonography compared with CT and radiography. Radiology. 1990;175:137–43.
25. Genereux GP, Howie JL. Normal mediastinal lymph node size and number: CT and anatomic study. AJR Am J Roentgenol. 1984;142:1095–100.
26. Glazer GM, Gross BH, Quint LE, Francis IR, Bookstein FL, Orringer MB. Normal mediastinal lymph nodes: number and size according to American Thoracic Society mapping. AJR Am J Roentgenol. 1985;144:261–5.
27. Quint LE, Glazer GM, Orringer MB, Francis IR, Bookstein FL. Mediastinal lymph node detection and sizing at CT and autopsy. AJR Am J Roentgenol. 1986;147:469–72.
28. Dietrich CF, Liesen M, Wehrmann T, Kirchner J, Caspary WF. Mediastinalsonographie, eine neue Bewertung der Befunde. Endoskopie heute. 1995;4:278–94.
29. Dietrich CF, Liesen M, Buhl R, Herrmann G, Kirchner J, Caspary WF, Wehrmann T. Detection of normal mediastinal lymph nodes by ultrasonography. Acta Radiol. 1997;38:965–9.
30. Hirche TO, Wagner TO, Dietrich CF. Mediastinal ultrasound: technique and possible applications. Med Klin. 2002;97:472–9.
31. Dietrich CF, Mathis G, Cui XW, Ignee A, Hocke M, Hirche TO. Ultrasound of the pleurae and lungs. Ultrasound Med Biol. 2015;41:351–65.

32. Dietrich CF, Mathis G, Blaivas M, Volpicelli G, Sebel A, Wastl D, Atkinson NS, Cui XW, Fan M, Dong Y. Lung B-line artefacts and their use. J Thorac Dis. 2016;8:1356–65.
33. Dietrich CF, Hirche TO, Schreiber DG, Wagner TOF. Ultrasonography of pleura and lung. Ultraschall Med. 2003;24:311.
34. Hirche TO, Hirche H, Cui XW, Wagner TO, Dietrich CF. Ultrasound evaluation of mediastinal lymphadenopathy in patients with sarcoidosis. Med Ultrason. 2014;16:194–200.
35. Dietrich CF, Chichakli M, Bargon J, Wehrmann T, Wiewrodt R, Buhl R, Caspary WF. Mediastinal lymph nodes demonstrated by mediastinal sonography: activity marker in patients with cystic fibrosis. J Clin Ultrasound. 1999;27:9–14.
36. Dietrich CF, Chichakli M, Hirche TO, Bargon J, Leitzmann P, Wagner TO, Lembcke B. Sonographic findings of the hepatobiliary-pancreatic system in adult patients with cystic fibrosis. J Ultrasound Med. 2002;21:409–16.
37. Dietrich CF, Viel K, Braden B, Caspary WF, Zeuzem S. [Mediastinal lymphadenopathy: an extrahepatic manifestation of chronic hepatitis C?]. Z Gastroenterol. 2000;38:143–52.
38. Wernecke K, Vassallo P, Rutsch F, Peters PE, Potter R. Thymic involvement in Hodgkin disease: CT and sonographic findings. Radiology. 1991;181:375–83.
39. Prosch H, Strasser G, Sonka C, Oschatz E, Mashaal S, Mohn-Staudner A, Mostbeck GH. Cervical ultrasound (US) and US-guided lymph node biopsy as a routine procedure for staging of lung cancer. Ultraschall Med. 2007;28:598–603.
40. Wernecke K, Diederich S. Sonographic features of mediastinal tumors. AJR Am J Roentgenol. 1994;163:1357–64.
41. Dietrich CF. Ultraschall-Kurs. 6 Auflage ed. Cologne: Deutscher Ärzteverlag; 2012.
42. Jenssen C, Gottschalk U, Schachschal G, Dietrich DF. Kursbuch Endosonografie. Stuttgart: Thieme; 2013.
43. Dietrich CF, Hocke M. Mediastinum. In: Dietrich CF, editor. Endosonographie. Stuttgart: Thieme Verlag; 2008. p. 422–32.
44. Alraiyes AH, Almeida FA, Mehta AC. Pericardial recess through the eyes of endobronchial ultrasound. Endosc Ultrasound. 2015;4:162–3.
45. Gdeedo A, Van Schil P, Corthouts B, Van Mieghem F, Van Meerbeeck J, Van Marck E. Prospective evaluation of computed tomography and mediastinoscopy in mediastinal lymph node staging. Eur Respir J. 1997;10:1547–51.
46. Dillemans B, Deneffe G, Verschakelen J, Decramer M. Value of computed tomography and mediastinoscopy in preoperative evaluation of mediastinal nodes in non-small cell lung cancer. A study of 569 patients. Eur J Cardiothorac Surg. 1994;8:37–42.
47. Gdeedo A, Van Schil P, Corthouts B, Van Mieghem F, Van Meerbeeck J, Van Marck E. Comparison of imaging TNM [(i)TNM] and pathological TNM [pTNM] in staging of bronchogenic carcinoma. Eur J Cardiothorac Surg. 1997;12:224–7.
48. Gould MK, Kuschner WG, Rydzak CE, Maclean CC, Demas AN, Shigemitsu H, Chan JK, et al. Test performance of positron emission tomography and computed tomography for mediastinal staging in patients with non-small-cell lung cancer: a meta-analysis. Ann Intern Med. 2003;139:879–92.
49. Dales RE, Stark RM, Raman S. Computed tomography to stage lung cancer. Approaching a controversy using meta-analysis. Am Rev Respir Dis. 1990;141:1096–101.
50. Arita T, Matsumoto T, Kuramitsu T, Kawamura M, Matsunaga N, Sugi K, Esato K. Is it possible to differentiate malignant mediastinal nodes from benign nodes by size? Reevaluation by CT, transesophageal echocardiography, and nodal specimen. Chest. 1996;110:1004–8.
51. Dhooria S, Agarwal R, Aggarwal AN, Gupta N, Gupta D, Behera D. Agreement of mediastinal lymph node size between computed tomography and endobronchial ultrasonography: a study of 617 patients. Ann Thorac Surg. 2015;99:1894–8.
52. Udoji TN, Phillips GS, Berkowitz EA, Berkowitz D, Ross C, Bechara RI. Mediastinal and hilar lymph node measurements. Comparison of multidetector-row computed tomography and Endobronchial ultrasound. Ann Am Thorac Soc. 2015;12:914–20.
53. Rusch VW, Asamura H, Watanabe H, Giroux DJ, Rami-Porta R, Goldstraw P. The IASLC lung cancer staging project: a proposal for a new international lymph node map in the forthcoming seventh edition of the TNM classification for lung cancer. J Thorac Oncol. 2009;4:568–77.
54. Tournoy KG, Annema JT, Krasnik M, Herth FJ, van Meerbeeck JP. Endoscopic and endobronchial ultrasonography according to the proposed lymph node map definition in the seventh edition of the tumor, node, metastasis classification for lung cancer. J Thorac Oncol. 2009;4:1576–84.
55. Wernecke K, Vassallo P, Peters PE, von Bassewitz DB. Mediastinal tumors: biopsy under US guidance. Radiology. 1989;172:473–6.
56. Vilmann P, Krasnik M, Larsen SS, Jacobsen GK, Clementsen P. Transesophageal endoscopic ultrasound-guided fine-needle aspiration (EUS-FNA) and endobronchial ultrasound-guided transbronchial needle aspiration (EBUS-TBNA) biopsy: a combined approach in the evaluation of mediastinal lesions. Endoscopy. 2005;37:833–9.
57. Talebian Yazdi M, Egberts J, Schinkelshoek MS, Wolterbeek R, Nabers J, Venmans BJ, Tournoy KG, et al. Endosonography for lung cancer staging: predictors for false-negative outcomes. Lung Cancer. 2015;90:451–6.
58. Dooms C, Tournoy KG, Schuurbiers O, Decaluwe H, De Ryck F, Verhagen A, Beelen R, et al. Endosonography for mediastinal nodal staging of clinical N1 non-small cell lung cancer: a prospective multicenter study. Chest. 2015;147:209–15.

59. Goeckenjan G, Sitter H, Thomas M, Branscheid D, Flentje M, Griesinger F, Niederle N, et al. Prevention, diagnosis, therapy, and follow-up of lung cancer. Interdisciplinary guideline of the German Respiratory Society and the German Cancer Society—abridged version. Pneumologie. 2011;65:e51–75.
60. Felip E, Garrido P, Trigo JM, Lopez-Brea M, Paz-Ares L, Provencio M, Isla D. SEOM guidelines for the management of non-small-cell lung cancer (NSCLC). Clin Transl Oncol. 2009;11:284–9.
61. Tournoy KG, Keller SM, Annema JT. Mediastinal staging of lung cancer: novel concepts. Lancet Oncol. 2012;13:e221–9.
62. Peric R, Schuurbiers OC, Veselic M, Rabe KF, van der Heijden HF, Annema JT. Transesophageal endoscopic ultrasound-guided fine-needle aspiration for the mediastinal staging of extrathoracic tumors: a new perspective. Ann Oncol. 2010;21: 1468–71.
63. Tournoy KG, Govaerts E, Malfait T, Dooms C. Endobronchial ultrasound-guided transbronchial needle biopsy for M1 staging of extrathoracic malignancies. Ann Oncol. 2011;22:127–31.
64. Navani N, Nankivell M, Woolhouse I, Harrison RN, Munavvar M, Oltmanns U, Falzon M, et al. Endobronchial ultrasound-guided transbronchial needle aspiration for the diagnosis of intrathoracic lymphadenopathy in patients with extrathoracic malignancy: a multicenter study. J Thorac Oncol. 2011;6:1505–9.
65. Sanz-Santos J, Cirauqui B, Sanchez E, Andreo F, Serra P, Monso E, Castella E, et al. Endobronchial ultrasound-guided transbronchial needle aspiration in the diagnosis of intrathoracic lymph node metastases from extrathoracic malignancies. Clin Exp Metastasis. 2013;30:521–8.
66. Fritscher-Ravens A, Sriram PV, Bobrowski C, Pforte A, Topalidis T, Krause C, Jaeckle S, et al. Mediastinal lymphadenopathy in patients with or without previous malignancy: EUS-FNA-based differential cytodiagnosis in 153 patients. Am J Gastroenterol. 2000;95:2278–84.
67. Fritscher-Ravens A, Ghanbari A, Topalidis T, Pelling M, Kon OM, Patel K, Arlt A, et al. Granulomatous mediastinal adenopathy: can endoscopic ultrasound-guided fine-needle aspiration differentiate between tuberculosis and sarcoidosis? Endoscopy. 2011;43:955–61.
68. Puri R, Vilmann P, Sud R, Kumar M, Taneja S, Verma K, Kaushik N. Endoscopic ultrasound-guided fine-needle aspiration cytology in the evaluation of suspected tuberculosis in patients with isolated mediastinal lymphadenopathy. Endoscopy. 2010;42:462–7.
69. Sun J, Teng J, Yang H, Li Z, Zhang J, Zhao H, Garfield DH, et al. Endobronchial ultrasound-guided transbronchial needle aspiration in diagnosing intrathoracic tuberculosis. Ann Thorac Surg. 2013;96:2021–7.
70. von Bartheld MB, Dekkers OM, Szlubowski A, Eberhardt R, Herth FJ, in 't Veen JC, de Jong YP, et al. Endosonography vs conventional bronchoscopy for the diagnosis of sarcoidosis: the GRANULOMA randomized clinical trial. JAMA. 2013;309:2457–64.
71. Oki M, Saka H, Kitagawa C, Kogure Y, Murata N, Ichihara S, Moritani S. Prospective study of endobronchial ultrasound-guided transbronchial needle aspiration of lymph nodes versus transbronchial lung biopsy of lung tissue for diagnosis of sarcoidosis. J Thorac Cardiovasc Surg. 2012;143:1324–9.
72. Yasuda I, Goto N, Tsurumi H, Nakashima M, Doi S, Iwashita T, Kanemura N, et al. Endoscopic ultrasound-guided fine needle aspiration biopsy for diagnosis of lymphoproliferative disorders: feasibility of immunohistological, flow cytometric, and cytogenetic assessments. Am J Gastroenterol. 2012;107:397–404.
73. von Bartheld MB, Veselic-Charvat M, Rabe KF, Annema JT. Endoscopic ultrasound-guided fine-needle aspiration for the diagnosis of sarcoidosis. Endoscopy. 2010;42:213–7.
74. Agarwal R, Srinivasan A, Aggarwal AN, Gupta D. Efficacy and safety of convex probe EBUS-TBNA in sarcoidosis: a systematic review and meta-analysis. Respir Med. 2012;106:883–92.
75. Navani N, Molyneaux PL, Breen RA, Connell DW, Jepson A, Nankivell M, Brown JM, et al. Utility of endobronchial ultrasound-guided transbronchial needle aspiration in patients with tuberculous intrathoracic lymphadenopathy: a multicentre study. Thorax. 2011;66:889–93.
76. Mehmood S, Loya A, Yusuf MA. Clinical utility of endoscopic ultrasound-guided fine-needle aspiration in the diagnosis of mediastinal and intra-abdominal lymphadenopathy. Acta Cytol. 2013;57:436–42.
77. Moonim MT, Breen R, Fields PA, Santis G. Diagnosis and subtyping of de novo and relapsed mediastinal lymphomas by endobronchial ultrasound needle aspiration. Am J Respir Crit Care Med. 2013;188:1216–23.
78. Nunez AL, Jhala NC, Carroll AJ, Mikhail FM, Reddy VV, Xian RR, Jhala DN. Endoscopic ultrasound and endobronchial ultrasound-guided fine-needle aspiration of deep-seated lymphadenopathy: analysis of 1338 cases. Cytojournal. 2012;9:14.
79. Dietrich CF. Endosonographie: Lehrbuch und Atlas des endoskopischen Ultraschalls. Stuttgart: Thieme; 2008.
80. Dietrich CF. Endoscopic ultrasound, an introductory manual and atlas. 2nd ed. Stuttgart: Thieme; 2011.
81. Dietrich CF, Nuernberg D. Lehratlas der interventionellen Sonographie. Stuttgart: Thieme; 2011.
82. Dietrich CF, Ponnudurai R, Bachmann NM. [Is there a need for new imaging methods for lymph node evaluation?]. Ultraschall Med. 2012;33:411–4.
83. Fujiwara T, Yasufuku K, Nakajima T, Chiyo M, Yoshida S, Suzuki M, Shibuya K, et al. The utility of sonographic features during endobronchial

ultrasound-guided transbronchial needle aspiration for lymph node staging in patients with lung cancer: a standard endobronchial ultrasound image classification system. Chest. 2010;138:641–7.
84. Dietrich CF, Averkiou MA, Correas JM, Lassau N, Leen E, Piscaglia F. An EFSUMB introduction into dynamic contrast-enhanced ultrasound (DCE-US) for quantification of tumour perfusion. Ultraschall Med. 2012;33:344–51.
85. Piscaglia F, Nolsoe C, Dietrich CF, Cosgrove DO, Gilja OH, Bachmann NM, Albrecht T, et al. The EFSUMB guidelines and recommendations on the clinical practice of contrast enhanced ultrasound (CEUS): update 2011 on non-hepatic applications. Ultraschall Med. 2012;33:33–59.
86. Nakajima T, Anayama T, Shingyoji M, Kimura H, Yoshino I, Yasufuku K. Vascular image patterns of lymph nodes for the prediction of metastatic disease during EBUS-TBNA for mediastinal staging of lung cancer. J Thorac Oncol. 2012;7:1009–14.
87. Nakajima T, Anayama T, Koike T, Shingyoji M, Castle L, Kimura H, Yoshino I, et al. Endobronchial ultrasound doppler image features correlate with mRNA expression of HIF1-alpha and VEGF-C in patients with non-small-cell lung cancer. J Thorac Oncol. 2012;7:1661–7.
88. Herth FJ, Yasufuku K, Eberhardt R, Hoffmann H, Krasnik M, Ernst A. Resistance index in mediastinal lymph nodes: a feasibility study. J Thorac Oncol. 2008;3:348–50.
89. Dietrich CF. [Elastography, the new dimension in ultrasonography]. Praxis (Bern 1994). 2011;100:1533–42.
90. Dietrich CF. Real-time tissue elastography. Multiple clinical applications. Multiple clinical solutions. Endoskopie heute. 2012;24:177–212.
91. Janssen J, Dietrich CF, Will U, Greiner L. Endosonographic elastography in the diagnosis of mediastinal lymph nodes. Endoscopy. 2007;39:952–7.
92. Dietrich CF, Jenssen C, Herth FJ. Endobronchial ultrasound elastography. Endosc Ultrasound. 2016;5:233–8.
93. Jenssen C, Hocke M, Fusaroli P, Gilja OH, Buscarini E, Havre RF, Ignee A, et al. EFSUMB guidelines on interventional ultrasound (INVUS), part IV—EUS-guided interventions: general aspects and EUS-guided sampling (long version). Ultraschall Med. 2016;37:E33–76.
94. Yan JH, Pan L, Chen XL, Chen JW, Yan LM, Liu B, Guo YZ. Endobronchial ultrasound versus conventional transbronchial needle aspiration in the diagnosis of mediastinal lymphadenopathy: a meta-analysis. Springerplus. 2016;5:1716.
95. Skov BG, Baandrup U, Jakobsen GK, Kiss K, Krasnik M, Rossen K, Vilmann P. Cytopathologic diagnoses of fine-needle aspirations from endoscopic ultrasound of the mediastinum: reproducibility of the diagnoses and representativeness of aspirates from lymph nodes. Cancer. 2007;111:234–41.
96. von Bartheld MB, van Breda A, Annema JT. Complication rate of endosonography (endobronchial and endoscopic ultrasound): a systematic review. Respiration. 2014;87:343–51.
97. von Bartheld MB, Annema JT. Endosonography-related mortality and morbidity for pulmonary indications: a nationwide survey in the Netherlands. Gastrointest Endosc. 2015;82:1009–15.
98. Nakajima T, Yasufuku K, Fujiwara T, Chiyo M, Sekine Y, Shibuya K, Hiroshima K, et al. Endobronchial ultrasound-guided transbronchial needle aspiration for the diagnosis of intrapulmonary lesions. J Thorac Oncol. 2008;3:985–8.
99. Tournoy KG, Rintoul RC, van Meerbeeck JP, Carroll NR, Praet M, Buttery RC, van Kralingen KW, et al. EBUS-TBNA for the diagnosis of central parenchymal lung lesions not visible at routine bronchoscopy. Lung Cancer. 2009;63:45–9.
100. Annema JT, Veselic M, Rabe KF. EUS-guided FNA of centrally located lung tumours following a non-diagnostic bronchoscopy. Lung Cancer. 2005;48:357–61.
101. Bugalho A, Ferreira D, Eberhardt R, Dias SS, Videira PA, Herth FJ, Carreiro L. Diagnostic value of endobronchial and endoscopic ultrasound-guided fine needle aspiration for accessible lung cancer lesions after non-diagnostic conventional techniques: a prospective study. BMC Cancer. 2013;13:130.
102. Cui XW, Jenssen C, Saftoiu A, Ignee A, Dietrich CF. New ultrasound techniques for lymph node evaluation. World J Gastroenterol. 2013;19:4850–60.
103. Cui XW, Hocke M, Jenssen C, Ignee A, Klein S, Schreiber-Dietrich D, Dietrich CF. Conventional ultrasound for lymph node evaluation, update 2013. Z Gastroenterol. 2014;52:212–21.
104. Koenig SJ, Narasimhan M, Mayo PH. Thoracic ultrasonography for the pulmonary specialist. Chest. 2011;140:1332–41.
105. Koegelenberg CF, von Groote-Bidlingmaier F, Bolliger CT. Transthoracic ultrasonography for the respiratory physician. Respiration. 2012;84:337–50.
106. Detterbeck FC, Jantz MA, Wallace M, Vansteenkiste J, Silvestri GA. Invasive mediastinal staging of lung cancer: ACCP evidence-based clinical practice guidelines (2nd edition). Chest. 2007;132:202S–20S.
107. Hahn M, Faigel DO. Frequency of mediastinal lymph node metastases in patients undergoing EUS evaluation of pancreaticobiliary masses. Gastrointest Endosc. 2001;54:331–5.
108. Ardengh JC, Bammann RH, Giovani M, Venco F, Parada AA. Endoscopic ultrasound-guided biopsies for mediastinal lesions and lymph node diagnosis and staging. Clinics (Sao Paulo). 2011;66:1579–83.
109. Ozgul MA, Cetinkaya E, Tutar N, Ozgul G, Onaran H, Bilaceroglu S. Endobronchial ultrasound-guided transbronchial needle aspiration for the diagnosis of intrathoracic lymphadenopathy in patients with extrathoracic malignancy: a study in a tuberculosis-endemic country. J Cancer Res Ther. 2013;9:416–21.

110. Senturk A, Kilic H, Hezer H, Karaduman YF, Hasanoglu HC. Endobronchial ultrasound-guided transbronchial needle biopsy for the diagnosis of mediastinal lymphadenopathy in patients with extrathoracic malignancies. Turk J Med Sci. 2014;44:989–95.
111. Parmaksiz ET, Caglayan B, Salepci B, Comert SS, Kiral N, Fidan A, Sarac G. The utility of endobronchial ultrasound-guided transbronchial needle aspiration in mediastinal or hilar lymph node evaluation in extrathoracic malignancy: benign or malignant? Ann Thorac Med. 2012;7:210–4.
112. Agarwal B, Gogia S, Eloubeidi MA, Correa AM, Ho L, Collins BT. Malignant mediastinal lymphadenopathy detected by staging EUS in patients with pancreaticobiliary cancer. Gastrointest Endosc. 2005;61:849–53.
113. Sobel JM, Lai R, Mallery S, Levy MJ, Wiersema MJ, Greenwald BD, Gunaratnam NT. The utility of EUS-guided FNA in the diagnosis of metastatic breast cancer to the esophagus and the mediastinum. Gastrointest Endosc. 2005;61:416–20.
114. Mortensen MB, Pless T, Durup J, Ainsworth AP, Plagborg GJ, Hovendal C. Clinical impact of endoscopic ultrasound-guided fine needle aspiration biopsy in patients with upper gastrointestinal tract malignancies. A prospective study. Endoscopy. 2001;33:478–83.
115. Hassan H, Vilmann P, Sharma V. Impact of EUS-guided FNA on management of gastric carcinoma. Gastrointest Endosc. 2010;71:500–4.
116. Wildi SM, Fickling WE, Day TA, Cunningham CD III, Schmulewitz N, Varadarajulu S, Roberts SS, et al. Endoscopic ultrasonography in the diagnosis and staging of neoplasms of the head and neck. Endoscopy. 2004;36:624–30.
117. Giovannini M, Bernardini D, Seitz JF, Moutardier V, Hoevenaeghel G, Monges G, Delpero JR. Value of endoscopic ultrasonography for assessment of patients presenting elevated tumor marker levels after surgery for colorectal cancers. Endoscopy. 1998;30:469–76.
118. Agarwal B, Gogia S, Eloubeidi MA, Correa AM, Ho L, Collins BT. Malignant mediastinal lymphadenopathy detected by staging EUS in patients with pancreaticobiliary cancer. Gastrointest Endosc. 2005;61:849–53.
119. Hahn M, Faigel DO. Frequency of mediastinal lymph node metastases in patients undergoing EUS evaluation of pancreaticobiliary masses. Gastrointest Endosc. 2001;54:331–5.
120. Sobel JM, Lai R, Mallery S, Levy MJ, Wiersema MJ, Greenwald BD, Gunaratnam NT. The utility of EUS-guided FNA in the diagnosis of metastatic breast cancer to the esophagus and the mediastinum. Gastrointest Endosc. 2005;61:416–20.
121. Mortensen MB, Pless T, Durup J, Ainsworth AP, Plagborg GJ, Hovendal C. Clinical impact of endoscopic ultrasound-guided fine needle aspiration biopsy in patients with upper gastrointestinal tract malignancies. A prospective study. Endoscopy. 2001;33:478–83.
122. Hassan H, Vilmann P, Sharma V. Impact of EUS-guided FNA on management of gastric carcinoma. Gastrointest Endosc. 2010;71:500–4.
123. Wildi SM, Fickling WE, Day TA, Cunningham CD 3rd, Schmulewitz N, Varadarajulu S, Roberts SS, et al. Endoscopic ultrasonography in the diagnosis and staging of neoplasms of the head and neck. Endoscopy. 2004;36:624–30.
124. Giovannini M, Bernardini D, Seitz JF, Moutardier V, Hoevenaeghel G, Monges G, Delpero JR. Value of endoscopic ultrasonography for assessment of patients presenting elevated tumor marker levels after surgery for colorectal cancers. Endoscopy. 1998;30:469–76.
125. Yasuda I, Goto N, Tsurumi H, Nakashima M, Doi S, Iwashita T, Kanemura N, et al. Endoscopic ultrasound-guided fine needle aspiration biopsy for diagnosis of lymphoproliferative disorders: feasibility of immunohistological, flow cytometric, and cytogenetic assessments. Am J Gastroenterol. 2012;107:397–404.
126. Yang B, Li F, Shi W, Liu H, Sun S, Zhang G, Jiao S. Endobronchial ultrasound-guided transbronchial needle biopsy for the diagnosis of intrathoracic lymph node metastases from extrathoracic malignancies: a meta-analysis and systematic review. Respirology. 2014;19:834–41.
127. Wernecke K, Vassallo P, Hoffmann G, Peters PE, Poetter R, Rummeny E, Koch P. Value of sonography in monitoring the therapeutic response of mediastinal lymphoma: comparison with chest radiography and CT. AJR Am J Roentgenol. 1991;156:265–72.
128. Grosu HB, Iliesiu M, Caraway NP, Medeiros LJ, Lei X, Jimenez CA, Morice RC, et al. Endobronchial ultrasound-guided transbronchial needle aspiration for the diagnosis and subtyping of lymphoma. Ann Am Thorac Soc. 2015;12:1336–44.
129. Jin M, Wakely PE Jr. Endoscopic/endobronchial ultrasound-guided fine needle aspiration and ancillary techniques, particularly flow cytometry, in diagnosing deep-seated lymphomas. Acta Cytol. 2016;60:326–35.
130. Wahidi MM, Herth F, Yasufuku K, Shepherd RW, Yarmus L, Chawla M, Lamb C, et al. Technical aspects of endobronchial ultrasound-guided transbronchial needle aspiration: CHEST guideline and expert panel report. Chest. 2016;149:816–35.
131. Jenssen C, Dietrich CF. Kontraindikationen, Komplikationen, Komplikationsmanagment. In: Dietrich CF, Nurnberg D, editors. Interventionelle Sonographie. Stuttgart: Thieme; 2011. p. 127–60.
132. Popescu A, Saftoiu A. Can elastography replace fine needle aspiration? Endosc Ultrasound. 2014;3:109–17.
133. Iglesias-Garcia J, Lindkvist B, Larino-Noia J, Dominguez-Munoz JE. Endoscopic ultrasound elastography. Endosc Ultrasound. 2012;1:8–16.

134. Navani N, Booth HL, Kocjan G, Falzon M, Capitanio A, Brown JM, Porter JC, et al. Combination of endobronchial ultrasound-guided transbronchial needle aspiration with standard bronchoscopic techniques for the diagnosis of stage I and stage II pulmonary sarcoidosis. Respirology. 2011;16:467–72.
135. Trisolini R, Lazzari AL, Tinelli C, De Silvestri A, Scotti V, Patelli M. Endobronchial ultrasound-guided transbronchial needle aspiration for diagnosis of sarcoidosis in clinically unselected study populations. Respirology. 2015;20:226–34.
136. Geake J, Hammerschlag G, Nguyen P, Wallbridge P, Jenkin GA, Korman TM, Jennings B, et al. Utility of EBUS-TBNA for diagnosis of mediastinal tuberculous lymphadenitis: a multicentre Australian experience. J Thorac Dis. 2015;7:439–48.
137. Barreiros AP, Braden B, Schieferstein-Knauer C, Ignee A, Dietrich CF. Characteristics of intestinal tuberculosis in ultrasonographic techniques. Scand J Gastroenterol. 2008;43:1224–31.
138. Jenssen C, Moeller K, Sarbia M, Wagner S. Endoscopic ultrasound-guided biopsy—indications, problems, pitfalls, troubleshooting, clinical impact. In: Dietrich CF, editor. Endoscopic ultrasound—an introductory manual and atlas. Stuttgart: Thieme; 2011.
139. Kennedy MP, Jimenez CA, Mhatre AD, Morice RC, Eapen GA. Clinical implications of granulomatous inflammation detected by endobronchial ultrasound transbronchial needle aspiration in patients with suspected cancer recurrence in the mediastinum. J Cardiothorac Surg. 2008;3:8.
140. Depew ZS, Gonsalves WI, Roden AC, Bungum AO, Mullon JJ, Maldonado F. Granulomatous inflammation detected by endobronchial ultrasound-guided transbronchial needle aspiration in patients with a concurrent diagnosis of cancer: a clinical conundrum. J Bronchol Interv Pulmonol. 2012;19:176–81.
141. Dietrich CF, Stryjek-Kaminska D, Teuber G, Lee JH, Caspary WF, Zeuzem S. Perihepatic lymph nodes as a marker of antiviral response in patients with chronic hepatitis C infection. AJR Am J Roentgenol. 2000;174:699–704.
142. Dietrich CF, Leuschner MS, Zeuzem S, Herrmann G, Sarrazin C, Caspary WF, Leuschner UF. Perihepatic lymphadenopathy in primary biliary cirrhosis reflects progression of the disease. Eur J Gastroenterol Hepatol. 1999;11:747–53.
143. Dietrich CF, Lee JH, Herrmann G, Teuber G, Roth WK, Caspary WF, Zeuzem S. Enlargement of perihepatic lymph nodes in relation to liver histology and viremia in patients with chronic hepatitis C. Hepatology. 1997;26:467–72.
144. Jenssen C, Brkljacic B, Hocke M, Ignee A, Piscaglia F, Radzina M, Sidhu PS, et al. EFSUMB guidelines on interventional ultrasound (INVUS), part VI—ultrasound-guided vascular interventions. Ultraschall Med. 2016;37:473–6.
145. Dietrich CF, Horn R, Morf S, Chiorean L, Dong Y, Cui XW, Atkinson NS, et al. Ultrasound-guided central vascular interventions, comments on the European Federation of Societies for Ultrasound in Medicine and Biology Guidelines on Interventional Ultrasound. J Thorac Dis. 2016;8:E851–68.
146. Dietrich CF, Horn R, Morf S, Chiorean L, Dong Y, Cui XW, Atkinson N, et al. US-guided peripheral vascular interventions, comments on the EFSUMB guidelines. Med Ultrason. 2016;18:231–9.

Part III

Applications

9 The Application of Ultrasound in the Diagnosis of Neonatal Lung Diseases

Jing Liu

9.1 Introduction

Recently, ultrasound has been used in the diagnosis of many kinds of neonatal lung diseases, including respiratory distress syndrome (RDS), transient tachypnea of the newborn (TTN), infectious pneumonia of the newborn (IPN), meconium aspiration syndrome (MAS), pulmonary atelectasis of the newborn (PAN), pneumothorax, etc. As an accurate, reliable, low-cost, simple, and free of radiation damage, lung ultrasound (LUS) has been extensively used in neonatal wards for the diagnosis and differential diagnosis of neonatal respiratory distress. The aim of this chapter is to introduce the ultrasonic features of neonatal common lung diseases and to improve the application of LUS in the neonatal field.

9.2 Terminology of Lung Ultrasound

1. *Pleural line and lung sliding*: The pleural line is formed by the echo reflection of the pleural-lung surface interface, which is a thin, smooth regular hyperechogenic line. Under the time-motion mode, the pleura can be observed moving in a to-and-from pattern, which is synchronized with respiration and is striking because the surrounding structures are motionless. This movement is known as lung sliding [1]. Pleural line abnormalities include significantly thickening, disappearance, exists of subpleural consolidation, and irregular or coarse appearance of the pleural line [2].
2. *A-line*: An A-line is one kind of reverberation artifact caused by the pleural line. Under ultrasound, A-lines present with a series of echogenic parallel lines, equidistant from one another, below the pleural line [3].
3. *B-line and Comet-tail artifacts*: The linearly high-echo reflection of pseudomorphism is caused by an ultrasound wave encountering the alveolar gas-liquid interface. B-line arises from the pleural line, with which it is roughly vertical, spreading to the edge of the screen without fading and synchronously moving with lung sliding and respiratory movements [4].

   The comet-tail artifact is also a result of an ultrasound wave that, upon encountering the alveolar gas-liquid interface, produces multiple reflections arising from the pleural line [5]. These are gradually weakening and paralleling lines that resemble the tail of a comet. Both B-lines and comet-tail artifact

J. Liu (✉)
Department of Neonatology and NICU, Beijing Chaoyang District Maternal and Child Health Care Hospital, Beijing, China

F. Feletti et al. (eds.), *Thoracic Ultrasound and Integrated Imaging*,
https://doi.org/10.1007/978-3-319-93055-8_9

are synchronously moving with lung sliding and respiratory movements. Previously, lines reaching the edge of the screen without fading can be labeled "B-lines," while those that do not reach the edge of the screen can be labeled "comet tails." But now, we generally call them B-lines because they have the same clinical significance. There are no B-lines or comet tails in normal children or adult lungs, but they can be found in some normal newborn infants within 1 week (even 2 weeks in extremely premature infants) after birth, since the lungs still have sufficient liquid.

4. *Lung consolidation*: Those lung tissues look like hepatization under ultrasound, determined with air or fluid bronchograms [5]. The bronchogram shows air or fluid inclusions in the bronchial tree and trapped consolidation areas; it presents with echoic (air) or anechoic (fluid) images, either linear or lentil sized. The air bronchograms can show inspiratory centrifugal movement when in real-time ultrasound, which is known as dynamic air bronchograms.
5. *Shred sign*: The shred sign appears when the border of aerated lung and consolidated lung is not sharp [6].
6. *Lung pulse*: When exists of severe, large area of lung consolidation, under real-time ultrasound, lung sliding disappearing, the consolidated lung tissues can be found pulsating following the heart activity; this kind of movement of consolidated lung tissues is called lung pulse [7].
7. *Alveolar-interstitial syndrome (AIS)*: AIS is defined as two or more sequential intercostal spaces with confluent B-lines in any scanning area,the commonest cause is pulmonary edema [8].
8. *White lung*: The presence of compact B-lines in all six areas, without spared regions, is known as white lung or bilateral white lung [2].
9. *Lung point*: A fleeting appearance of a normal lung pattern is replaced by an abnormal lung pattern in a particular location on the chest wall [9]. Lung point is the specific ultrasound sign for the diagnosis of pneumothorax [9].
10. *Double lung point*: Due to a difference in severity or nature of pathological changes in different areas of the lung, a longitudinal scan shows a clear difference between upper and lower lung fields, and the sharp cutoff point is known as a "double lung point" [10].

9.3 The Probes

Generally, a high-frequency linear-array probe should be used when diagnosing neonatal lung diseases, which is generally more than 10.0 MHz; according to appearance, a probe with the frequency of 12–14 MHz is much better.

9.4 Operational Method

When in quiet state, the infant is placed in supine, side, or prone position. Each side of lung field is divided into three areas by the anterior and posterior axillary line. Each region of the bilateral lung is scanned with the probe, which should be vertical or parallel with the ribs.

9.5 Lung Ultrasound Appearance of Normal Newborn Infants

The normal lung field is hypoechoic (black), the pleural line and the A-line are hyperechoic; both of them are smooth and clear, equidistantly parallel with each other. Three days after birth, there should be few to no B-lines or comet-tail signs, no AIS, and no pleural effusion (Fig. 9.1).

9.6 The Ultrasonic Imaging Features of Neonatal Respiratory Distress Syndrome (NRDS)

Respiratory distress syndrome (RDS) is one of the most common causes of neonatal respiratory failure and neonatal mortality. The underlying pathogenesis of the disease involves developmental immaturity of the lungs, leading to the absence of pulmonary surfactant. Previously, the diagnosis of RDS is usually based on case history, clinical manifestations, arterial blood gas analysis, and chest X-rays. Recently, however, ultrasounds have been used successfully in the diagnosis of NRDS.

Both the sensitivity and specificity of diagnosing RDS by lung ultrasonography are almost 100%. According to our study and other studies [2, 11–13], the most important indicator of RDS under lung ultrasound is lung consolidation with air bronchograms, which can be seen in all RDS patients. Besides, pleural line abnormalities and A-line disappearance were also found in 100% of RDS patients. The other ultrasound manifestations including pleural effusion, AIS, and double lung point (in the acute stage of mild RDS and the recurring stage of severe RDS) (Fig. 9.2).

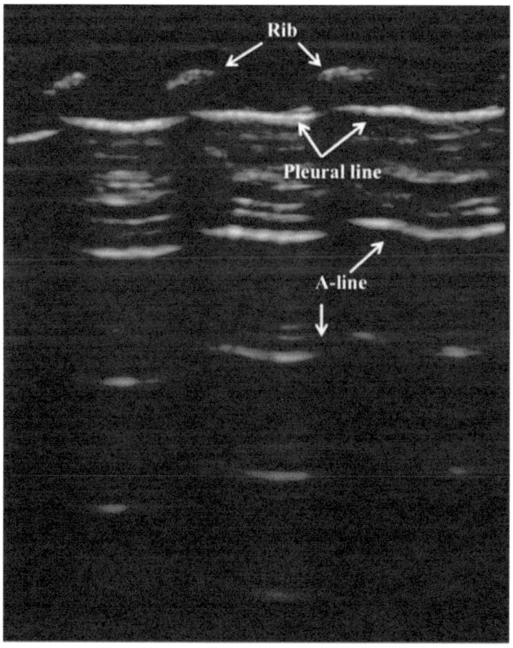

Fig. 9.1 Neonatal normal lung ultrasonic manifestation. Longitudinal scan showing the lung field was hypoechoic and the pleural lines and A-lines were smoothly, clearly, and regularly hyperechoic, which are paralleled lines, equidistant from one another

9.7 The Ultrasonic Imaging Features of Transient Tachypnea of the Newborn (TTN)

Transient tachypnea of the newborn (TTN), also known as wet lung, is one of the most common causes of dyspnea in newborns. Although TTN rarely leads to neonatal death, it must be accurately differentiated from other causes of dyspnea, especially RDS. It is difficult to differentiate TTN and RDS from medical history, clinical presentation, arterial blood gas analysis, and chest X-ray examination. However, LUS is much easier to be used for this.

The previous study showed that the presence of a double lung point is the specific sonographic characteristic of TTN; both the sensitivity and specificity are 100% [10, 12], but our recent large sample study confirms that severe TTN primarily manifests as white lung or a compact B-line, whereas mild TTN primarily manifests as AIS or a double lung point. The findings indicate that white lung/compact B-line had a sensitivity of 33.8% and a specificity of 91.3% for diagnosing

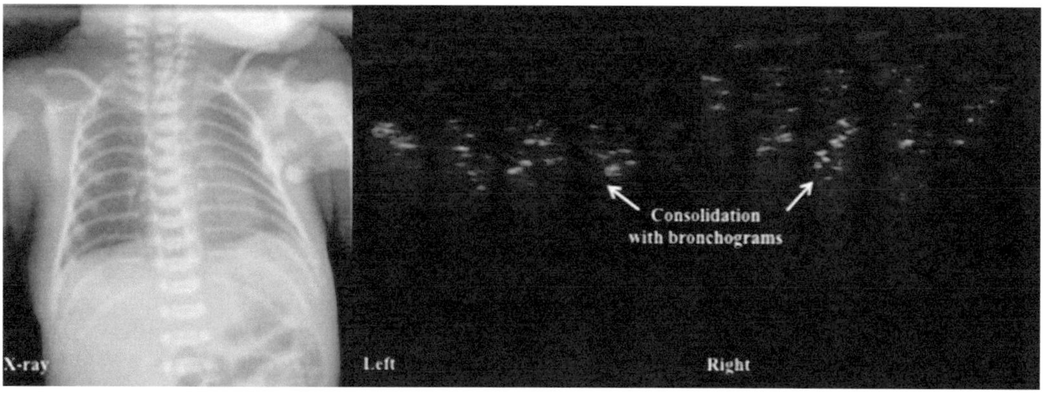

Fig. 9.2 Ultrasonic manifestation of RDS. This infant was admitted to the hospital after suffering from dyspnea for 4 h because of RDS. LUS showed a large area of lung consolidation with air bronchograms in lung fields and the disappearance of pleural lines and A-lines

TTN, whereas double lung point had a sensitivity of 45.6% and a specificity of 94.8% for diagnosing severe TTN [13]. Other common findings in TTN are pleural effusion, pleural line abnormalities, and A-line disappearance (Fig. 9.3).

9.8 The Ultrasonic Imaging Features of Infectious Pneumonia of the Newborn (IPN)

Infectious pneumonia (including intrauterine infection, hospital-acquired infection, community-acquired infection, as well as ventilator-associated pneumonia) of the newborn (IPN) is the most common infectious disease in neonates and is a significant cause of neonatal death. Ultrasound has been widely used in diagnosing infectious pneumonia in children and adults. The typical ultrasonic image features are hypoechoic areas (lung consolidation) of varying size and shape, irregular and serrated margins, air bronchograms or even dynamic air bronchograms in severe patients, AIS, pleural line abnormalities, and pleural effusion. In mild patients or the early stages of the diseases, however, it can only be manifested with AIS and small subpleural consolidation [14] (Fig. 9.4).

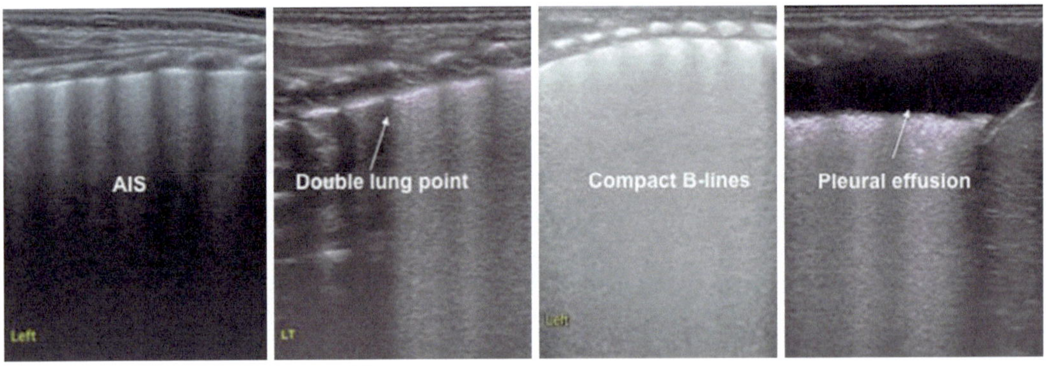

Fig. 9.3 Ultrasonic manifestation of TTN. This lung ultrasound image from a TTN neonate shows the double lung point, AIS, pleural effusion, pleural line abnormalities, and A-line disappearance

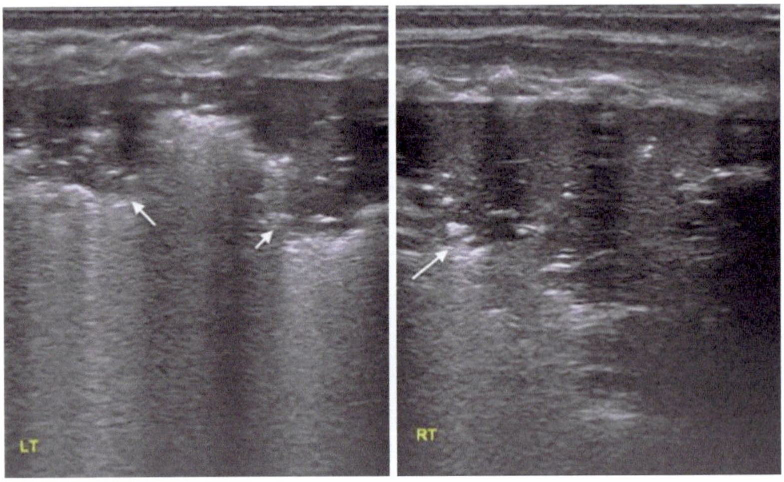

Fig. 9.4 Ultrasonic manifestation of pneumonia. Lung ultrasound image from neonatal infectious pneumonia, which shows large consolidation with irregular and serrated margins and air bronchograms (arrow)

9.9 The Ultrasonic Imaging Features of Meconium Aspiration Syndrome of the Newborn (MAS)

Meconium aspiration syndrome (MAS) is a common cause of severe respiratory distress in neonates especially in full-term or post-term infants, with an associated highly variable morbidity and mortality. MAS accounts for about 10% of all cases of respiratory failure with 39% mortality rate in developing and newly industrialized countries. Early diagnosis and early treatment are important for improving the prognosis. Recently, lung ultrasound has been used for the diagnosis of MAS [15, 16]. According to our study of 117 newborns enrolled with MAS, the main lung ultrasonographic findings in patients with MAS were as follows: (1) pulmonary consolidation with air bronchogram was found in all patients; (2) pleural line anomalies and the disappearance of the A-line were found in all patients; (3) atelectasis was found in 16.2% of severe cases, who demonstrated severe massive atelectasis and visible lung pulse; (4) pleural effusion was found in 13.7% of the patients; and (5) alveolar-interstitial syndrome or B-line in the non-consolidation area was found in all patients with MAS (Fig. 9.5).

9.10 The Ultrasonic Imaging Features of Pulmonary Hemorrhage of the Newborn (PHN)

Pulmonary hemorrhage of the newborn (PHN) is a common severe and critical disease in newborn infants, and it has complicated etiologies, rapid progression, and a high mortality rate. It was reported that the incidence rate of PHN was 1–12% of live births, and it increased to 50% in infants with high-risk factors. Until now, a diagnosis of PHN has been mainly based on the case history, typical clinical manifestations, arterial blood gas analysis, and chest X-rays findings, while lung ultrasound has not been applied in the diagnostic protocol. This study aimed to investigate the diagnostic value of lung ultrasonography for PHN. We have tried to use ultrasound to diagnose PHN, and we found that the main ultrasound findings included [17] lung consolidation with air bronchograms with an incidence of 82.5%, a shred sign with an incidence of 91.2%, pleural effusion with an incidence of 84.2% (pleurocentesis confirmed the fluid was really bleeding), atelectasis with an incidence of 33.3%, pleural line abnormalities as well as disappearing A-lines with an incidence of 100%, and 11.9% of these patients had the main manifestations of alveolar-interstitial syndrome (Fig. 9.6).

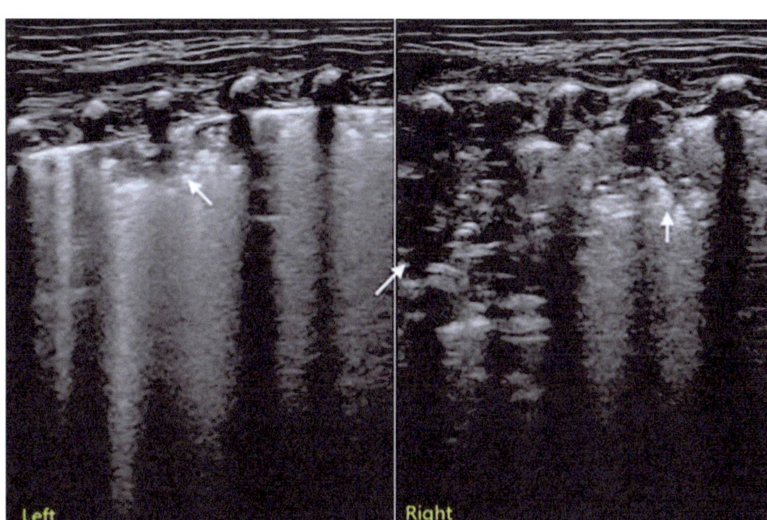

Fig. 9.5 Ultrasonic manifestation of MAS. Lung ultrasonography showed large areas of lung consolidation with air bronchogram and irregular edges in the lungs (more significantly in the right lung). The pleural line was abnormal, and the A-line disappeared in the consolidation area

9.11 The Ultrasonic Imaging Features of Neonatal Pulmonary Atelectasis (NPA)

Neonatal pulmonary atelectasis (NPA) is a common complication of a variety of lung diseases (such as RDS, pneumonia, sputum obstruction, etc.) and is one of the most common reasons for difficulty in weaning from mechanical ventilation. Early and accurate diagnosis of NPA is important for enabling appropriate treatment and improving the prognosis. The sensitivity of lung ultrasound in diagnosing neonatal atelectasis is 100% [18]. The main ultrasound imaging features of atelectasis are large lung consolidation with air bronchograms or paralleled air bronchogram. Other ultrasound signs of atelectasis include pleural line abnormalities and A-line disappearance. Lung pulse and lung sliding disappearance in large atelectasis can be monitored by real-time ultrasound. Vascular flow in the areas of consolidation can also be found by color or power Doppler imaging [18] (Fig. 9.7).

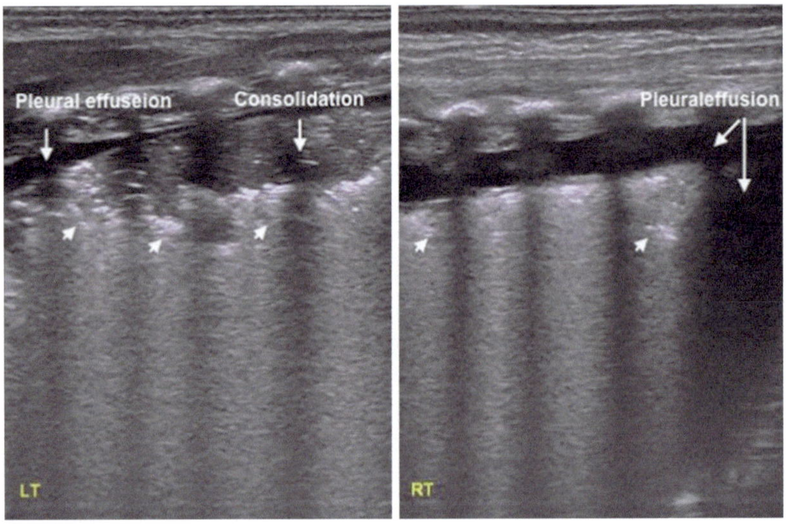

Fig. 9.6 Ultrasonic manifestation of pulmonary hemorrhage of the newborn (PHN). The lung ultrasound findings from a severe PHN patient. It showed a large area of lung consolidation with an air bronchogram in the left lung, significant shred sign (arrow), pleural effusion in both sides of the lungs (which was confirmed as bleeding by thoracocentesis), and a disappeared pleural line and A-lines

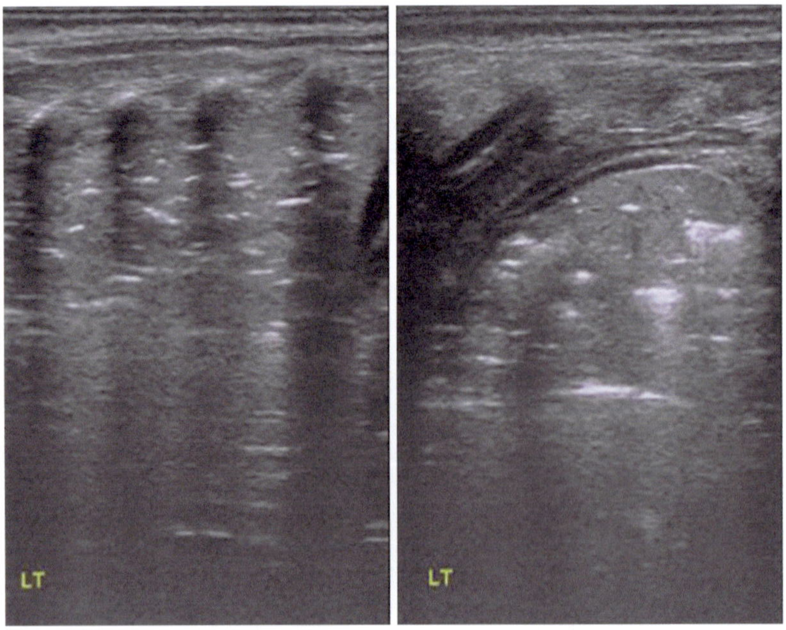

Fig. 9.7 Ultrasonic manifestation of neonatal pulmonary atelectasis (NPH). Lung ultrasound image from neonatal large area of atelectasis which shows large consolidation with regular margins and significant air bronchograms (left, the probe vertical with the ribs; right, the probe parallel with the ribs)

9.12 The Ultrasonic Imaging Features of Neonatal Pneumothorax

Pneumothorax is also one kind of common neonatal critical illness in clinics and is one of the common reasons for deaths among newborns and preterm infants. An early accurate and rapid diagnosis is the key for successful emergency treatment and saving the lives of infants. Lung ultrasound has been successfully used in the diagnosis of pneumothorax. According to a meta-analysis from Dr. Alrajab [19], ultrasonography had a pooled sensitivity of 78.6% (95% CI, 68.1–98.1) and a specificity of 98.4% (95% CI, 97.3–99.5), while chest radiography had a pooled sensitivity of 39.8% (95% CI, 29.4–50.3) and a specificity of 99.3% (95% CI, 98.4–100), which indicates that ultrasonography is more accurate than chest radiography for detection of pneumothorax. The lung point is a specific sign of pneumothorax, and the sensitivity and specificity of lung point in diagnosing pneumothorax are 66% and 100%, respectively [20]. Lung sliding disappearance is the most important ultrasound sign, which can rule out pneumothorax if existing, with a sensitivity and specificity of 95.3% and 91.1%, respectively. Moreover, its negative predictive value is 100% [1]. The negative predictive value of the comet-tail sign or B-line existence with pneumothorax is 99.2–100% [4, 21, 22]. In an extreme emergency, the absence of pleural line movement, coupled with the absence of B-lines, can be used in diagnosing pneumothorax promptly and safely, without the need to search for the lung point. According to the reports of Dr. Raimondi [23], the lung ultrasound accuracy in diagnosing neonatal pneumothorax was sensitivity 100%, specificity 100%, positive predictive value 100%, and negative predictive value 100% (Fig. 9.8).

9.13 Conclusions

There are many other applications in neonatal clinical practices, such as to help us to clarify the cause of long-term oxygen dependency in preterm babies, help to guide ventilator weaning, identify the atelectasis or thymus, etc. [23].

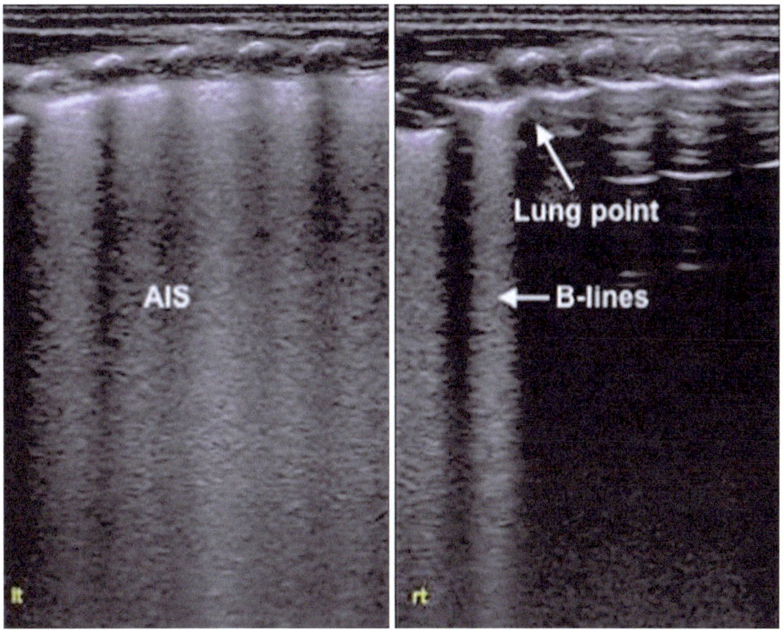

Fig. 9.8 Lung point in a patient with pneumothorax. Longitudinal scan of the anterior axillary line, supine. Left picture showed the AIS. The absence of exist of lung sliding under real-time ultrasound. Right picture defined the location of "lung point" and the transition from the B-lines area (left side) to a hypoechoic area with horizontal reverberations of the parietal pleura (right side)

Lung ultrasound has many advantages over X-ray; it is convenient to perform at the bedside; therefore, the chest X-ray should be replaced by lung sonography used as the first-line approach in the diagnosis of lung diseases and routine application in the neonatal intensive care unit [24, 25].

References

1. Lichtenstein DA, Menu Y. A bedside ultrasound sign ruling out pneumothorax in the critically III: lung sliding. Chest. 1995;108:1345–8.
2. Copetti R, Cattarossi L, Macagno F, et al. Lung ultrasound in respiratory distress syndrome: a useful tool for early diagnosis. Neonatology. 2008; 94:52–9.
3. Lichtenstein DA, Lascols N, Mezière G, et al. Ultrasound diagnosis of alveolar consolidation in the critically ill. Intensive Care Med. 2004;30:276–81.
4. Lichtenstein DA, Mezière G, Lascols N, et al. Ultrasound diagnosis of occult pneumothorax. Crit Care Med. 2005;33:1231–8.
5. Lichtenstein DA, Mezière G, Biderman P, et al. The comet-tail artifact: an ultrasound sign of alveolar-interstitial syndrome. Am J Respir Crit Care Med. 1997;156:1640–6.
6. Touw HRW, Tuinman PR, Gelissen HPMM, et al. Lung ultrasound: routine practice for the next generation of internists. Neth J Med. 2015;73(3):100–7.
7. Lichtenstein DA, Lascols N, Prin S, et al. The "lung pulse": an early ultrasound sign of complete atelectasis. Intensive Care Med. 2003;29:2187–92.
8. Liu J, Copetti R, Sorantin E, et al. Protocol and guidelines for point-of-care lung ultrasound in diagnosing neonatal pulmonary diseases based on international expert consensus. J Vis Exp. 2019;145(3):e58990. https://doi.org/10.3791/58990.
9. Lichtenstein DA, Meziere G, Biderman P, et al. The "lung point": an ultrasound sign specific to pneumothorax. Intensive Care Med. 2000;26:1434–40.
10. Copetti R, Cattarossi L. The "double lung point": an ultrasound sign diagnostic of transient tachypnea of the newborn. Neonatology. 2007;91:203–9.
11. Liu J, Cao HY, Wang HW, et al. The role of lung ultrasound in diagnosis of respiratory distress syndrome in newborn infants. Iran J Pediatr. 2014;24(2):147–54.
12. Liu J, Wang Y, Fu W, et al. The diagnosis of neonatal transient tachypnea and its differentiation from respiratory distress syndrome using lung ultrasound. Medicine. 2014;93(27):e197.
13. Liu J, Chen XX, Li XW, et al. Lung ultrasonography to diagnose transient tachypnea of the newborn. Chest. 2016;149(5):1269–75.
14. Liu J, Liu F, Liu Y, et al. Lung ultrasonography for the diagnosis of severe pneumonia of the newborn. Chest. 2014;146(2):483–8.
15. Piastra M, Yousef N, Brat R, et al. Lung ultrasound findings in meconium aspiration syndrome. Early Hum Dev. 2014;90(Suppl 2):S41–3.
16. Liu J, Cao HY, Fu W. Lung ultrasonography to diagnose meconium aspiration syndrome of the newborn. J Int Med Res. 2016;44(6):1534–42.
17. Ren XL, Fu W, Liu J, et al. Lung ultrasonography to diagnose pulmonary hemorrhage of the newborn. J Matern Fetal Neonatal Med. 2017;30(21):2601–6. https://doi.org/10.1080/14767058.2016.1256997.
18. Liu J, Chen SW, Liu F, et al. The diagnosis of neonatal pulmonary atelectasis using lung ultrasonography. Chest. 2015;147(4):1013–9.
19. Alrajab S, Youssef AM, Akkus NI, et al. Pleural ultrasonography versus chest radiography for the diagnosis of pneumothorax: review of the literature and meta-analysis. Crit Care. 2013;17:R208.
20. Volpicelli G. Sonographic diagnosis of pneumothorax. Intensive Care Med. 2011;37:224–32.
21. Husain LF, Hagopian L, Wayman D, et al. Sonographic diagnosis of pneumothorax. J Emerg Trauma Shock. 2012;5:76–81.
22. Raimondi F, Fanjul JR, Aversa S, et al. Lung ultrasound for diagnosing pneumothorax in the critically ill neonate. J Pediatr. 2016;175(8):74–78.e1.
23. Liu J, Cao HY, Wang XL, et al. The significance and the necessity of routinely performing lung ultrasound in the neonatal intensive care units. J Matern Fetal Neonatal Med. 2016;29(24):4025–30.
24. Cattarossi L, Copetti R, Poskurica B. Radiation exposure early in life can be reduced by lung ultrasound. Chest. 2011;139:730–1.
25. Chen SW, Fu W, Liu J, et al. Routine application of lung ultrasonography in the neonatal intensive care unit. Medicine. 2017;96(2):e5826.

10 Pediatrics

Ron Berant

10.1 Introduction

The use of thoracic ultrasound in the field of pediatrics for bedside diagnosis is a very appealing option for any physician who is treating children. The first reason is the lack of radiation in the exam. It has been the mainstay of radiologists and pediatricians for the last two decades to try and avoid unnecessary exposure to X-ray radiation since children are considerably more sensitive than adults, as demonstrated in epidemiologic studies of exposed populations [1]. In addition, children have a longer life expectancy than adults, resulting in a larger window of opportunity for expressing radiation damage. Lastly, children may receive a higher radiation dose than necessary if settings are not adjusted for their smaller body size [2].

Another consideration for choosing thoracic ultrasound instead of chest X-ray as the imaging modality is that children's body habitus has a thinner adipose tissue layer, thus making it possible to adequately demonstrate the lung parenchyma with a linear transducer, even if the transducer's depth is relatively superficial, and still benefit from high-resolution images.

In addition, thoracic ultrasound has the benefit of being a dynamic exam, and it would be more suitable for imaging babies and toddlers who would find it difficult to remain still for other imaging modalities such as chest X-ray, CT, or MRI. The operator can move the transducer over the child and compensate for his or her movements.

The dynamic quality of the exam allows demonstration of movement to further investigate conditions such as pneumothorax and diaphragm paralyses.

Finally, the use bedside, by the treating physician, without the necessity of consult from radiology has the potential to considerably hasten accurate diagnosis and appropriate treatment.

10.2 Technical Issues

As mentioned, while in adults the transducer of choice would be a phased array or curvilinear transducer, in children the physician may make use of a linear transducer as well as the aforementioned transducers.

The choice of transducer would be highly dependent on the application and the organ that the physician desires to scan. The transducers are the same as for in adults, i.e., linear and phased array, and if necessary a microconvex transducer may be chosen, taking advantage of its small footprint.

R. Berant (✉)
Pediatric Emergency Medicine, Schneider Children's Medical Center of Israel, Petah-Tikva, Israel

Sackler School of Medicine, Tel-Aviv University, Tel-Aviv, Israel
e-mail: ronbe@clalit.org.il

F. Feletti et al. (eds.), *Thoracic Ultrasound and Integrated Imaging*, https://doi.org/10.1007/978-3-319-93055-8_10

In most cases, in pediatrics, to scan for a pneumonia, a high-frequency linear transducer would suffice to generate high-quality images, since children are small with a thin adipose tissue and most pneumonias are peripheral. If the physician wishes to attempt to demonstrate the diaphragm's movement, it would be better to use a phased array or curvilinear transducer in M-mode. The transducer is placed in the RUQ and LUQ views, similar to the positions in the FAST exam. The scan line is placed over the diaphragm to demonstrate its movement. Movement of over 4 mm is considered normal.

Color Doppler mode may be used for the demonstration of pleural movement in investigating a pneumothorax or to further investigate mediastinal masses.

When examining the children, they may lie in bed, sit in a chair, or be held by their parents arms, as long as they are most comfortable and the examiner interrogates all relevant planes.

In most cases, scanning the child's chest in longitudinal and transverse orientation in three longitudinal planes, i.e., midclavicular, midaxillary, and posterior (Figs. 10.1, 10.2, and 10.3), per each lung would suffice to demonstrate the lungs and any potential pathology. When scanning in a longitudinal plane, the probe marker should be directed toward the head of the patient.

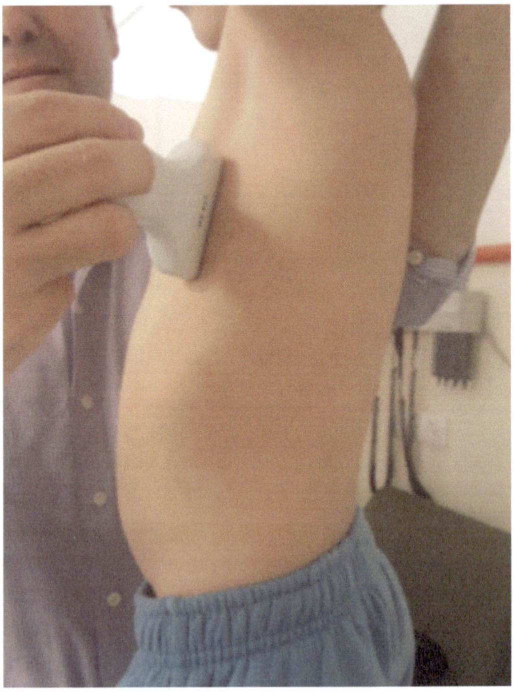

Fig. 10.1 Lung scan in midaxillary view

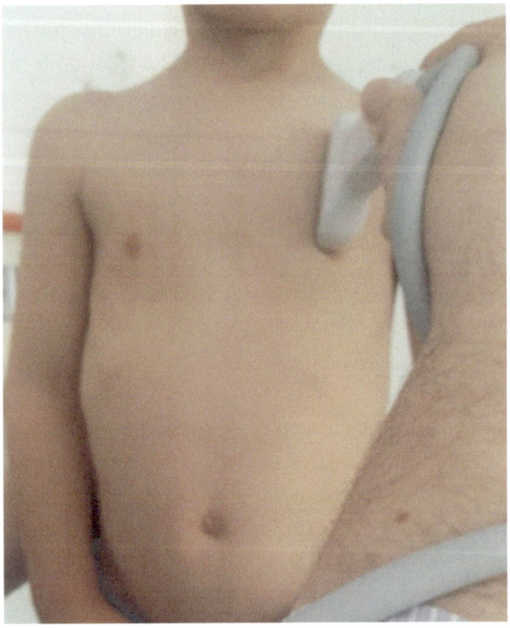

Fig. 10.2 Lung scan in midclavicular plane

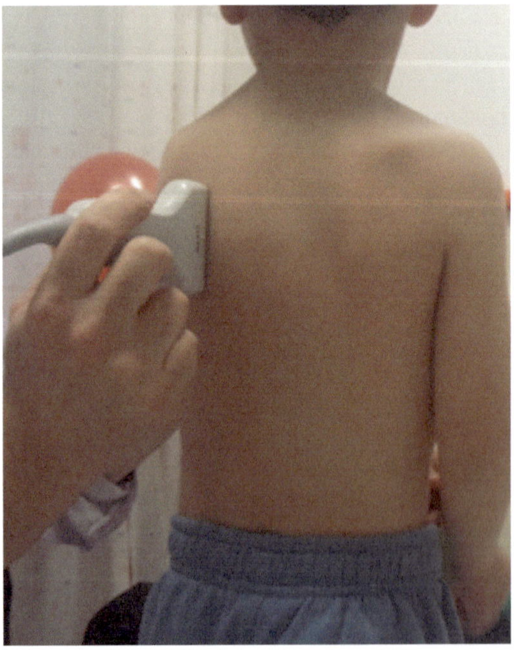

Fig. 10.3 Lung scan in posterior plane

A transverse plane, in between the ribs, may supplement the scans and add more information regarding the pathology initially demonstrated. When scanning in a transverse plane, the probe marker should be directed toward the patient's right. If scanning the chest wall for a focal finding, then a linear high-frequency transducer would be appropriate, and transducer orientation should be with probe marker either to the patient's right or head.

While in adults it is not very crucial, the use of warmed gel is highly recommended when examining children and infants to soothe the anxious child and not further agitate him or her. Commercially available gel warmers may be ordered specifically for this purpose.

10.3 The Chest Wall

The chest wall includes superficial echoic layer of the adipose tissue and underneath the hypoechoic layer of the intercostal muscles. The cortical surface of the ribs, clavicle, and sternum shall appear hyperechoic with intense shadowing.

In children, many soft tissue and vascular and musculoskeletal diagnoses may be facilitated by ultrasound.

10.3.1 Soft Tissue Pathology

10.3.1.1 Mastitis

Mastitis can appear in the neonatal period as well as in adolescents. Neonatal mastitis is an infection that usually occurs in term or near-term infants, while mastitis in adolescents originates from irritation of the skin (through shaving or nipple stimulation), trauma, a foreign body (e.g., piercing), ductal abnormality (such as ductal ectasia), or infection of an epidermal cyst. Mastitis is defined as evidence of breast inflammation with or without abscess. Sonographically increased echogenicity of the breast bud and hyperemia may be seen. Breast abscess shall be present as an avascular mass that would be hyperechoic or anechoic with increased through transmission and surrounding hyperemia (Fig. 10.4) [3].

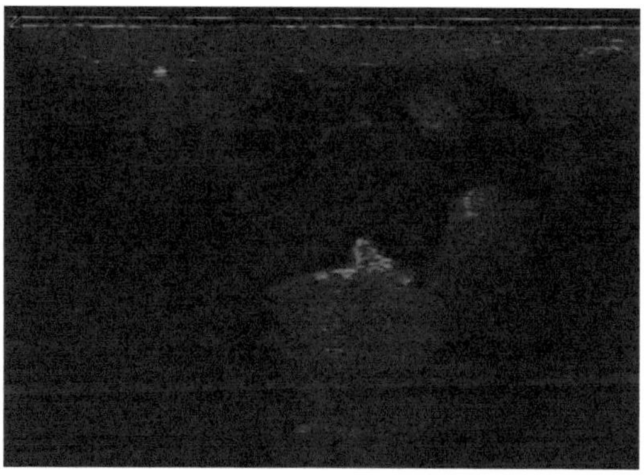

Fig. 10.4 An abscess and cellulitis in a child presenting with redness tenderness and local warmth of the left breast bud

10.3.1.2 Hemangiomas

Hemangiomas are a common soft tissue tumor and characterized by rapid growth for 8–12 months, followed by slow regression for the next 1–5 years [4]. Some of the hemangiomas fully regress, while others still leave a skin mark as a remnant of the original lesion. When the hemangioma is deep in the subcutaneous tissue, the overlying skin may appear normal and imaging might be needed. In gray-scale ultrasound, the hemangioma shall appear as a well-circumscribed homogenous solid mass. Color mode would assist in demonstrating the flow in the hemangioma, thus confirming the diagnosis [5]. Hemangiomas become more heterogeneous during the involuting phase and increased vascularity, containing arteries, veins, and even evidence of shunting, often seen on color Doppler, especially during the proliferative phase [6].

10.3.1.3 Vascular Malformations

Vascular malformations that may appear are lymphangiomas and venous malformations. These lesions are slow flowing by nature, and so color mode might not be helpful. The lymphangioma may appear as a cystic mass with internal septations, without internal flow or solid components (Fig. 10.5). Venous malformations typically appear as anechoic vascular channels which on Doppler mode shall show a venous flow pattern although many times the flow is so slow that it cannot be detected [7].

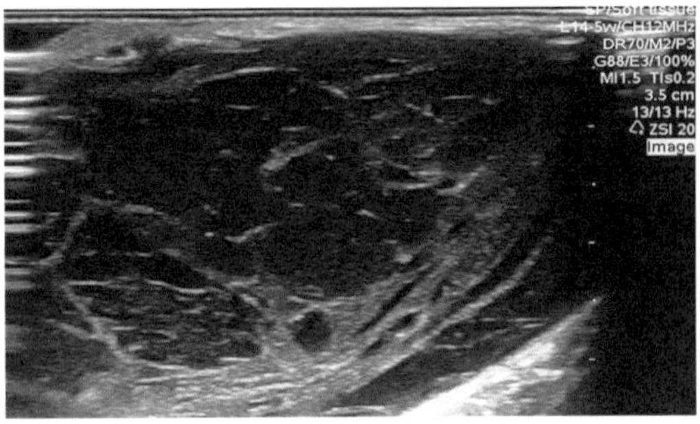

Fig. 10.5 Chest lymphangioma. Notice the internal septations within the mass

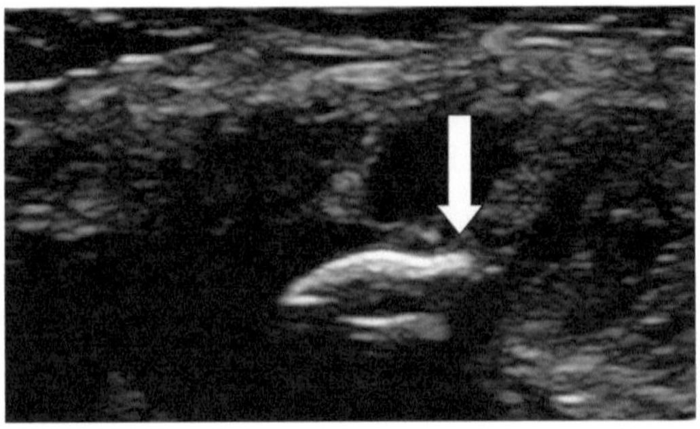

Fig. 10.7 The bony cortex is disrupted by the fracture (arrow)

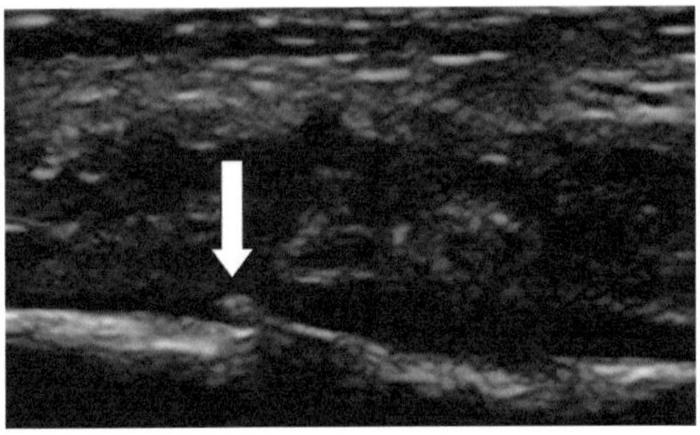

Fig. 10.6 Note the fracture line indicated by the arrow

10.3.2 Skeletal System

Clavicle fractures may be easily demonstrated by ultrasound. Clavicle fractures remain the most commonly fractured bone in children and represent approximately 10% of all fractures presenting to the ED [8]. With the use of point-of-care ultrasound, it has been demonstrated that a facture may be diagnosed with sensitivity and specificity of nearly 90% (Figs. 10.6 and 10.7). Given these exam characteristics if ultrasound is positive for fracture and the patient has no deficits or gross deformity, a confirmatory radiograph may be unnecessary [9].

Rib fractures diagnosed by thoracic ultrasound have been described in adult literature [10], but evidence in pediatrics is sparse [11]. Still the potential exists and should be considered especially when there are concerns of potential child abuse [12]. Fractures are demonstrated as discontinuation of the cortex or with periosteal thickening and subperiosteal hematoma. The boundaries of fractures may be highlighted by some artifacts such as the "chimney phenomenon" (see Chap. 2 in this book). As a fracture begins to heal, early hypoechoic callus becomes hyperechoic hard callus, which can eventually bridge the fracture gap or step-off deformity [13]. In addition, ultrasound may detect rib malformations such as focal anterior angulation, waviness, or hypertrophy [14].

10.4 Pleural Diseases

Pleural effusions can be readily detected by ultrasound. In children, the exam is performed in an upright sitting position evaluating the base of the lung with a high-resolution linear transducer, although if needed the exam may be performed with the child supine.

The most common cause of pleural effusion in children is bacterial pneumonia (50–70%), followed by heart failure (5–10%), while rheumatologic causes and metastatic intrathoracic malignancy are rare [15, 16]. In the setting of an observation of the "white" hemithorax on a chest radiograph, supine and decubitus X-ray views may not be helpful in differentiating between pleural fluid, lung consolidation, atelectasis, or other pathologies [17], yet an ultrasound exam may detect as little as 3–5 mL of fluid and help guide further investigations. In a child with pleural effusion, the hypoechoic fluid shall be noted above the diaphragm, while lung hepatization shall be noted in a lobar pneumonia (Fig. 10.8).

Effusions may be classified into simple or complex, i.e., free of echoes or loculated and full

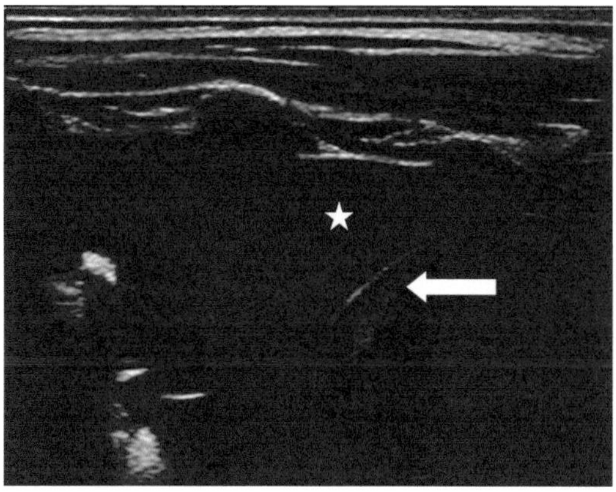

Fig. 10.8 Pleural effusion. The star notes the effusion, while the arrow indicates the double line of the diaphragm

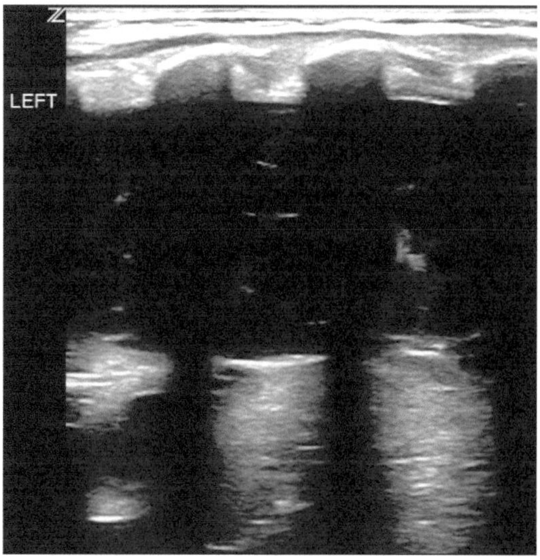

Fig. 10.9 A multiloculated pleural effusion with internal septations

of floating debris echoes, respectively. In simple pleural effusions, the fluid seen on sonography is uniformly anechoic or hypoechoic, and it changes in shape with respiration or position [18, 19]. Echogenic debris may be visualized within the pleural effusion in cases of exudates or hemothorax. Complicated fluid collections may be multiloculated and show internal septations (Fig. 10.9). The nature of the pleural fluid and the presence or absence of septations are helpful in determining whether the patient requires intervention.

It is noteworthy that ultrasound in children has been found to have similar ability as chest CT in detecting loculated effusion and lung necrosis or abscess resulting from complicated pneumonia. Fibrin strands were identified in patients with effusion on chest ultrasound, while they could not be clearly delineated on chest CT images. This makes the chest CT exam unnecessary and spares the child from exposure to high-dose radiation [20].

Pneumothorax is another condition that may be diagnosed with thoracic ultrasound. In pediatrics a pneumothorax may be primary, spontaneous, or secondary.

Primary pneumothorax occurs spontaneously in teenagers and young adults, mostly male. Commonly these patients are tall and thin. The common theory is that these patients have subpleural blebs which put them at risk for a pneumothorax. Patients with collagen synthesis defects, such as Ehlers-Danlos disease and Marfan syndrome, are unusually prone to the development of pneumothorax.

Secondary causes may be appear in patients with pneumonia, usually with empyema or secondary to pulmonary abscess, gangrene, infarct, rupture of a cyst or an emphysematous bleb (in asthma), or foreign bodies in the lung. It is found in $\approx 5\%$ of hospitalized asthmatic children and usually resolves without treatment [21].

In a meta-analysis it was found that thoracic ultrasound had a sensitivity of 90.9% and specificity of 98.2% to detect a pneumothorax with positive and negative likelihood ratios of 50.5 and 0.09, respectively [22]. The absence of B-lines and lung sliding, in the presence of A-lines, might raise the suspicion of a pneumothorax.

Further support of a pneumothorax would come from the stratosphere sign on M-mode (Fig. 10.10). Only the parietal pleura would be demonstrated and no lung parenchyma underneath the M-mode would show just straight lines, hence designating it as the "stratosphere sign." In a normal lung, the sliding of the pleura and the movement of the lung parenchyma would create on the bottom half of the screen a grainy appearance—the "Sea shore sign."

Using the color mode would also facilitate demonstration of the movement of the pleura on the normal lung, as opposed to the pneumothorax (Fig. 10.11).

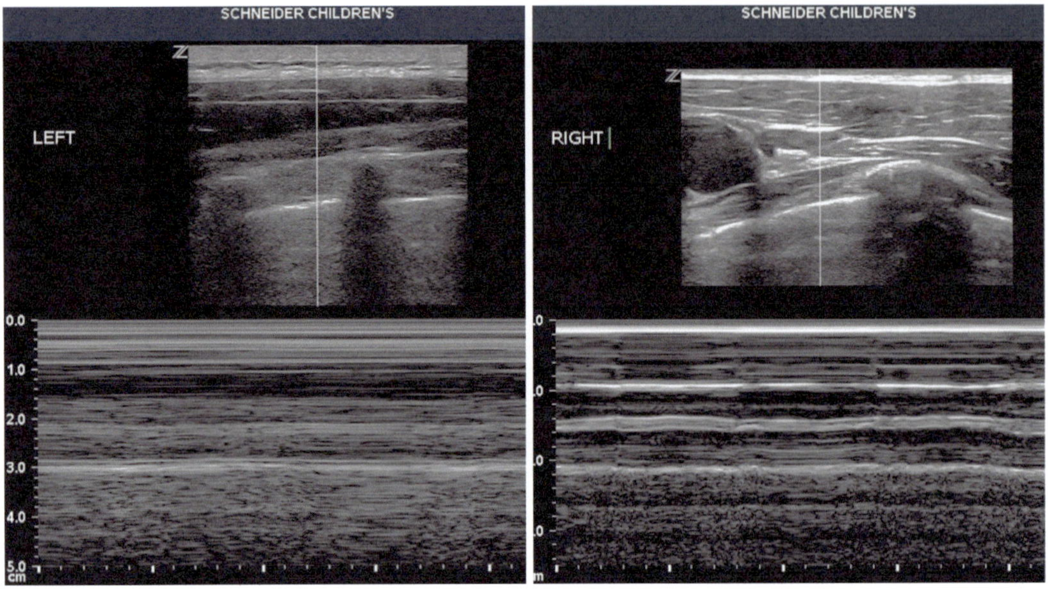

Fig. 10.10 M-mode view of the lungs with left pneumothorax. On the right the lower half of the screen has a grainy appearance giving the image a seashore resemblance; on the left only straight lines appear, designating this image—stratosphere sign

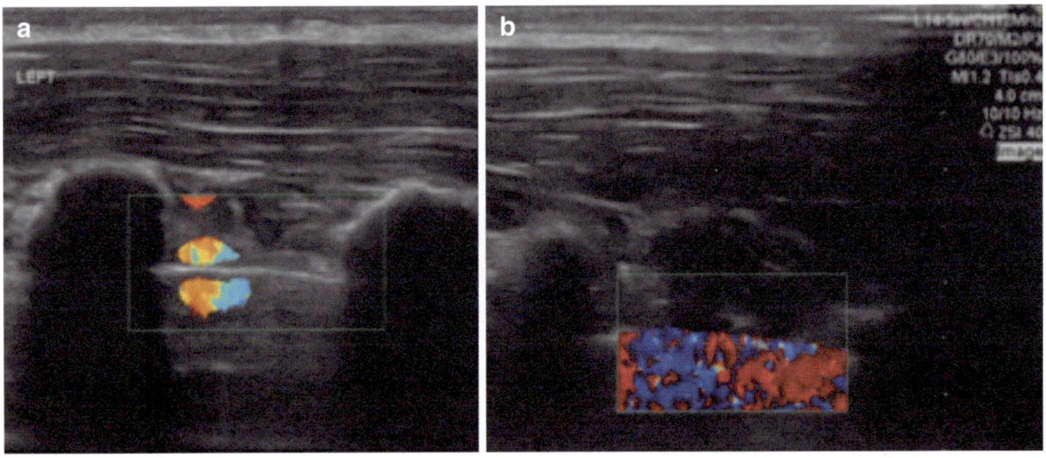

Fig. 10.11 Using color mode may demonstrate the movement of the pleura and lung parenchyma (**a**) versus no movement (**b**)

With demonstration of the lung point sign, the diagnosis may be confirmed. Using this approach if a patient is suspected clinically to have a pneumothorax, demonstration of no lung sliding, a stratosphere sign, and finally a lung point may diagnose a pneumothorax. While the pneumothorax can be diagnosed by thoracic ultrasound, a chest X-ray would still be necessary to correctly evaluate the extent of the pneumothorax. Only one study, in adults, demonstrated a possibility of semiquantifying the size of the pneumothorax, and even then thoracic US only reliably indicated the size of pneumothorax for diagnosing small pneumothoraxes [23].

10.5 Diseases of the Lung

10.5.1 Bronchiolitis

More than 100,000 children younger than 1 year old are hospitalized annually in the United States because of RSV infection [24]. The diagnosis of acute bronchiolitis is clinical, particularly in a previously healthy infant presenting with a first-time wheezing episode during a community outbreak. While chest radiography is not indicated in all patients with bronchiolitis, nevertheless many children undergo unnecessary X-rays [25]. Studies have demonstrated that in children with bronchiolitis, B-lines appear throughout the lung (Fig. 10.12), and the more severe the illness, the more B-lines would be visible on the thoracic ultrasound [26, 27]. Additional findings reported to be seen in bronchiolitis are subpleural consolidations, compact and isolated B-lines, and pleural line abnormalities [28].

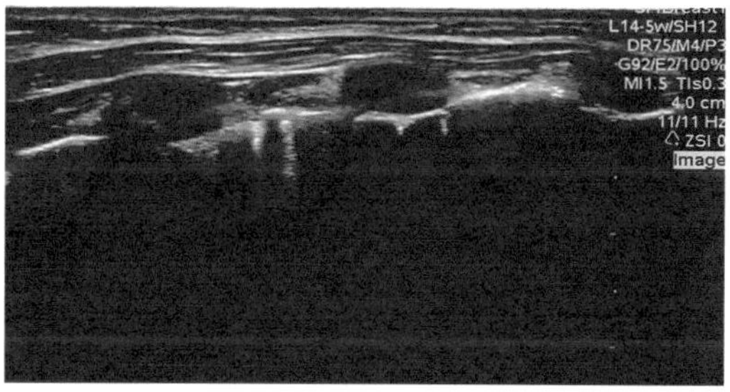

Fig. 10.12 Bronchiolitis in an 8-month-old infant. Note multiple B-lines extending from the pleura

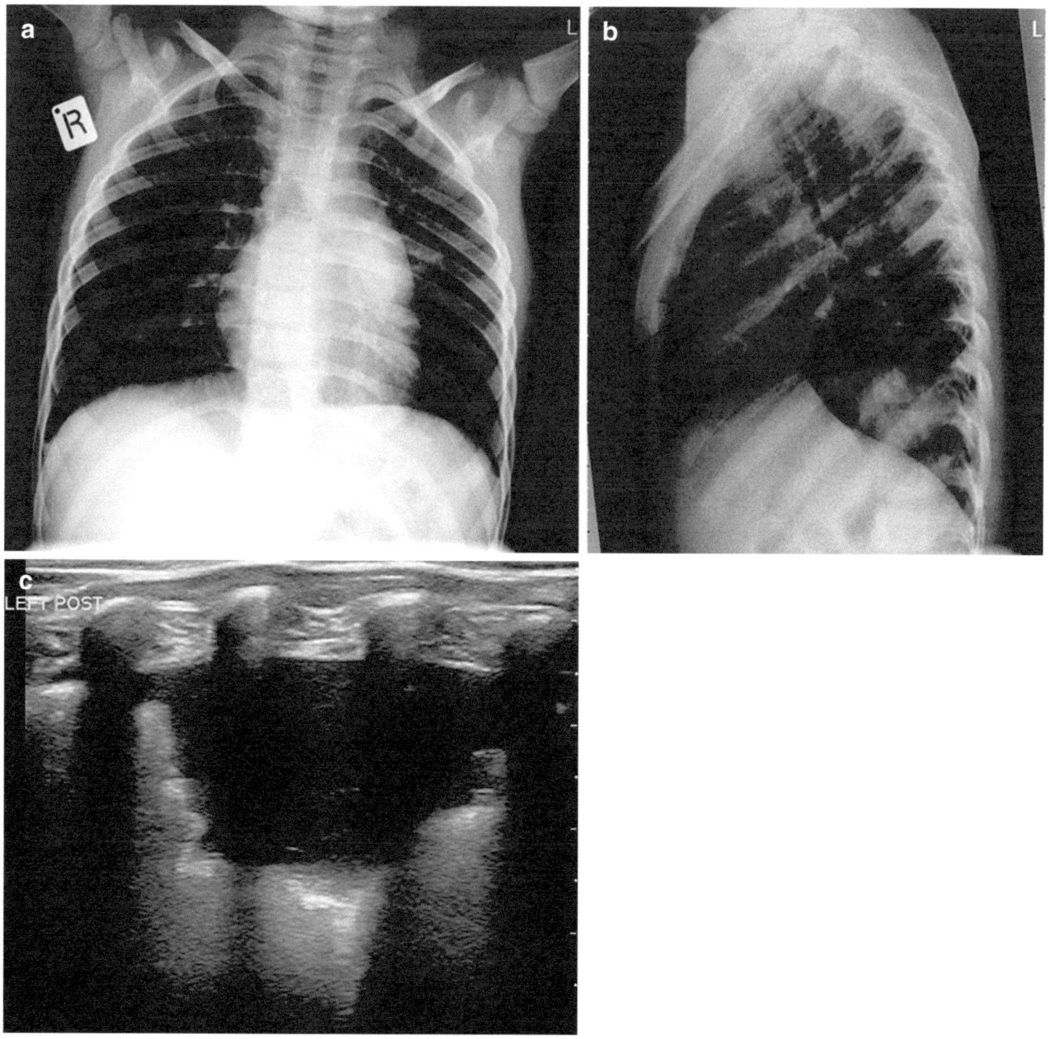

Fig. 10.13 Pneumonia. The consolidation was barely visible on X-ray but very clear on the TUS

10.5.2 Pneumonia

The diagnosis of pneumonia by thoracic ultrasound is one of the more studied topics. Pneumonia is the leading cause of death globally among children younger than age 5 years, accounting for an estimated one million (16% total) deaths annually [29, 30]. While diagnosis may be made by symptoms and signs found in clinical exam alone, many physicians choose to send the child for an X-ray exam. If the child has several febrile episodes, he may be exposed to repeated chest X-ray exams. Since most of children's febrile episodes are viral by nature, these exams lead to unnecessary exposure to X-ray radiation [31, 32].

Several studies have proved that the sensitivity and specificity of lung ultrasound are equal to chest X-ray [33] and may even surpass it [34] (Fig. 10.13a–c).

The main drawback of using ultrasound as a substitute for chest X-ray is higher rate of pneumonia diagnosis and higher prescription rate. This can be explained by the fact that lung ultrasound may find consolidations as small as 1 cm in length which are not visible on plain film.

Distinct from the shred sign of pneumonia as described in adults, the border between consolidated and aerated lung is irregular, fully opposed to the lung line [35]; children may present with a lung hepatization appearance and with dynamic air bronchograms—bright white lines that move with the child's respirations (Fig. 10.14). This dynamic appearance differs from static air bronchograms—bright white lines that do not move with respirations—that are thought to represent atelectasis [36].

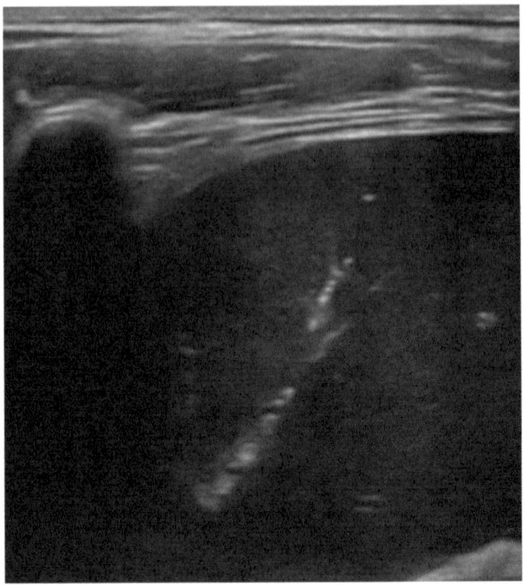

Fig. 10.14 Pneumonia in a 4.5-year-old child, not improving on antibiotics for 48 h. In this image lung hepatization as well as the bright white lines of air bronchograms are demonstrated

Sonographic features of an aspirated foreign body have been described as well. These include hepatization of the lung and confluent B-lines in the adjacent lung, suggesting an alveolar syndrome pattern consistent with lung inflammation or pneumonia. In addition, thoracic ultrasound showed an abnormal convex pleural line, which corresponded to the overinflated lung [37].

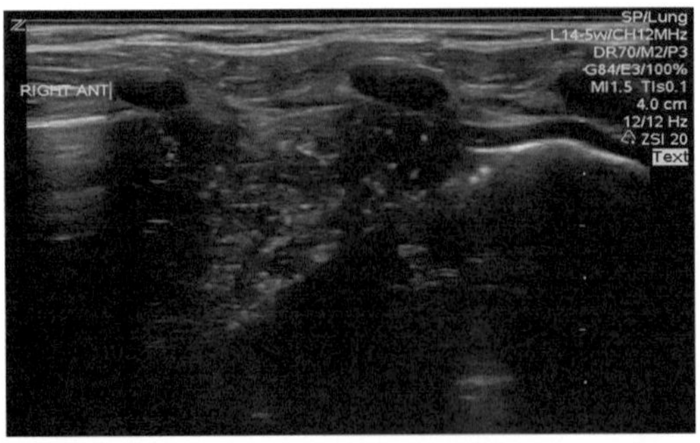

Fig. 10.15 Congenital pulmonary adenomatoid malformation. Instead of A-lines, a complex echogenic mass is noted

10.5.3 Congenital Pulmonary Lesions

Congenital pulmonary lesions are difficult to diagnose by ultrasound alone. Nevertheless, ultrasound may be useful as a primary assessment tool when encountering a chest X-ray with a whiteout lung [17]. For example, a congenital cystic adenomatoid malformation can present as either homogeneously solid lesion (microcystic) or as complex mass with cystic components (macrocystic or medium-sized cysts with solid components) (Fig. 10.15).

Congenital diaphragmatic hernia is another potential condition that its diagnosis may be facilitated by ultrasound. Desjardins et al. have described two cases of children presenting with history and symptoms suggestive of diaphragmatic hernia. Thoracic ultrasound was used at the bedside to demonstrate the presence of bowel in the thorax and accurately guided the care of these children [38]. In both patients they have demonstrated bowel with active peristalsis in the chest, and in one of the patients, an absence of the diaphragm at the junction of the IVC, right atrium, and liver.

10.6 Mediastinum

The use of sonography in evaluation of the mediastinum is limited. The posterior mediastinum is obscured by overlying anatomic structures, making it difficult for transthoracic sonography to characterize or evaluate posterior mediastinal masses. On the other hand, the anterior mediastinum is easily assessable, especially in young children, as the sternal ossification centers have not yet fused.

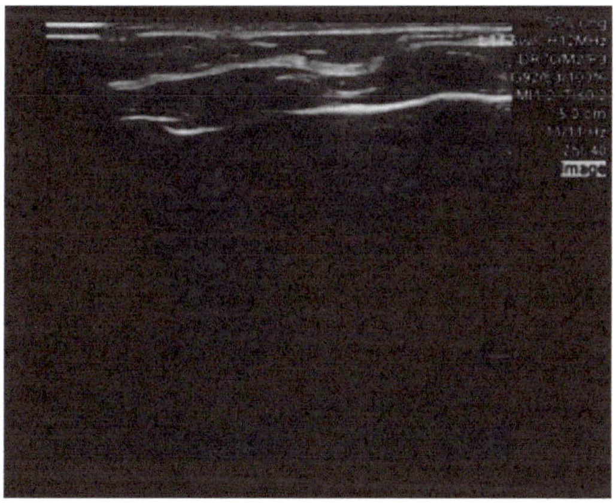

Fig. 10.16 A normal thymus adjacent to a normal lung

The thymus may be visualized in a normal, healthy child (Fig. 10.16). The thymus is larger compared with the rest of the thorax during the first year of life [39]. The thymus has a characteristic echotexture, with regular linear and punctate echogenicities that allows its confident recognition and differentiation from mediastinal pathology (Fig. 10.16).

10.6.1 Mediastinal Pathology

Sometimes mediastinal masses are identified after a suspicious chest radiograph. Although the imaging modality of choice should be a chest CT, ultrasound can be used as an initial imaging modality, because it quickly and easily differentiates thymic from other conditions and can analyze the compositions of the mass (solid, cystic, calcified, or complex) or vascularity or effect on adjacent vessels and thus allow an initial diagnosis or differential diagnosis helping to choose the appropriate further imaging [40] (Fig. 10.17).

10.7 Summary

Ultrasound can be used as an easy, bedside imaging tool to facilitate rapid diagnosis of diverse conditions in children presenting to the pediatri-

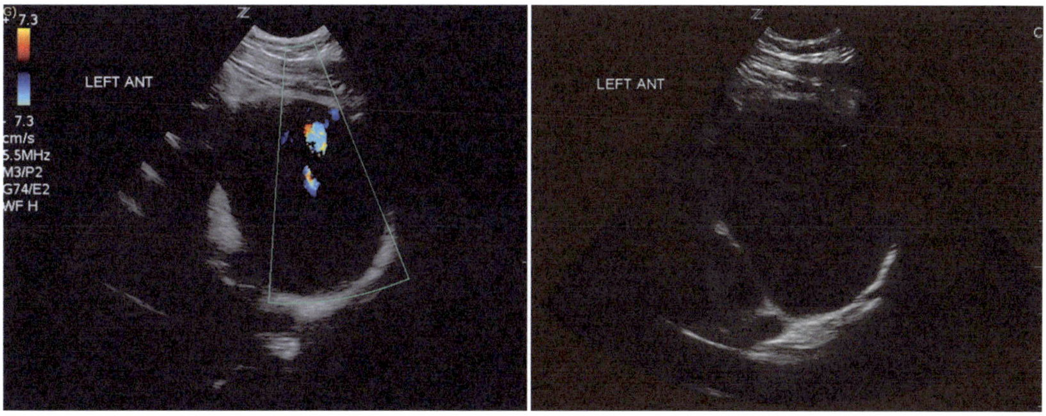

Fig. 10.17 Longitudinal scan of a child's anterior chest with and without color demonstrating a mass with vacularity within it

cian or emergency room, while sparing the child from unnecessary exposure to ionizing radiation. It should be noted that most of the applications are used based on studies from adults and case reports in pediatrics, and there is need for further research to establish the evidence.

References

1. Pearce MS, Salotti JA, Little MP, et al. Radiation exposure from CT scans in childhood and subsequent risk of leukaemia and brain tumours: a retrospective cohort study. Lancet. 2012;380:499–505.
2. Frush DP. CT dose and risk estimates in children. Pediatr Radiol. 2011;41(Suppl 2):483–7.
3. Borders H, Mychaliska G, Gebarski KS. Sonographic features of neonatal mastitis and breast abscess. Pediatr Radiol. 2009;39:955–8.
4. Léauté-Labrèze C, Harper JI, Hoeger PH. Infantile haemangioma. Lancet. 2017;390(10089):85–94.
5. Coley BD. Caffey's pediatric diagnostic imaging, 12e, Chapter 59. New York: Elsevier; 2013. p. 633–46.
6. Coley BD. Chest sonography in children: current indications, techniques, and imaging findings. Radiol Clin North Am. 2011;49(5):825–46.
7. Paltiel HJ, Burrows PE, Kozakewich HP, et al. Soft-tissue vascular anomalies: utility of US for diagnosis. Radiology. 2000;214(3):747–54.
8. Lien J. Pediatric orthopedic injuries: evidence-based management in the emergency department. Pediatr Emerg Med Pract. 2017;14(9):1–28.
9. Chien M, Bulloch B, Garcia-Filion P, et al. Bedside ultrasound in the diagnosis of pediatric clavicle fractures. Pediatr Emerg Care. 2011;27(11):1038–41.
10. Turk F, Kurt AB, Saglam S. Evaluation by ultrasound of traumatic rib fractures missed by radiography. Emerg Radiol. 2010;17(6):473–7.
11. Orth RC, Laor T. Isolated costal cartilage fracture: an unusual cause of an anterior chest mass in a toddler. Pediatr Radiol. 2009;39(9):985–7.
12. Kelloff J, Hulett R, Spivey M. Acute rib fracture diagnosis in an infant by US: a matter of child protection. Pediatr Radiol. 2009;39(1):70–2.
13. Craig JG, Jacobson JA, Moed BR. Ultrasound of fracture and bone healing. Radiol Clin North Am. 1999;37(4):737–51, ix.
14. Donnelly LF, Frush DP. Abnormalities of the chest wall in pediatric patients. AJR Am J Roentgenol. 1999;173(6):1595–601.
15. Kleigman RM, Stanton BF, St Geme J, et al. Nelson textbook of pediatrics. 20th ed. Philadelphia: Elsevier; 2016. p. 2131.
16. Efrati O, Barak A. Pleural effusions in the pediatric population. Pediatr Rev. 2002;23(12):417–26.
17. Berant R, Kwan C, Fischer J. Emergency point-of-care ultrasound assessment of whiteout lung in the pediatric emergency department. Pediatr Emerg Care. 2015;31(12):872–5.
18. Doniger SJ. Pediatric emergency and critical care ultrasound, Ch. 7. Cambridge: Cambridge University Press; 2013. p. 109.
19. Prina E, Torres A, Carvalho C. Lung ultrasound in the evaluation of pleural effusion. J Bras Pneumol. 2014;40(1):1–5.
20. Kurian J, Levin TL, Han BK, et al. Comparison of ultrasound and CT in the evaluation of pneumonia complicated by parapneumonic effusion in children. AJR Am J Roentgenol. 2009;193(6):1648–54.
21. Kleigman RM, Stanton BF, St Geme J, et al. Nelson textbook of pediatrics, Ch. 411. 20th ed. Philadelphia: Elsevier; 2016. p. 2135–6.
22. Raja AS, Jacobus CH. How accurate is ultrasonography for excluding pneumothorax? Ann Emerg Med. 2013;61(2):207–8.
23. Volpicelli G, Boero E, Sverzellati N, et al. Semi-quantification of pneumothorax volume by lung ultrasound. Intensive Care Med. 2014;40(10):1460–7.
24. Kleigman RM, Stanton BF, St Geme J, et al. Nelson textbook of pediatrics, Ch. 391. 20th ed. Philadelphia: Elsevier; 2016. p. 2045.
25. Florin TA, Plint AC, Zorc JJ. Viral bronchiolitis. Lancet. 2017;389(10065):211–24.
26. Basile V, Di Mauro A, Scalini E, et al. Lung ultrasound: a useful tool in diagnosis and management of bronchiolitis. BMC Pediatr. 2015;15:63.
27. Cohen JS, Hughes N, Tat S, Chamberlain JM, Teach SJ, Boniface K. The utility of bedside lung ultrasound findings in bronchiolitis. Pediatr Emerg Care. 2017;33(2):97–100.
28. Caiulo VA, Gargani L, Caiulo S, et al. Lung ultrasound in bronchiolitis: comparison with chest X-ray. Eur J Pediatr. 2011;170(11):1427–33.
29. Rudan I, Tomaskovic L, Boschi-Pinto C, et al.; WHO Child Health Epidemiology Reference Group. Global estimate of the incidence of clinical pneumonia among children under five years of age. Bull World Health Organ. 2004;82(12):895–903.
30. World Health Organization. Pneumonia. Fact sheet no. 331. www.who.int/mediacentre/factsheets/fs331/en/. Accessed 1 Dec 2017.
31. Harris M, Clark J, Coote N, et al. British Thoracic Society guidelines for the management of community acquired pneumonia in children: update 2011. British Thoracic Society Standards of Care Committee. Thorax. 2011;66(Suppl 2):ii1.
32. Jain S, Williams DJ, Arnold SR, et al. Community-acquired pneumonia requiring hospitalization among U.S. children CDC EPIC Study Team. N Engl J Med. 2015;372(9):835.
33. Pereda MA, Chavez MA, Hooper-Miele CC, et al. Lung ultrasound for the diagnosis of pneumonia in children: a meta-analysis. Pediatrics. 2015;135:714.
34. Jones BP, Tay ET, Elikashvili I, et al. Feasibility and safety of substituting lung ultrasound for chest X-ray when diagnosing pneumonia in children: a randomized controlled trial. Chest. 2016;150(1):131–8.

35. Lichtenstein D. Lung ultrasound in the critically ill. Ann Intensive Care. 2014;4:1.
36. Goh Y, Kapur J. Sonography of the pediatric chest. J Ultrasound Med. 2016;35(5):1067–80.
37. Weerdenburg KD, Kwan CW, Fischer JW, et al. Point-of-care ultrasound findings associated with foreign body aspiration in the pediatric emergency department. Pediatr Emerg Care. 2016;32:486–8.
38. Desjardins MP, Weerdenburg KD, Fischer JW. Emergency point-of-care ultrasound diagnosis of diaphragmatic hernia in the pediatric emergency department. Pediatr Emerg Care. 2016;32(10):685–7.
39. Yekeler E, Tambag A, Tunaci A, et al. Analysis of the thymus in 151 healthy infants from 0 to 2 years of age. J Ultrasound Med. 2004;23:1321–6.
40. Trinavarat P, Riccabona M. Potential of ultrasound in the pediatric chest. Eur J Radiol. 2014;83:1507–18.

Lung Ultrasound in Critical Care and Trauma

11

Jung-Un Choi, Abdulrahman Alharthy, Dimitrios Karakitsos, and Lawrence M. Gillman

11.1 Introduction

The management of critically ill patients is complex yet requires rapid decision-making and action, often in the setting of limited information and in a population who may be too ill to give further history or to transport for definitive investigations. Point-of-care ultrasound (POCUS) is appealing in this patient population as it offers a noninvasive bedside tool that can be used to gather important patient data utilizing a rapid and easily repeatable assessment technique. Initial studies of POCUS compared its findings to existing definitive diagnostic modalities including chest X-rays [1–4] and computed tomography (CT) scans [5–8]. However, this puts ultrasound at an unfair disadvantage and is not really consistent with the modern philosophy of bedside ultrasound. Instead POCUS should be considered another tool in the clinician's assessment armamentarium, and in place of a definitive test, it should be an extension of the physical examination with the results being integrated into the clinicians overall patient assessment [9, 10].

With this shift in philosophy comes a different way of classifying ultrasound assessments. Once considered as a system-based assessment, i.e., lung ultrasound, abdominal ultrasound, cardiac ultrasound, and so on, modern POCUS for critical care is better understood by incorporating pieces of these systems into a holistic problem-based approach, such as assessment of shock, or cardio-respiratory failure, as described in the literature [11]. Thus, despite the fundamental goal of this text, it is impossible to discuss lung ultrasound's role in critical care without discussing how the assessment can be integrated with other body system assessments, taking a more holistic and less fragmented approach to the patient.

11.2 Acute Respiratory Failure: The BLUE Protocol

Acute respiratory failure represents one of the most common reasons for ICU admission. Identifying the cause of deterioration is however

Electronic Supplementary Material The online version of this chapter (https://doi.org/10.1007/978-3-319-93055-8_11) contains supplementary material, which is available to authorized users.

J.-U. Choi
Department of Surgery, University of Manitoba, Winnipeg, MB, Canada

A. Alharthy
King Saud Medical City, Riyadh, Kingdom of Saudi Arabia

D. Karakitsos
King Saud Medical City, Riyadh, Kingdom of Saudi Arabia

University of Southern California, Keck Medical School, Los Angeles, CA, USA

L. M. Gillman (✉)
Winnipeg, MB, Canada
e-mail: Lawrence.Gillman@umanitoba.ca

F. Feletti et al. (eds.), *Thoracic Ultrasound and Integrated Imaging*,
https://doi.org/10.1007/978-3-319-93055-8_11

not always immediately obvious, and physical exam and portable radiography may be unreliable in establishing a diagnosis [1, 12].

These limitations, coupled with the increasing interest in lung ultrasound, led to the development of the BLUE protocol by Daniel Lichtenstein in 2008 [13]. Developed initially for ICU use, POCUS can provide a fast and accurate diagnosis and subsequent management plan. The BLUE protocol utilizes a systematic assessment of lung sliding, presence of lung artifacts, and venous assessment to classify patients into seven distinct profiles. The lung component is performed in three stages investigating the (1) anterior, (2) lateral, and (3) posterior aspects of each hemithorax. These are termed upper BLUE, lower BLUE, and PLAPS (posterior and/or lateral alveolar and/or pleural syndrome) points, respectively. At each point one looks for (1) lung sliding abolition (present or not), (2) lung rockets (B-lines) (present or absent), and (3) posterior and/or lateral alveolar and/or pleural syndrome (PLAPS) (present or absent) (Fig. 11.1, Video 11.1). This forms the basis for classification into seven profiles and their corresponding diagnoses (Fig. 11.2) [14].

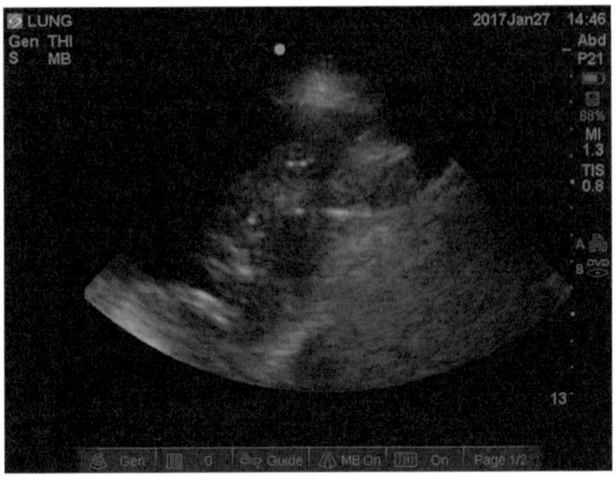

Fig. 11.1 Sonographic view from the PLAPS (posterior and/or lateral alveolar and/or pleural syndrome) point in a patient with a pleural effusion and consolidated lung. Hyperechoic areas within the lung represent sonographic air bronchograms

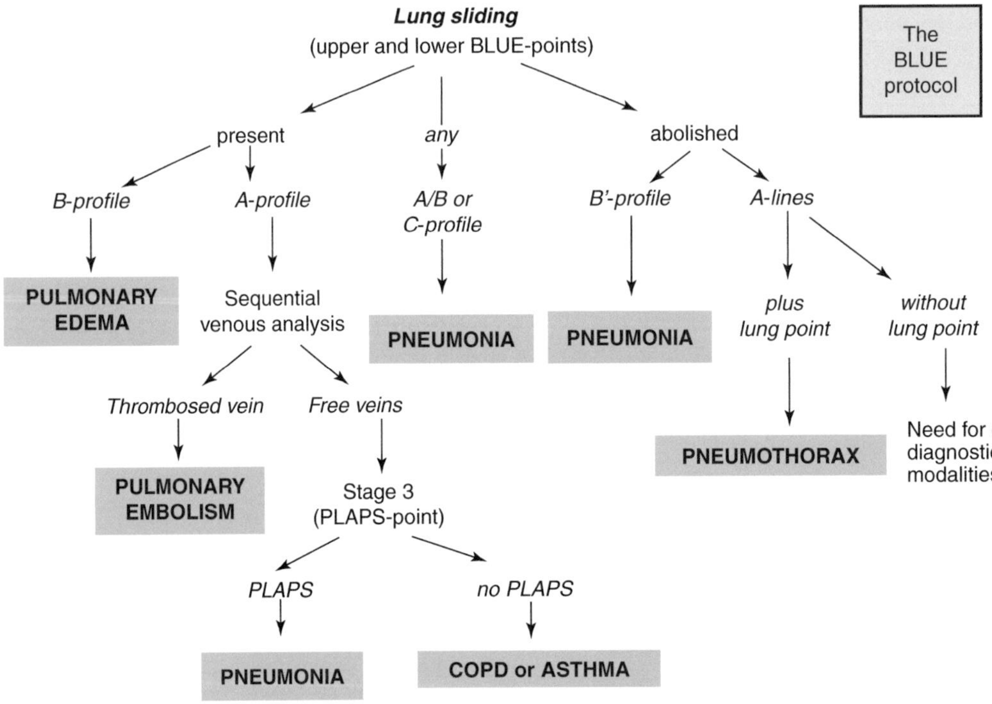

Fig. 11.2 Decision tree for BLUE protocol. Reprinted from Chest, 134(1), Lichtenstein DA, Mezière GA, Relevance of Lung Ultrasound in the Diagnosis of Acute Respiratory Failure: The BLUE Protocol, 117–125, Copyright 2008, with permission from Elsevier

The BLUE protocol was developed based on a study which included 300 patients with acute respiratory failure [15]. It has been noted that BLUE protocol provides 90% accuracy ranging between 81 and 100% of the profiles [15].

11.3 Shock: Fluid Administration Limited by Lung Sonography (FALLS) Protocol

Acute circulatory failure or shock is another common reason for ICU admission. As in respiratory failure, the etiology of shock is not always clear on presentation. The FALLS protocol was developed as a tool for management of unexplained shock. It is based on an adaptation from the BLUE protocol whereby lung US profiles are used in conjunction with basic cardiac sonography [16].

Weil's classification of shock forms the basis of the FALLS protocol. The assessment begins with a brief bedside ultrasound cardiac exam to search for pericardial effusion and right ventricular dilatation. In the absence of these, the next assessment is for the presence of lung sliding to rule out tension pneumothorax. The absence of any abnormal findings in this quick assessment essentially rules out obstructive shock. Next one searches for B-lines. Although B-lines are not specific to left heart failure, the absence of B-profile in a patient in shock may exclude cardiogenic shock from left heart failure as a cause and, in that sense, render the possibility of sepsis due to lung infection and/or ARDS [17, 18].

The FALLS protocol is most useful for the next causes of shock: hypovolemic and distributive shock. The lung US is useful as a patient with A-profiles, which indicates dry lungs, would benefit from fluid therapy. As one can see, the FALLS protocol is a useful tool to expedite the diagnosis and allows earlier fluid therapy especially in hypovolemic shock. If the shock persists despite fluid therapy, the fluid will ultimately penetrate the lung and result in interstitial edema. This will be apparent on ultrasound at earlier stages by the transformation of A-lines to B-lines. This transformation not only provides an endpoint for fluid therapy but in the presence of ongoing hypotension may be also indicative of the presence of distributive shock. In summary, the FALLS protocol provides the advantage of early and guided fluid therapy on admission, before confirmation of sepsis, and aims to decrease the mortality rate from septic shock [15, 16, 18].

Despite the advantages of using the FALLS protocol in shock patients, there are some limitations. One of the main limitations is that the FALLS protocol is dynamic and looks at transformation on US. If there is evidence of the B-profile on admission, it would be impossible to detect any transformation from A-lines to B-lines [18]. In addition, despite the FALLS protocol focusing on acute circulatory failure, it is not useful for monitoring cardiac output changes [18]. Further validation of the FALLS protocol is necessary.

11.4 Extravascular Lung Water

Extravascular lung water (EVLW) is a common finding in critically ill patients. It is defined as the amount of fluid that accumulates in the interstitial and alveolar spaces. Increased EVLW is potentially life threatening due to reduction in lung compliance and impairment of gas exchange. Its etiology may be secondary to aggressive fluid resuscitation, capillary damage related to sepsis, acute respiratory distress syndrome (ARDS), and/or left heart failure (mixed type of pulmonary edema). In critically ill patients, it has been associated with organ dysfunction and increased mortality [19]. Accordingly, clinicians need to be able to detect excessive EVLW. Previously EVLW was assessed via transpulmonary thermodilution. Recently, ultrasound assessment of the lungs has been used to quantify EVLW, detect fluid accumulation, and guide resuscitation. Pulmonary congestion is often seen and evident by presence of both air and fluid leading to B-line formation on ultrasound. Increases in extravascular lung water cause changes in lung ultrasound findings on a continuum from no B-lines to multiple B-lines and finally the white lung (Fig. 11.3, Video 11.2) as fluid progressively

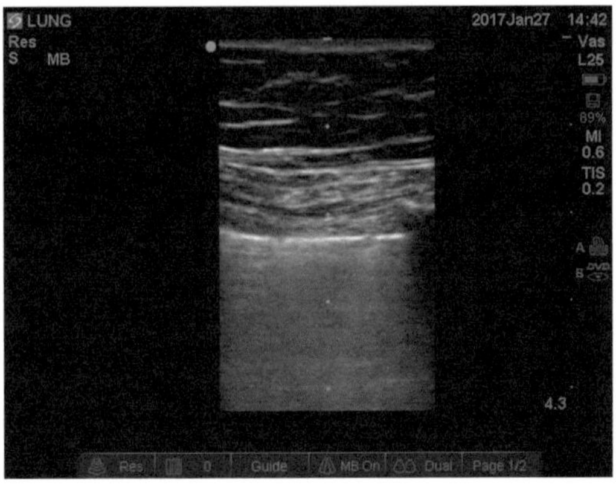

Fig. 11.3 Sonographic view of a "white lung" consisting of innumerable overlapping B-lines

accumulates. Multiple studies have demonstrated strong correlation between lung ultrasound finding and EVLW detected by transpulmonary thermodilution [20–23].

A number of standardized techniques have been developed for the ultrasound quantification of EVLW including:

1. Total B-line scores (TBS) [24]
   The anterior and lateral chest, parasternal, midclavicular, anterior axillary, and midaxillary lines are scanned in 3 rib spaces on the right and 4 on the left for a total of 28 sites. At each site the number of B-lines is counted and added together to yield the TBS.
2. Four-zone examination [13, 15]
   In this examination four sites are scanned (two from each hemithorax). A scan with at least three B-lines at each point is considered abnormal.
3. Eight-zone examination [25]
   Finally in this protocol, each hemithorax is divided into four areas (two anterior, two lateral). For a scan to be considered abnormal, it must meet the following criteria: (1) multiple artifacts per scan (at least three), (2) positive findings in more than one scan per side, and (3) positive findings bilaterally.

   To our knowledge these protocols have not been prospectively validated or compared head to head. This represents another area in need of further research.

11.5 Trauma (E-FAST)

Trauma has been one of the major causes of morbidity and mortality in North America. The management of trauma patients is highly complex as many patients arrive with multiple injuries and shock. FAST has been incorporated into ATLS guidelines as a noninvasive test that can be done rapidly at the patient's bedside to address major life-threatening injuries. FAST was initially designed to quickly evaluate for the presence of free fluid in the abdomen, pelvis, and pericardium.

In approximately half of all trauma patients with thoracic injury, pneumothorax and hemothorax have been reported. Given the nature of the chaotic trauma setting, it is almost impossible to appreciate the findings of pneumothorax and/or hemothorax on clinical examination. In cases where the patient is unable to sit up, supine chest X-ray does not provide good evidence of pneumothorax nor hemothorax.

In many institutions, extended fast (E-FAST) is now an accepted standard of care in the resuscitation of injured patients [26]. E-FAST is an extension of FAST, whereby US is used to assess for hemothorax and/or pneumothorax. The simplest extension of the basic FAST is to shift the probe cephalad when examining the left and right upper quadrants and examine for hemothorax seen as fluid above the diaphragm. Studies suggest as little as 25 cm^3 of fluid may be detected [27]. Lung ultrasound has also shown sensitivity of 97.5% and specificity of 99.7% for diagnosing acute hemothorax since its first use in 1993 [28].

By adding an additional view on the anterior chest (second or third interspace midclavicular line), lung sliding can be quickly evaluated. While the absence of lung sliding requires further confirmation before a pneumothorax can be confidently diagnosed, the presence of lung sliding effectively rules out pneumothorax under the applied ultrasound probe. In the absence of thoracic adhesions from previous surgery, infection, or chronic lung disease, this single view in a supine patient can essentially rule out a significant pneumothorax. The sensitivity and specificity of this sign has varied, but reported values have been as high as 99–100% [7, 23, 29–35].

11.6 Pleural Effusions and Procedural Guidance

Pleural effusions are extremely common in ICU patients and are generally related to a combination of resuscitation fluids and "third spacing" due to hypoalbuminemia and capillary leak. While often treated conservatively, they do at times require either aspiration or drainage for diagnostic or therapeutic reasons. Ultrasound guidance has been shown to increase success rate and reduce complications, including reducing injury to surrounding structures [36, 37]. We generally advocate using a low-frequency phased array transducer to localize and quantify the effusion (Video 11.3) followed by a high-frequency linear transducer to then choose the specific site of puncture (Video 11.3). While it can be performed under direct ultrasound guidance, many use ultrasound to landmark and choose a puncture site for the subsequent thoracentesis ensuring the patient does not move after the spot has been marked but not necessarily performing the procedure under direct guidance [38].

Lichtenstein suggested three sonographic criteria to ensure safe thoracentesis [39]:

1. Use the presence of a sinusoid sign to confirm the correct diagnosis of a pleural effusion.
2. Ensure an interpleural distance of 15 mm, visible over three adjacent intercostal spaces on full inspiration.
3. Ensure there is no interposition of the lung, aorta, heart, liver, or spleen, especially on inspiration.

11.7 Conclusion

The use of ultrasound in the intensive care unit and trauma bay allows for a fast and accurate evaluation of the causes of acute respiratory failure and shock. The routine use of ultrasound is an attractive alternative to other costly and time-consuming imaging modalities, i.e., CT scan as it is noninvasive, safe, and easily performed. The integration of lung ultrasound in the initial assessment of patients provides an advantageous diagnostic and monitoring tool in critical care and trauma settings that could further improve diagnosis and clinical management.

References

1. Lichtenstein D, Goldstein I, Mourgeon E, Cluzel P, Grenier P, Rouby JJ. Comparative diagnostic performances of auscultation, chest radiography, and lung ultrasonography in acute respiratory distress syndrome. Anesthesiology. 2004;100(1):9–15.
2. Knudtson JL, Dort JM, Helmer SD, Smith RS. Surgeon-performed ultrasound for pneumothorax in the trauma suite. J Trauma. 2004;56(3):527–30.
3. Eibenberger KL, Dock WI, Ammann ME, Dorffner R, Hörmann MF, Grabenwöger F. Quantification of pleural effusions: sonography versus radiography. Radiology. 1994;191(3):681–4.
4. Volpicelli G, Caramello V, Cardinale L, Mussa A, Bar F, Frascisco MF. Detection of sonographic B-lines in patients with normal lung or radiographic alveolar consolidation. Med Sci Monit. 2008;14(3):CR122–8.
5. Lichtenstein DA, Lascols N, Mezière G, Gepner A. Ultrasound diagnosis of alveolar consolidation in the critically ill. Intensive Care Med. 2004;30(2):276–81.
6. Reissig A, Heyne JP, Kroegel C. Sonography of lung and pleura in pulmonary embolism: sonomorphologic characterization and comparison with spiral CT scanning. Chest. 2001;120(6):1977–83.
7. Lichtenstein D, Mezière G, Biderman P, Gepner A. The "lung point": an ultrasound sign specific to pneumothorax. Intensive Care Med. 2000;26(10):1434–40.
8. Soldati G, Testa A, Silva FR, Carbone L, Portale G, Silveri NG. Chest ultrasonography in lung contusion. Chest. 2006;130(2):533–8.
9. Gillman LM, Kirkpatrick AW. Portable bedside ultrasound: the visual stethoscope of the 21st century. Scand J Trauma Resusc Emerg Med. 2012;20:18. https://doi.org/10.1186/1757-7241-20-18. Review.
10. Coşkun F, Akıncı E, Ceyhan MA, Sahin Kavaklı H. Our new stethoscope in the emergency department: handheld ultrasound. Ulus Travma Acil Cerrahi Derg. 2011;17(6):488–92. https://doi.org/10.5505/tjtes.2011.89914.
11. Neri L, Storti E, Lichtenstein D. Toward an ultrasound curriculum for critical care medicine. Crit Care Med. 2007;35(5 Suppl):S290–304.
12. Greenbaum DM, Marschall KE. The value of routine daily chest x-rays in intubated patients in the medical intensive care unit. Crit Care Med. 1982;10(1):29–30.
13. Lichtenstein DA, Mezière GA. Relevance of lung ultrasound in the diagnosis of acute respiratory failure: the BLUE protocol. Chest. 2008;134(1):117–25. https://doi.org/10.1378/chest.07-2800.
14. Lichtenstein DA. Chapter 20. Basic applications of lung ultrasound in the critically ill: 2—the ultra-

sound approach of an acute respiratory failure: the BLUE protocol. In: Lichtenstein DA, editor. Whole body ultrasonography in the critically ill. New York: Springer; 2016.
15. Lichtenstein DA. BLUE-protocol and FALLS-protocol: two applications of lung ultrasound in the critically ill. Chest. 2015;147(6):1659–70. https://doi.org/10.1378/chest.14-1313.
16. Lichtenstein DA. Lung ultrasound in the critically ill. Ann Intensive Care. 2014;4(1):1. https://doi.org/10.1186/2110-5820-4-1.
17. Lichtenstein DA, Mezière GA, Lagoueyte JF, Biderman P, Goldstein I, Gepner A. A-lines and B-lines: lung ultrasound as a bedside tool for predicting pulmonary artery occlusion pressure in the critically ill. Chest. 2009;136(4):1014–20. https://doi.org/10.1378/chest.09-0001.
18. Lichtenstein D, Karakitsos D. Integrating lung ultrasound in the hemodynamic evaluation of acute circulatory failure (the fluid administration limited by lung sonography protocol). J Crit Care. 2012;27(5):533. https://doi.org/10.1016/j.jcrc.2012.03.004.
19. Sakka SG, Klein M, Reinhart K, Meier-Hellmann A. Prognostic value of extravascular lung water in critically ill patients. Chest. 2002;122(6):2080–6.
20. Enghard P, Rademacher S, Nee J, Hasper D, Engert U, Jörres A, Kruse JM. Simplified lung ultrasound protocol shows excellent prediction of extravascular lung water in ventilated intensive care patients. Crit Care. 2015;19:36. https://doi.org/10.1186/s13054-015-0756-5.
21. Agricola E, Bove T, Oppizzi M, Marino G, Zangrillo A, Margonato A, Picano E. "Ultrasound comet-tail images": a marker of pulmonary edema: a comparative study with wedge pressure and extravascular lung water. Chest. 2005;127(5):1690–5.
22. Volpicelli G, Skurzak S, Boero E, Carpinteri G, Tengattini M, Stefanone V, Luberto L, Anile A, Cerutti E, Radeschi G, Frascisco MF. Lung ultrasound predicts well extravascular lung water but is of limited usefulness in the prediction of wedge pressure. Anesthesiology. 2014;121(2):320–7. https://doi.org/10.1097/ALN.0000000000000300.
23. Lichtenstein D, Mézière G, Biderman P, Gepner A, Barré O. The comet-tail artifact. An ultrasound sign of alveolar-interstitial syndrome. Am J Respir Crit Care Med. 1997;156(5):1640–6.
24. Jambrik Z, Monti S, Coppola V, Agricola E, Mottola G, Miniati M, Picano E. Usefulness of ultrasound lung comets as a nonradiologic sign of extravascular lung water. Am J Cardiol. 2004;93(10):1265–70.
25. Volpicelli G, Mussa A, Garofalo G, Cardinale L, Casoli G, Perotto F, Fava C, Frascisco M. Bedside lung ultrasound in the assessment of alveolar-interstitial syndrome. Am J Emerg Med. 2006;24(6):689–96.
26. Kirkpatrick AW, Sirois M, Laupland KB, Liu D, Rowan K, Ball CG, Hameed SM, Brown R, Simons R, Dulchavsky SA, Hamiilton DR, Nicolaou S. Hand-held thoracic sonography for detecting post-traumatic pneumothoraces: the extended focused assessment with sonography for trauma (EFAST). J Trauma. 2004;57(2):288–95.
27. Lichtenstein DA. Ultrasound in the management of thoracic disease. Crit Care Med. 2007;35(5 Suppl):S250–61.
28. Sisley AC, Rozycki GS, Ballard RB, Namias N, Salomone JP, Feliciano DV. Rapid detection of traumatic effusion using surgeon-performed ultrasonography. J Trauma. 1998;44(2):291–6; discussion 296–7.
29. Ku BS, Fields JM, Carr B, Everett WW, Gracias VH, Dean AJ. Clinician-performed beside ultrasound for the diagnosis of traumatic pneumothorax. West J Emerg Med. 2013;14(2):103–8. https://doi.org/10.5811/westjem.2012.12.12663.
30. Blaivas M, Lyon M, Duggal S. A prospective comparison of supine chest radiography and bedside ultrasound for the diagnosis of traumatic pneumothorax. Acad Emerg Med. 2005;12(9):844–9.
31. Rowan KR, Kirkpatrick AW, Liu D, Forkheim KE, Mayo JR, Nicolaou S. Traumatic pneumothorax detection with thoracic US: correlation with chest radiography and CT—initial experience. Radiology. 2002;225(1):210–4.
32. Targhetta R, Bourgeois JM, Chavagneux R, Marty-Double C, Balmes P. Ultrasonographic approach to diagnosing hydropneumothorax. Chest. 1992;101(4):931–4.
33. Targhetta R, Bourgeois JM, Chavagneux R, Balmes P. Diagnosis of pneumothorax by ultrasound immediately after ultrasonically guided aspiration biopsy. Chest. 1992;101(3):855–6.
34. Goodman TR, Traill ZC, Phillips AJ, Berger J, Gleeson FV. Ultrasound detection of pneumothorax. Clin Radiol. 1999;54(11):736–9.
35. Dulchavsky SA, Hamilton DR, Diebel LN, Sargsyan AE, Billica RD, Williams DR. Thoracic ultrasound diagnosis of pneumothorax. J Trauma. 1999;47(5):970–1.
36. Rozycki GS, Pennington SD, Feliciano DV. Surgeon-performed ultrasound in the critical care setting: its use as an extension of the physical examination to detect pleural effusion. J Trauma. 2001;50(4):636–42.
37. Jones PW, Moyers JP, Rogers JT, Rodriguez RM, Lee YC, Light RW. Ultrasound-guided thoracentesis: is it a safer method? Chest. 2003;123(2):418–23.
38. Lichtenstein DA. Chapter 15. Pleural effusion. In: Lichtenstein DA, editor. Whole body ultrasonography in the critically ill. New York: Springer; 2016.
39. Lichtenstein D, Hulot JS, Rabiller A, Tostivint I, Mezière G. Feasibility and safety of ultrasound-aided thoracentesis in mechanically ventilated patients. Intensive Care Med. 1999;25(9):955–8.

Ultrasound-Guided Procedures 12

Alexander P. Brueder, Samira Shojaee, and A. Christine Argento

12.1 Introduction

The first use of ultrasound as a diagnostic medical tool was by the Austrian neurologist Dr. Karl Theo Dussik, who first presented his work at Mount Sinai Hospital in 1951 and was able to successfully diagnose brain tumors and evaluate the ventricles [1].

Dr. Pell was the first to use ultrasound to examine the thorax of a patient with pleural effusion both before and after thoracentesis in 1964 [2]. In 1967, Dr. Joyner successfully used the ultrasound to accurately locate puncture sites for thoracentesis in 15 patients who had a diagnosis of a pleural effusion by chest roentgenography (CXR) [3].

Ultrasound has since evolved to identify many forms of pleural and parenchymal pathology. Ultrasound characteristics of pneumothorax were first described in 1986 [4]. Studies have since shown ultrasound is more sensitive than CXR and similar to our current gold standard, computerized tomography (CT) for evaluation of anatomy, pleural effusion, pneumothorax, and parenchymal lesions [5–10].

Currently, thoracic ultrasonography is invaluable in pulmonary medicine. It is readily available in most hospitals, portable, and accurate, provides immediate results, and imparts little to no risk to the patient in the hands of an experienced clinician. Newer technology with higher definition and smaller devices continues to increase ultrasound's breadth of utility [11, 12].

In this chapter, we will discuss the utility of ultrasound in pleural and pulmonary procedures. This chapter is organized into three sections: (1) Ultrasound-Guided Pleural Catheter Procedures, including thoracentesis, chest tube, and indwelling pleural catheters, (2) Ultrasound-Guided Needle Biopsy, and (3) Ultrasound-Guided Thoracoscopy.

A. P. Brueder
Section of Pulmonary and Critical Care, Department of Medicine, Northwestern University Feinberg School of Medicine, Chicago, IL, USA

S. Shojaee
Section of Pulmonary and Critical Care, Department of Medicine, Virginia Commonwealth University, Richmond, VA, USA
e-mail: samira.shojaee@vcuhealth.org

A. C. Argento (✉)
Section of Pulmonary and Critical Care, Department of Medicine, Northwestern University Feinberg School of Medicine, Chicago, IL, USA

Division of Pulmonary, Allergy and Critical Care Medicine, Northwestern University, Interventional Pulmonology, Chicago, IL, USA
e-mail: Angela.argento@nm.org, cargento@northwestern.edu

F. Feletti et al. (eds.), *Thoracic Ultrasound and Integrated Imaging*,
https://doi.org/10.1007/978-3-319-93055-8_12

12.2 Equipment

The three primary transducers used for the procedures are the linear (high frequency, 10–15 MHz, providing low penetration and high resolution), curvilinear (low frequency, 1–8 MHz, providing high penetration and low resolution), and phased array probes (5–7 MHz, with increased resolution at deeper penetration). See Figs. 12.1, 12.2, and 12.3. They all contain piezoelectric crystals but differ in crystal arrangement as well as in the size and shape of the imaging surface.

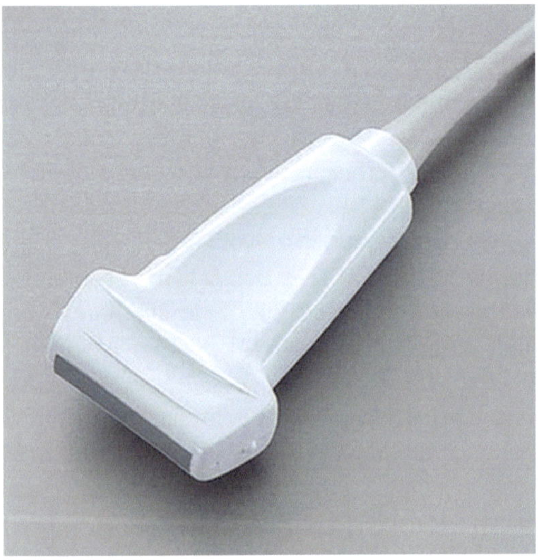

Fig. 12.1 Linear or high-frequency ultrasound probe

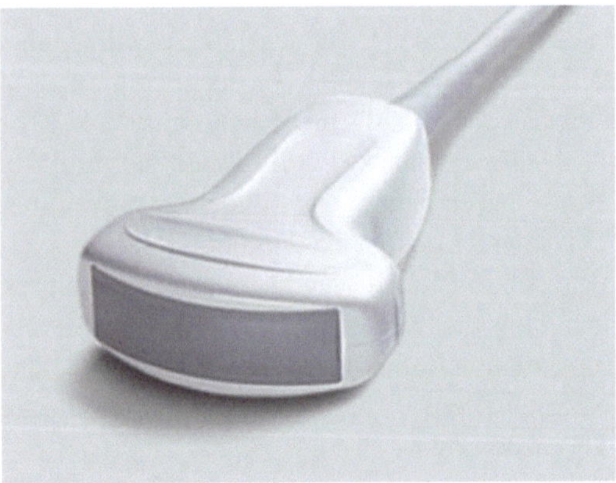

Fig. 12.2 Curvilinear or low-frequency ultrasound probe

All ultrasound probes have an indicator that corresponds to a dot on the screen. By convention, thoracic ultrasound places the dot on the upper left and the indicator on the probe oriented cephalad. Using a phased array probe with this setup will have the apices of the lungs on the left of the screen and the bases/diaphragm on the right (Fig. 12.4) [13].

12.3 Image Quality

There are several functions on every ultrasound that can be manipulated to assist with image quality. The first is depth. The depth is denoted by dashed lines that represent centimeters, typically found on the right side of the screen. The depth can be adjusted with the goal of having the target area in the middle of the screen. The second is gain. Changing the gain will change the brightness on the screen. It does not change the resolution or definition. Doppler is the third which can help distinguish soft tissue from vascular structures which can be helpful when selecting a procedural site [13]

12.4 Limitations

Although ultrasound can access most of the pleura (–70%), there are some areas difficult to visualize with ultrasound because of the bony

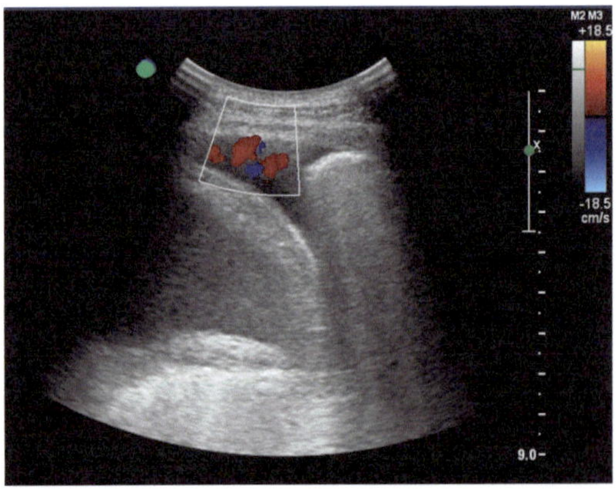

Fig. 12.3 Phased array ultrasound probe

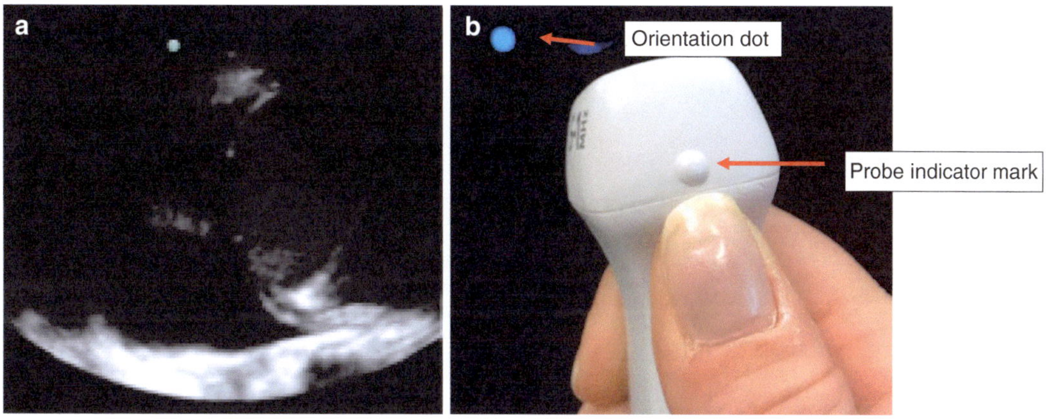

Fig. 12.4 Ultrasound image orientation. (**a**) The green dot indicates cephalad and corresponds to (**b**) the indicator on the ultrasound probe

thoracic cage [14]. A large body habitus can also preclude adequate visualization of structures with ultrasound.

Furthermore, because ultrasound waves do not travel through air, certain conditions with bullae or extensive subcutaneous air make it difficult to sonographically examine the pleural surface. This also, at times, limits the visualization of the normal lung parenchyma. Another potential limitation is in patients who have undergone pleurodesis or those who have trapped lung. Finally, ultrasound image acquisition and interpretation require operator skills and experience. The American College of Chest Physicians/Sociétè de Reanimation de Langue Française have published guidelines for thoracic ultrasound competence in pulmonary/critical care [15].

12.4.1 Ultrasound-Guided Pleural Catheter Procedures

12.4.1.1 Thoracentesis

Thoracentesis is percutaneous aspiration of the pleural space and is divided into two categories: diagnostic and therapeutic. Diagnostic thoracentesis is aspiration of a small volume of pleural fluid (10–100 cm^3) for the exclusive purpose of fluid analysis. In contrast, a therapeutic thoracentesis is aspiration of a larger volume of pleural fluid to achieve symptomatic relief, for assessment of lung parenchyma obscured secondary to a pleural effusion or, finally, for evacuation of an infected pleural space. Often, a procedure will be for both diagnostic and therapeutic purposes.

On ultrasound, a pleural effusion will appear as one of four different categories of pleural effusions based on ultrasound characteristics: echo-free, complex non-septated, complex septated, and homogeneous echogenic (Fig. 12.5a–d) [16–18]. It is important to distinguish echo-free from the latter three as studies have shown that the latter three patterns of effusion are always exudative, while echo-free effusions can be exudative or transudative [18]. In addition to characterizing the effusion, ultrasound can be effective in determining the quantity of fluid in the collection [19, 20].

Ultrasound to identify the puncture site immediately prior to a thoracentesis is now the standard of care [11, 12] as this has repeatedly shown a decrease in procedure-related complications and cost [21–24]. Another alternative that is equally effective would be to use real-time ultrasoundguidance and use the ultrasound with a sterile sheath (Fig. 12.6). On the contrary, using the "X marks the spot" technique where a patient is brought down to radiology, puncture site is marked with an X, and patient

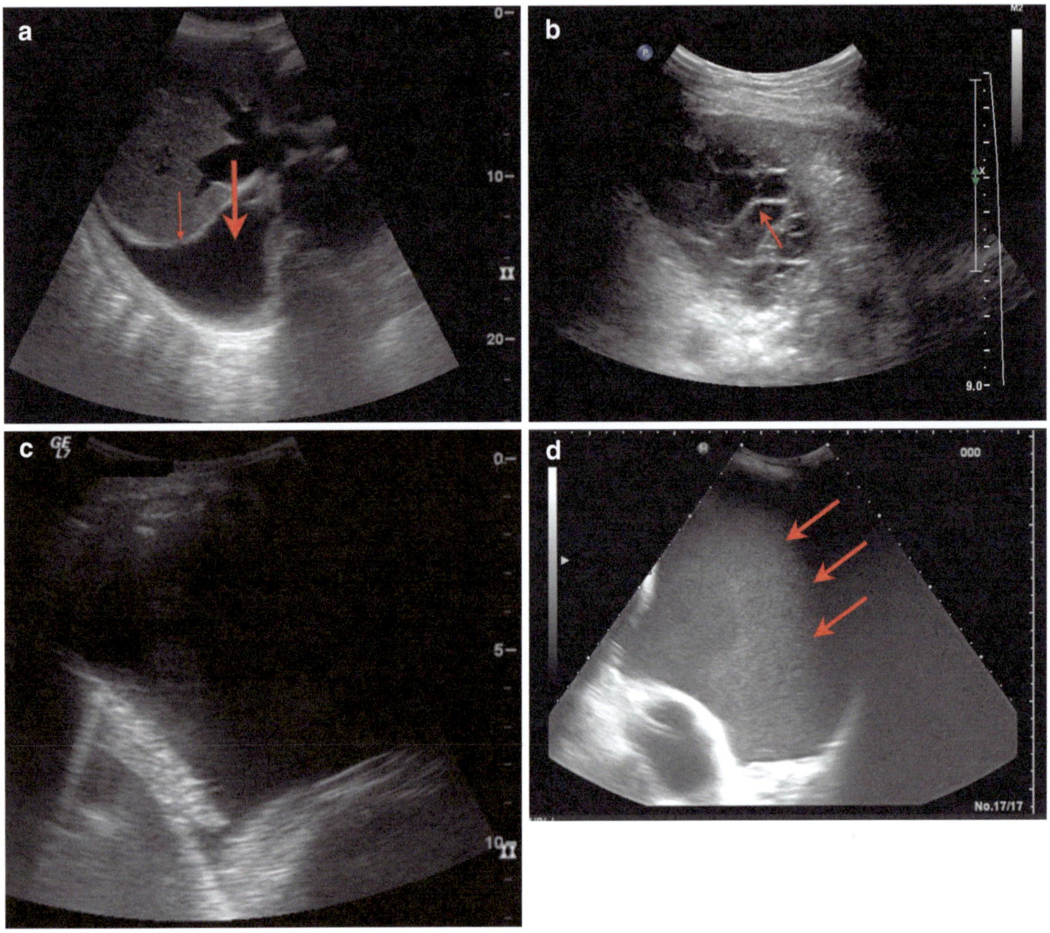

Fig. 12.5 (**a**) Simple, echo-free effusion with small arrow at the diaphragm and larger arrow indicating the effusion. (**b**) Complex-septated effusion where fibrinous strands (arrow) are seen in an otherwise hypoechoic space. (**c**) Complex non-septated effusion: echogenic spaces heterogeneously scatted in hypoechoic fluid. (**d**) Homogeneous echogenic effusion: homogeneously echogenic fluid that is sometimes difficult to distinguish from surrounding organs

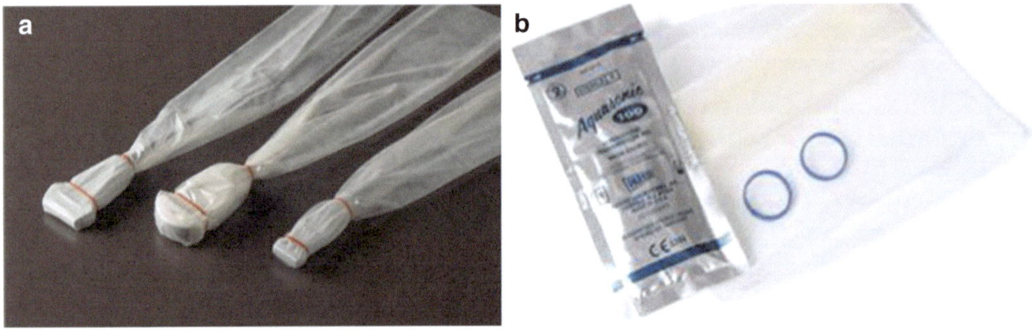

Fig. 12.6 (**a**) Sterile sheath/cover for use with all ultrasound probes; (**b**) the kit comes with sterile ultrasound gel, the sterile probe sheath/cover, and sterile elastic bands to keep the sheath/cover in place during use

is sent back to their room for a procedure at a later time has shown to have no improvement in pneumothorax rate compared to thoracentesis without ultrasound guidance [23]. Despite the evidence, the appropriate use of pre-procedural ultrasound guidance is still not universal. An audit by the British Thoracic Society (BTS) in 2013 showed that only 70% of pleural aspiration procedures used appropriate ultrasound guidance. This is an increase from 52% in the 2010 audit [12].

Indications

The indications for thoracentesis include any new, undiagnosed pleural effusion or a pleural effusion with a known cause that is causing symptoms such as dyspnea, fatigue, or pain.

Contraindications

There are no absolute contraindications to performing a thoracentesis. Relative contraindications to thoracentesis are increased risk of bleeding, skin lesions at the insertion site, and morbid obesity. Risk factors for bleeding include inherent disorders of coagulation or clot formation, renal dysfunction and patients who are therapeutically anticoagulation. There is mounting evidence to suggest, however, that a thoracentesis can safely be performed despite a risk of bleeding [25–28], though this has not yet been proven for all operators in large cohorts of patients, so this is to be done by experienced proceduralists with caution. See Tables 12.1 and 12.2 for guidelines on standard lab parameters and length of time to hold various anticoagulant medications prior to ultrasound-guided procedures.

Table 12.1 Ideal anticoagulation parameters for procedures; multiple abnormalities will likely increase the risk of bleeding complications

Procedure	INR	Platelet	BUN	Creatinine
Thoracentesis	<2	50	<50	<6
Chest tube-Seldinger				
Chest tube-blunt dissection or trocar	<1.5			
Indwelling pleural catheters				
Transthoracic needle biopsy				
Medical thoracoscopy				

Table 12.2 How long to hold medications prior to ultrasound-guided procedures

Medication	Time to hold with normal renal function	Time to hold with abnormal renal function	When to resume
ASA	Don't hold	7 days	12–24 h
Heparin	4.5–6 h	4.5–6 h	
LMWH	24 h	Should not be used in patients with renal failure	
Bivalirudin	2.5 h	5 h	
Argatroban	5 h	5 h	
Warfarin	5–7 days	5–7 days	
Clopidogrel	5–7 days	5–7 days	
Prasugrel	7 days	7 days	
Dabigatran	2 days	3 days	
Apixaban	2 days	2 days	
Rivaroxaban	2 days	Should not be used in patients with renal failure	
Edoxaban	2–3 days	2–3 days	
Ticagrelor	5 days	5 days	
NSAIDs	Controversial, 0–10 days	7–10 days	

LMWH low molecular weight heparin, *NSAIDs* nonsteroidal anti-inflammatory drugs
You should always consult with the prescribing physician prior to discontinuation of any medications that you are not managing

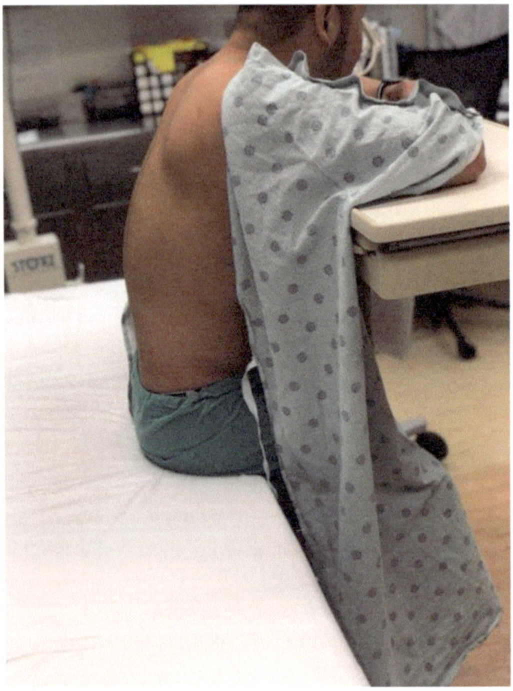

Fig. 12.7 Thoracentesis position (sitting)

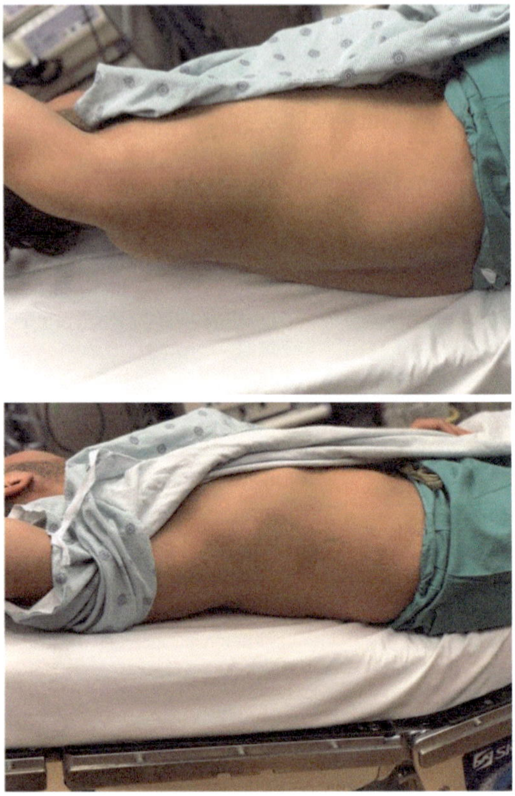

Fig. 12.8 Thoracentesis position (supine)

Technique

Thoracentesis is performed either at bedside or in a procedural suite. There are three options for optimal patient positioning. The first is to have the patient sitting on the edge of the bed with their arms and head resting on a table with one or more pillows (Fig. 12.7). This allows for the patient to sit comfortably and for free-flowing fluid to rest on the diaphragm in a gravity-dependent position. For patients that cannot sit up, they can lie supine, the head of the bed can be elevated, and the patient's ipsilateral arm secured above their head (Fig. 12.8). In this position, free-flowing effusions will rest on the posterior chest wall. The third option is to have the patient in the lateral decubitus position with the effusion side up.

Once consent is obtained, the patient is positioned appropriately, a time-out is performed, and the site of thoracentesis is either marked with ultrasound guidance, immediately cephalic to the superior edge of the rib, or the ultrasound probe is covered with a sterile sheath/cover in order to be used for real-time guidance of the needle. If marking the skin and not using real-time guidance, the mark can be made with either a marking pen (though this is often removed with the chlorhexidine or betadine used for cleaning) or by using pressure from the tip of a syringe or other sterile device to make a small indentation on the skin. The operator must take notice of the angle of the ultrasound when marking the patient, as this should be the angle of entry to the pleural space and perpendicular to the patient. The operator then undergoes aseptic precautions. The next focus is local anesthesia with lidocaine. The most sensitive areas encountered are the epidermal nerve endings, rib periosteum, and parietal pleura. The subcutaneous tissue is injected first using a finder needle on a 10 cm^3 syringe filled with lidocaine to create a "wheel" (Fig. 12.9). The finder needle is then withdrawn and several seconds allowed for the area to become appropriately numb. The operator should again palpate the superior edge of the rib or continue to moni-

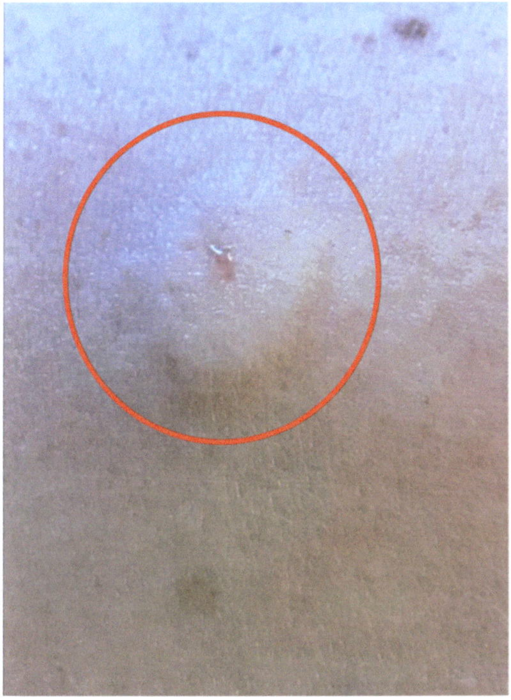

Fig. 12.9 Lidocaine wheel

tor with ultrasound. The site of entry of the finder needle should be at the same angle as the ultrasound and should be just above the rib. Using continuous aspiration, the needle is inserted until fluid is obtained. The rib periosteum should be avoided, but if it is contacted, the anesthetic can be injected and the needle readjusted to enter the pleural space above the rib. After fluid is obtained, the finder needle is withdrawn until fluid aspiration stops. That is the site of the sensitive parietal pleura and should be generously anesthetized with 5–10 cm^3 of lidocaine. The finder needle is then withdrawn.

If premarking the space and marking immediately prior to puncture rather than using continuous ultrasound guidance and obtaining the fluid is unsuccessful, the ultrasound probe should be covered with a sterile sheath/cover and used throughout the procedure to verify the location and direction of the needle under real-time guidance. The finder needle is then removed.

A small incision the width of the catheter is then made to facilitate entry through the skin. The catheter over a needle is then advanced through the same track as the finder needle, again using continuous aspiration, and can be directly observed with ultrasound. Once fluid is aspirated, the catheter and needle should be advanced another 1–2 mm. This allows the catheter tip to enter the pleural space. The catheter is then inserted fully into the pleural space using seldinger technique and the needle removed. The catheter is then attached to a drainage system. Manual aspiration of the pleural fluid is preferred over removal with a vacuum bottle as this creates less negative pressure and should lead to less cases of pain and re-expansion pulmonary edema and pneumothorax. Manual drainage also allows performance of manometry which can be done based on symptoms or more commonly at 200–250 mL increments of pleural fluid removal. There are three methods of performing pleural manometry. The first is with an electronic transducer (Fig. 12.10a). In this method, the electronic transducer is flushed with sterile saline and subsequently connected to the three-way stopcock using arterial line tubing. Using an IV pole with an adjustable clamp, the transducer is positioned level to the thoracentesis catheter insertion site. The transducer is then zeroed to atmospheric pressure and then allowed to take measurements.

The second method is using a U-tube manometer (Fig. 12.10b), whereby the thoracentesis catheter tubing is held perpendicular to the patient's back and the level is adjusted up or down from the thoracentesis catheter insertion site until the pleural fluid is free-flowing. The distance up (positive) or down (negative) from the thoracentesis catheter insertion site is then measured in centimeters, and you get a pleural pressure measurement in cm H_2O. The last method is using a digital pleural manometer (Fig. 12.10c) which is placed in line with the thoracentesis catheter and will produce a numeric display [29, 30]. The pleural pressures can be used to understand pleural physiology and are particularly useful when removing large volumes of fluid and plotting pleural pressure (*Y*-axis) and volume of pleural fluid removed (*X*-axis) to determine the slope of your elastance graph which will then allow you to determine if the patient has normal, entrapped, or trapped lung physiology. Once the

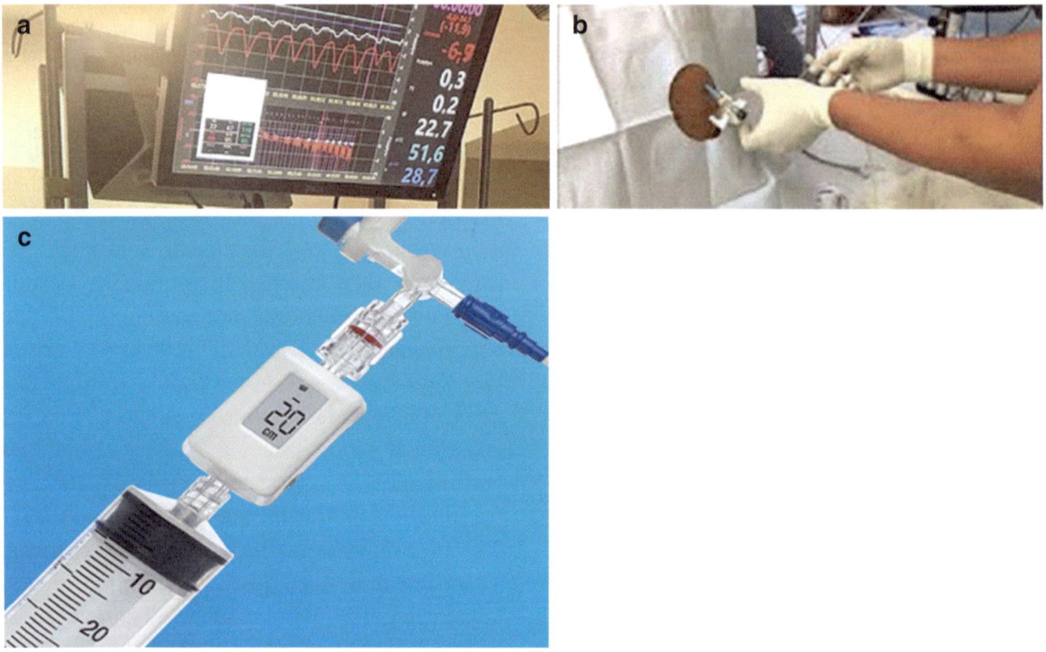

Fig. 12.10 (**a**) Electronic transducer, (**b**) U-tube manometer, (**c**) digital pleural manometer

drainage is complete, the operator should instruct the patient to perform a maneuver that increases intrathoracic pressure (such as a breath hold or continuous humming) as the catheter is removed and a bandage applied.

Complications

Diacon et al. showed that the precision of identifying the puncture site using physical exam and chest X-ray is suboptimal when compared with ultrasound use [21]. In their study, the planned location by exam and chest X-ray was verified with ultrasound performed by pulmonologists and showed that 15% of the time the marked location was inaccurate and 10% of the marked areas were over a solid organ.

Pneumothorax is the most common complication of thoracentesis. Other complications associated with thoracentesis are hemorrhage, infection, cough, chest pain, and injury to the liver, spleen, or kidneys. It is shown that the incidence of pneumothorax is much less when the procedure is guided with ultrasound [22–24].

Ultrasound-guided thoracentesis has shown to be a safer and more efficient method when compared with thoracentesis without ultrasound use. Ultrasound guidance results in a lower rate of pneumothorax and an overall more efficient procedure [21, 31].

Patel et al. in a retrospective study comparing 8824 thoracenteses without ultrasound and 10,510 thoracenteses with ultrasound found that the risk of pneumothorax was significantly lower in the ultrasound group (3.9% vs. 4.6%) [24]. Raptopoulos showed that the risk of pneumothorax dropped from 18 to 3% when ultrasound use was initiated. Air can enter the pleural space from the alveoli by injuring the lung tissue with the thoracentesis needle or if the pleural catheter is allowed to be open to the atmosphere while the patient is inhaling. Another less common occurrence is the presence of loculated air after thoracentesis, often in the setting of trapped lung where lung re-expansion is delayed and negative intrapleural pressure ensues [32]. Real-time pleural space manometry (described above) while draining the pleural fluid is thought to decrease the risk of pneumothorax ex vacuo by preventing pleural pressure decrements of −20 mm Hg [33–35].

Duncan and colleagues proposed a new practice model which included a group of pulmonologists with expertise in pleural diseases as instructors, ultrasound use for all thoracentesis, and structured proficiency and competency standards for training proceduralists [36]. Once implemented, they showed that the rate of iatrogenic pneumothorax decreased from 8.6 to 1.1%.

There is also sufficient evidence to show that routine chest X-ray is not necessary after each thoracentesis and a chest X-ray should only be obtained if the patient develops symptoms [37–39]. Jones and colleagues [40] showed that if patient is asymptomatic and a pneumothorax is not suspected, the likelihood of a pneumothorax requiring tube thoracostomy is low (3 in 907 cases).

Infection of the pleural space can result from thoracentesis if the procedure is not performed with strictly sterile technique, although in one study of 2489 thoracenteses, there were no reports of infection [41].

Hemothorax as a result of intercostal artery injury is another known complication of thoracentesis, especially in the older patient population where the path of the arteries is more tortuous and may be within the intercostal space as opposed to underneath the inferior aspect of the rib [42]. Risk of bleeding and alterations in coagulation are higher in patients with thrombocytopenia and those with renal dysfunction, particularly when creatinine is >6 mg/dL [26]. However, in one study of 321 patients with increased risk of bleeding, defined as platelet count <50,000, International Normalized Ratio (INR) > 1.5 with liver disease or on warfarin, and renal disease, no significant change in hematocrit was noted in pre-procedure and post-procedure testing [27]. In a study of 25 patients undergoing thoracentesis while on clopidogrel (Plavix), the risk of bleeding was noted to be low with one patient having a hemothorax requiring 2 units of blood transfusion. In larger randomized trials, the safety of thoracentesis in this patient population needs to be evaluated [25, 27].

Re-expansion pulmonary edema (REPE) is a rare but potentially fatal complication of thoracentesis as it could be accompanied by hypotension and hypoxemic respiratory failure [43]. REPE is thought to be secondary to rapid reinflation of the lung that has been collapsed due to pleural effusion or pneumothorax and can happen in approximately 0.2–1% per thoracentesis. In 1979, Pavlin and colleagues noted that REPE was more severe when rabbit lungs had been collapsed for a longer period of time and when pleural pressure dropped as low as −40 mmHg, while pleural pressure of more than −20 mmHg did not suffer from such severe edema [44]. By real-time measurement of pleural pressure throughout the procedure, one may be able to avoid REPE if a drop in pleural pressure below −20 mmHg is avoided or stopping the procedure if symptoms such as worsening chest pain or intractable cough develop when pleural manometry is not performed [40, 45].

12.4.1.2 Chest Tubes

Chest Tube

Tube thoracostomy is used to evacuate air or fluid from the pleural cavity. The first description of its use was in the fifth century BC for the treatment of empyema by Hippocrates [46]. Later, Trousseau was the first to develop a water-sealed drainage system in 1850 where the distal end of the drain was submerged in the fluid being drained. In 1867, Hiller adjusted the design to include an underwater seal drainage for children, though its widespread use was popularized in 1972 by Playfair. Hewett included the use of continuous chest drainage with a closed water-sealed system in 1876, and Bülau used the closed water-sealed drainage for empyema as early as 1875 and published his technique in 1891 [47, 48].

Indications

Indications for chest tube placement include pneumothorax, penetrating or blunt chest trauma, hemothorax, symptomatic pleural effusion, complicated parapneumonic effusion or empyema, and postoperative use in thoracic/cardiac surgery [49–51].

Contraindications

Contraindications to thoracostomy placement are all relative and include previous history of pleurodesis, patients at risk of bleeding, or patients with extensive pulmonary blebs or fibrosis.

Technique

Three techniques for chest tube placement are:

- Blunt dissection
- Seldinger technique
- Trocar

For all the three techniques, the patient is placed in the lateral decubitus position with the affected side facing upward. Sterile technique and ultrasound guidance should be utilized.

Blunt dissection is the traditional method of chest tube insertion and is often referred to as a "surgical chest tube." This includes making an incision in the skin parallel to the rib, dissecting down to the pleural space which is entered using a Kelly clamp. The pleural space is digitally palpated to ensure that there are no adhesions and that lung is felt, and then a chest tube is inserted with the use of the clamp into the desired position [11].

Seldinger technique is a stepwise approach whereby the pleural space is first accessed with a seeker needle through which a guidewire is inserted. The needle is removed, and sequential dilators are used over the guidewire until the chest tube can be inserted into the pleural space over the guidewire. Typically, a blunt stylet is used to stiffen the chest tube to improve entry into the pleural space. Once into the pleural space, the stylet is removed with the guidewire and the tube is secured.

Trocar method starts with a small incision in the skin after which the chest tube which has been loaded onto a sharp-tipped rod is inserted and pierces its way into the pleural space. Once in the pleural space, the trocar is removed and the tube is secured. This method has a higher risk of complications such as puncture of the lung and surrounding organs; thus it is not recommended [13].

Chest tubes should be inserted into the "triangle of safety," an area bordered anteriorly by the lateral border of the pectoralis major, posteriorly by the lateral border of the latissimus dorsi, and inferiorly by a horizontal line at the level of the fifth intercostal space [40, 52]. Staying in this triangle prevents injury to underlying vessels and organs. For pneumothorax, the tube is often aimed anterior and apically; for drainage of fluid, it is often directed posterior and basilarly. For loculated effusions, the chest tube placement may be dictated by the location of the fluid as identified on ultrasound. Although physical examination, fluoroscopy, and CT scan can be used to guide chest tube placement, ultrasound is becoming increasingly popular for guidance. Ultrasound improves successful placement of the chest tube, especially in loculated pockets of fluid [40, 53–56]. The BTS pleural disease guidelines strongly recommend the use of ultrasound guidance for chest tube placement [11]. Potential complications include abdominal, thoracic, or vascular injury, fistula formation, recurrent pneumothorax, insertion site infection, and nonfunctioning or malpositioned chest tubes [57].

Size of Chest Tube

French (Fr) is a unit of measurement first proposed by the French surgical instrument maker Joseph-Frederic-Benoit Charrie in the 1800s. Fr refers to the outer diameter of the cylindrical tube. A unit of Fr is equivalent to 0.333 mm [58]. Small-bore chest tubes are those that are 14 Fr or smaller, and large-bore chest tubes are those larger than 14 Fr. Chest tubes come in a variety of sizes based on the external diameter, ranging from 6 to 40 Fr, and they may be straight or coiled at the end ("pigtailed").

It was initially thought that large-bore chest tubes are needed to drain anything other than simple fluid, but more recent data contradict this notion and would support a trial of small-bore chest tube initially for most indications and progressing to a large-bore chest tube only if the small one fails. The small-bore catheters have lower flow rates, so a larger-bore tube should be utilized when large air leaks are expected such as with patients on mechanical ventilation [59]. In a series of 1092 patients with size 12 Fr catheters placed for benign or malignant pleural effusion or pneumothorax, Cafarotti et al. found them to be safe, effective, and less painful than larger-bore chest tubes. They did note that, in the case of empyema, these tubes were often obstructed and required exchange for a larger-bore chest tube [60]. However, other groups have maintained successful drainage and catheter patency if the tube is flushed with saline regularly [61].

With respect to chest tube complications, the incidence of injury with large-bore versus small-bore tube was 1.4% versus 0.2%. The incidence of malposition was 6.5% versus 0.6%, while the incidence of empyema was 1.4% versus 0.2%. However, the incidence of catheter obstruction was 5.2% with large tubes, while it was 8.1% with small tubes [62].

Indwelling Pleural Catheters

Indwelling pleural catheters (IPC) are tunneled, fenestrated, silicone catheters that terminate at the distal end with a one-way valve. First approved by the FDA in 1997, they offer a long-term solution for pleural access in patients that require intermittent pleural drainage. These catheters were initially developed for patients with malignant pleural effusion (MPE) who could not tolerate surgical pleurodesis or who failed a prior pleurodesis attempt. More recent data, however, has questioned the efficacy and safety of talc pleurodesis with a trend toward using IPCs as a first-line therapy [63]. The concerns of pleurodesis and preference for use of an IPC are well outlined by Lui et al. They include:

1. A significant proportion of patients with MPE do not have an expandable lung.
2. The rate of failure of pleurodesis in patients who do have an expandable lung.
3. More hospital days required for surgical pleurodesis.
4. Increased inflammation created as a result of pleurodesis [64].

Finally, IPC are the only option for management of symptomatic, recurrent effusions in patients with trapped lung [64].

Indications

IPC is indicated for the intermittent, long-term drainage of any recurrent, symptomatic pleural effusion, including MPE. There is some evidence even for its use in congestive heart failure. Herlihy et al. reported their experience with five patients who received an IPC for congestive heart failure. The patients overall had improvement in New York Heart Association functional class and quality of life. There were, however, complications with loculated effusions as well as an empyema [65].

Technique

The procedure can be performed as an inpatient or outpatient with or without sedation. With the patient in the lateral decubitus position and the ipsilateral arm raised, the insertion site, typically in the fifth to seventh intercostal space in the anterior or mid axillary line, is identified, marked, and confirmed with ultrasound. Another site is then marked 5 cm anterior and inferior to the insertion site as the exit site for the catheter. Using sterile technique, local anesthesia is used with lidocaine similar to thoracentesis and chest tube insertion. A tunnel is created between the insertion and exit sites of the skin and also anesthetized with lidocaine. A seeker needle is inserted into the pleural space, above the rib, and the periosteum and parietal pleura are anesthetized as well with lidocaine. Once fluid is found, a 1 cm incision at both the insertion and exit site is created with the scalpel. A 16-gauge needle is then introduced into the pleural space just superior to the rib. A guidewire is introduced through the needle, and the needle is removed while the wire is left in place. The IPC is then attached to a tunneling device and is tunneled from the exit site to the insertion site. Sequential dilators are used over the guidewire, and finally a "peel-away" sheath is then inserted into the pleural space using a dilator through which the IPC is introduced. It is important all the fenestrations on the IPC are within the pleural space. The "peel-away" catheter is then removed, and the insertion and exit sites are sutured with a sterile dressing then applied.

Complications

Complications related to IPC can be divided into two categories: those related to insertion and those related to the catheter itself. The complications related to insertion are the same as for thoracentesis and chest tube, described in detail above.

While IPC are generally well tolerated, there are some complications that must be reviewed. The first is IPC-related pleural infection. A large, 11 center reviews of 1021 patients with IPC found an infection rate of 4.8% [66]. In this study, infections were typically mild, with a mortality <1%. Most infections resolve with antibiotics, and the IPC generally does not require removal in case of infection, though larger studies are needed to confirm this result [67]. Similar to non-tunneled chest tubes, intrapleural t-PA and DNase can be inserted to help clear the infection [66].

Another concern is the potential for catheter tract metastasis (CTM). Patients will typically present with a new subcutaneous mass near the insertion site. The incidence of CTM varies widely between different studies, which could be related to the difference in the primary malignancies in the studies, and treatment is a dose of localized radiation to the area [64].

Other complications include symptomatic loculations whereby occasionally patients require additional fluid drainage with thoracentesis or chest tube placement. Fracture upon removal of the catheter is rare but can necessitate another incision or surgical removal. Catheter blockage happens intermittently with some frequency, particularly if the pleural fluid is proteinaceous, and lytics can be used to re-establish patency. Finally, chest pain that can be temporary or long-lasting, usually mild, and will improve with either local heat or cold therapy but on rare occasions requires narcotics for symptomatic relief.

12.4.2 Ultrasound-Guided Needle Biopsy

Ultrasound-guided needle placement for biopsy of thoracic lesions was first described by Chandrasekhar et al. in 1976 [68]. Multiple studies were performed in the 1990s that increased its validity [69–77]. The obvious advantages of using ultrasonography are decreased radiation exposure, real-time evaluation of respiratory excursion, and flexibility to be performed either in a procedural suite or at the bedside. Despite these advantages, the bias remains toward using CT or fluoroscopic guidance for peripherally located or pleural lesions [78]. Multiple studies have suggested these modalities are equivalent, but others have shown ultrasound-guided procedures to be superior. One recent study by Jarmakani et al. showed that ultrasound-guided procedures derived a definitive diagnosis in 98% of patients (54 of 55) versus 87% (113 of 130) in CT-guided procedures. The rate of pneumothorax requiring treatment was also lower in the ultrasound group (2% vs. 5%) [79].

12.4.2.1 Indications

There are many indications for diagnostic ultrasound-guided percutaneous needle biopsy of the thorax:

- First, peripheral pulmonary nodules or masses identified on CT where there is a low chance the needle would have to traverse a significant amount of aerated lung. Success rates range from 89 to 98% with relatively low complication rates [74, 80, 81].
- Next, masses of the anterior, superior, and posterior mediastinum. For anterior mediastinal masses, they must extend lateral to the parasternal region to be accessed using this technique. Posterior mediastinal masses must extend laterally, posteriorly, and abut the pleura. Most superior mediastinal masses are easily accessible. Success rates for mediastinal masses range from 71 to 100% again with low complication rates [70, 82–86].
- Other indications are lesions of either the pleura or chest wall.

12.4.2.2 Contraindications

Centrally located lesions that are surrounded by aerated lung are better accessed by CT guidance or bronchoscopically rather than by transthoracic ultrasound guidance. Ultrasound waves do not penetrate the aerated lung very well and make visualization difficult if not impossible when there is no acoustic window generated by either adjacent pleural fluid or atelectasis. Coagulopathy is another contraindication and should be corrected prior to the procedure.

12.4.2.3 Technique

Ultrasound-guided transthoracic biopsies are typically performed by interventional radiologists or interventional pulmonologists. All patients should have a pre-biopsy CT so that the most accessible lesion for biopsy can be identified as well as the most appropriate technique and trajectory selected.

Two techniques for needle insertion are freehand guidance and the use of a needle guide. This is largely based on experience and preference. A needle guide allows a more predictable needle path but decreases flexibility. Figure 12.11a–d shows the needle guide and the accessory kit that comes with it.

Patient positioning is determined by the location of the lesion. Needle size is determined by type of biopsy (fine-needle aspiration or core biopsy). Moderate sedation with local analgesia is most commonly used though some cases require general anesthesia.

The ultrasound probe should be oriented parallel to the intercostal space. This minimizes rib shadowing and allows better needle visualization. Linear, curvilinear, and phased array ultrasound transducers can all be used. The linear and curvilinear probes have higher resolution proximally, which provide better visualization of the shallow structures; however, they have a larger footprint. This forces a steeper angle of the needle to the lesion. The phased array probe has a smaller footprint but decreased resolution. Some proceduralists will use a combination of two

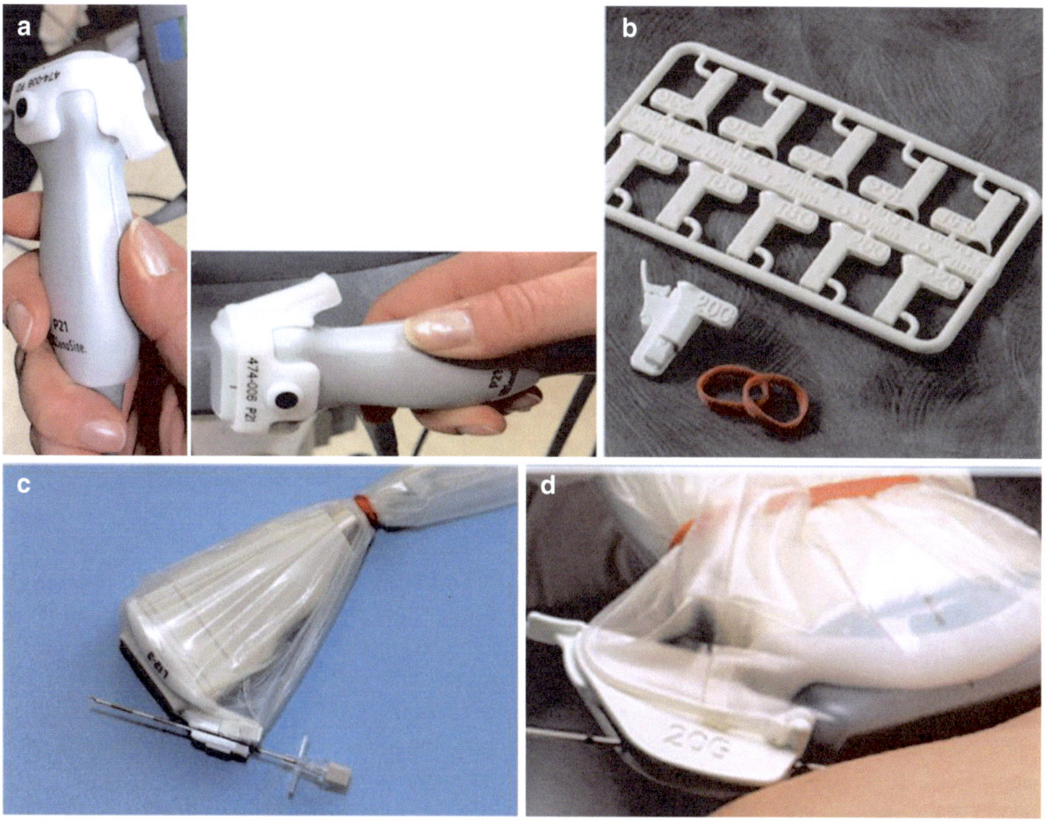

Fig. 12.11 (**a**) Ultrasound probe with needle guide. (**b**) Kit for the needle guide that comes with adapters for various needle types; (**c**, **d**) ultrasound probe with needle guide and needle attached with sterile sheath as would be used for ultrasound-guided needle aspiration or core needle biopsy

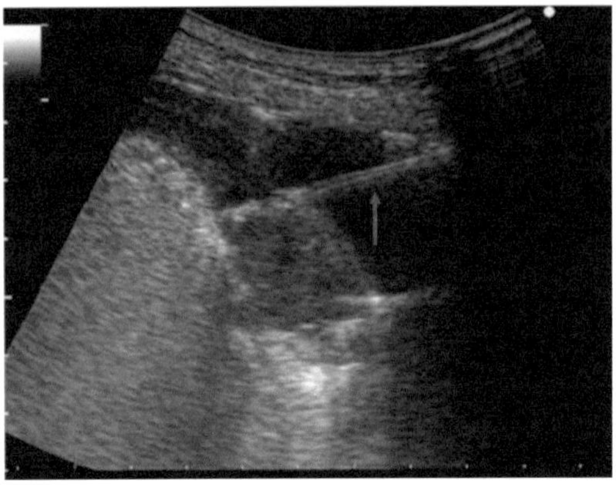

Fig. 12.12 Transthoracic ultrasound-guided needle biopsy demonstrating the needle (arrow) in the lesion

probes. The needle is advanced into the lesion under direct visualization for biopsy, and often several passes are performed (Fig. 12.12).

12.4.2.4 Complications

Complications, as stated above, occur in less than 5% of patients. The most common is pneumothorax followed by hemoptysis. Very rarely, these require intervention and/or transfer to an ICU for monitoring [75–77, 79–81, 84–86].

12.4.3 Ultrasound-Guided Thoracoscopy

Direct visualization of the parietal pleura or thoracic wall for biopsy can be accomplished with thoracoscopy performed with local anesthesia, designated medical thoracoscopy (MT), or with video-assisted thoracoscopic surgery (VATS), typically performed under general anesthesia.

MT is used for the diagnosis and treatment of a variety of pleural diseases, benign or malignant. MT was first used as a tool to diagnose and treat tuberculosis. Jacobaeus, sometimes called "the father of thoracoscopy," used a thoracoscope to induce a pneumothorax as well as to lyse adhesions [87]. This practice largely ended in the 1950s with the advent of anti-mycobacterial medications; however the indications for MT have continued to expand since that time.

Ultrasonography was first used in conjunction with MT by Macha et al. in 1992. Prior to this, if there was not a significant pleural effusion, to facilitate safe entry of the trocar into the pleural space, a pneumothorax was induced which took approximately 20–30 min. This had to be confirmed with fluoroscopy or chest roentgenography prior to starting the procedure. Macha et al. were the first to use ultrasound to safely find an entry point in 687 cases without requiring pneumothorax induction and with avoidance of areas of adhesion [88]. In 2003, this use was expanded by Hersh et al., and ultrasound was used to safely identify entry sites for MT even in the presence of adhesions [89]. Finally, in 2015 Marchetti et al. published a series whereby even patients without pleural effusion could have a safe entry point identified using ultrasound for MT to obtain pleural biopsies [90].

12.4.3.1 Indications

The indications for MT can be divided into diagnostic and therapeutic. Diagnostic indications include pleural effusions that remain undiagnosed despite less invasive measures such as thoracentesis. Valsecchi et al. performed a 30-year retrospective review of 2752 thoracoscopies performed at their institution and found an overall diagnostic yield of 71% [89]. In that series, more than half were diagnostic of cancer with malignant pleural mesothelioma and lung cancer metastases being the two most common [91]. Tuberculosis was the most common benign disease but was much less common due to the high diagnostic yield of less invasive measures [92]. Since then, diagnostic yield has improved further and is reported more recently from 89 to 95% [93, 94].

The most common therapeutic indication for MT is for drainage of a recurrent pleural effusion, most commonly malignant, with pleurodesis via talc poudrage. Otherwise, MT can be used for lysis of adhesions and loculations. Success rates for therapeutic indications are variable, and there is a trend toward using indwelling pleural catheters as a first line.

12.4.3.2 Contraindications

Dense adhesions can prevent exploration of the pleural space and thus are the most common contraindication to MT [90]. Other contraindications include the inability to lie flat, severe cardiac disease, and coagulopathy [95].

12.4.3.3 Technique

Ultrasonography prior to MT should include evaluation of the pleural space, size of pleural effusion, diaphragm location, as well as evidence of pleural sliding. Lack of pleural sliding classically is a sign of pneumothorax; however, in the study by Cassanelli et al., they were able to demonstrate that visceral sliding less than 2 cm had a sensitivity of 80.6% and a specificity of 96.1% for identification of pleural adhesions [96].

Once a safe location that is free from adhesions is determined and marked, the patient is sterilely prepped and draped. A 10 mm incision is made over the superior edge of the rib. Blunt dissection is performed with hemostats down through the parietal pleura. A trocar is then placed, taking care to avoid the lung. The thoracoscope is then inserted via the trocar. Pleural fluid is evacuated; biopsies can be obtained from the parietal pleura or the chest wall. Talc poudrage is then often performed. The procedure is completed, and most patients are discharged home the same or the following day.

12.4.3.4 Complications

When performed by experienced clinicians, complication rates from MT are very low with mortality <0.1% and empyema 2–3% [97–100]. Brims et al. performed a 12-month retrospective review of their thoracoscopies and found a rate of hospital-acquired infection (HAI) in 10.5% of patients [101]. Other complications include persistent air leak as well as subcutaneous emphysema. The most common complaint post procedure is chest wall pain at the site of trocar insertion.

12.5 Conclusions

Thoracic ultrasonography is safe, relatively inexpensive, portable, and superior to chest radiographs and chest CT scans for real-time procedure guidance and examination of the pleura. Training has become a part of pulmonary and critical care medicine programs in many universities around the world and particularly in the USA as ultrasound-guided procedures have become a part of ACGME requirements. The new generation of pulmonary and critical care specialists will hopefully have a much broader and consistent exposure to ultrasound use to elevate their pleural and thoracic procedural skills.

References

1. Shampo MA, Kyle RA. Karl Theodore Dussik—pioneer in ultrasound. Mayo Clin Proc. 1995;70:1136.
2. Pell R. Ultrasound for routine clinical investigation. Ultrasonics. 1964;2:87–9.
3. Joyner CR Jr, Herman RJ, Reid JM. Reflected ultrasound in the detection and localization of pleural effusion. JAMA. 1967;200:399–402.
4. Rantanen NW. Diseases of the thorax. Vet Clin North Am Equine Pract. 1986;2:49–66.
5. Alrajhi K, Woo MY, Vaillancourt C. Test characteristics of ultrasonography for the detection of pneumothorax: a systematic review and meta-analysis. Chest. 2012;141:703–8.
6. Lichtenstein D, Meziere G. A lung ultrasound sign allowing bedside distinction between pulmonary edema and COPD: the comet-tail artifact. Intensive Care Med. 1998;24:1331–4.
7. Lichtenstein D, Meziere G, Biderman P, Gepner A. The comet-tail artifact: an ultrasound sign ruling out pneumothorax. Intensive Care Med. 1999;25:383–8.
8. Lichtenstein D, Meziere G, Biderman P, Gepner A. The "lung point": an ultrasound sign specific to pneumothorax. Intensive Care Med. 2000;26:1434–40.
9. Rowan KR, Kirkpatrick AW, Liu D, Forkheim KE, Mayo JR, Nicolaou S. Traumatic pneumothorax detection with thoracic US: correlation with chest radiography and CT—initial experience. Radiology. 2002;225:210–4.
10. Soldati G, Testa A, Sher S, Pignataro G, La Sala M, Silveri NG. Occult traumatic pneumothorax: diagnostic accuracy of lung ultrasonography in the emergency department. Chest. 2008;133:204–11.
11. Havelock T, Teoh R, Laws D, Gleeson F, Group BTSPDG. Pleural procedures and thoracic ultrasound: British Thoracic Society pleural disease guideline 2010. Thorax. 2010;65(Suppl 2):ii61–76.
12. Hooper CE, Welham SA, Maskell NA, British Thoracic Society. Pleural procedures and patient safety: a national BTS audit of practice. Thorax. 2015;70:189–91.
13. Shojaee S, Argento AC. Ultrasound-guided pleural access. Semin Respir Crit Care Med. 2014;35:693–705.
14. Mathis G. [Thoraxsonography—part 1: chest wall and pleura]. Praxis (Bern 1994). 2004;93:615–21.

15. Mayo PH, Beaulieu Y, Doelken P, Feller-Kopman D, Harrod C, Kaplan A, Oropello J, Vieillard-Baron A, Axler O, Lichtenstein D, Maury E, Slama M, Vignon P. American College of Chest Physicians/La Societe de reanimation de langue Francaise statement on competence in critical care ultrasonography. Chest. 2009;135:1050–60.
16. Koenig SJ, Narasimhan M, Mayo PH. Thoracic ultrasonography for the pulmonary specialist. Chest. 2011;140:1332–41.
17. Light RW. Pleural diseases. Curr Opin Pulm Med. 2003;9:251–3.
18. Yang PC, Luh KT, Chang DB, Wu HD, Yu CJ, Kuo SH. Value of sonography in determining the nature of pleural effusion: analysis of 320 cases. AJR Am J Roentgenol. 1992;159:29–33.
19. Balik M, Plasil P, Waldauf P, Pazout J, Fric M, Otahal M, Pachl J. Ultrasound estimation of volume of pleural fluid in mechanically ventilated patients. Intensive Care Med. 2006;32:318–21.
20. Roch A, Bojan M, Michelet P, Romain F, Bregeon F, Papazian L, Auffray JP. Usefulness of ultrasonography in predicting pleural effusions > 500 mL in patients receiving mechanical ventilation. Chest. 2005;127:224–32.
21. Diacon AH, Brutsche MH, Soler M. Accuracy of pleural puncture sites: a prospective comparison of clinical examination with ultrasound. Chest. 2003;123:436–41.
22. Patel PA, Ernst FR, Gunnarsson CL. Ultrasonography guidance reduces complications and costs associated with thoracentesis procedures. J Clin Ultrasound. 2012;40:135–41.
23. Raptopoulos V, Davis LM, Lee G, Umali C, Lew R, Irwin RS. Factors affecting the development of pneumothorax associated with thoracentesis. AJR Am J Roentgenol. 1991;156:917–20.
24. Wrightson JM, Fysh E, Maskell NA, Lee YC. Risk reduction in pleural procedures: sonography, simulation and supervision. Curr Opin Pulm Med. 2010;16:340–50.
25. Mahmood K, Shofer SL, Moser BK, Argento AC, Smathers EC, Wahidi MM. Hemorrhagic complications of thoracentesis and small-bore chest tube placement in patients taking clopidogrel. Ann Am Thorac Soc. 2014;11:73–9.
26. McVay PA, Toy PT. Lack of increased bleeding after paracentesis and thoracentesis in patients with mild coagulation abnormalities. Transfusion. 1991;31:164–71.
27. Puchalski JT, Argento AC, Murphy TE, Araujo KL, Pisani MA. The safety of thoracentesis in patients with uncorrected bleeding risk. Ann Am Thorac Soc. 2013;10:336–41.
28. Patel MD, Joshi SD. Abnormal preprocedural international normalized ratio and platelet counts are not associated with increased bleeding complications after ultrasound-guided thoracentesis. AJR Am J Roentgenol. 2011;197:W164–8.
29. Lee HJ, Yarmus L, Kidd D, Ortiz R, Akulian J, Gilbert C, Hughes A, Thompson RE, Arias S, Feller-Kopman D. Comparison of pleural pressure measuring instruments. Chest. 2014;146:1007–12.
30. Walter JM, Matthay MA, Gillespie CT, Corbridge T. Acute hypoxemic respiratory failure after large-volume thoracentesis. Mechanisms of pleural fluid formation and reexpansion pulmonary edema. Ann Am Thorac Soc. 2016;13:438–43.
31. Gordon CE, Feller-Kopman D, Balk EM, Smetana GW. Pneumothorax following thoracentesis: a systematic review and meta-analysis. Arch Intern Med. 2010;170:332–9.
32. Ponrartana S, Laberge JM, Kerlan RK, Wilson MW, Gordon RL. Management of patients with "ex vacuo" pneumothorax after thoracentesis. Acad Radiol. 2005;12:980–6.
33. Feller-Kopman D. Therapeutic thoracentesis: the role of ultrasound and pleural manometry. Curr Opin Pulm Med. 2007;13:312–8.
34. Feller-Kopman D, Berkowitz D, Boiselle P, Ernst A. Large-volume thoracentesis and the risk of reexpansion pulmonary edema. Ann Thorac Surg. 2007;84:1656–61.
35. Feller-Kopman D, Walkey A, Berkowitz D, Ernst A. The relationship of pleural pressure to symptom development during therapeutic thoracentesis. Chest. 2006;129:1556–60.
36. Duncan DR, Morgenthaler TI, Ryu JH, Daniels CE. Reducing iatrogenic risk in thoracentesis: establishing best practice via experiential training in a zero-risk environment. Chest. 2009;135:1315–20.
37. Aleman C, Alegre J, Armadans L, Andreu J, Falco V, Recio J, Cervera C, Ruiz E, Fernandez de Sevilla T. The value of chest roentgenography in the diagnosis of pneumothorax after thoracentesis. Am J Med. 1999;107:340–3.
38. Capizzi SA, Prakash UB. Chest roentgenography after outpatient thoracentesis. Mayo Clin Proc. 1998;73:948–50.
39. Doyle JJ, Hnatiuk OW, Torrington KG, Slade AR, Howard RS. Necessity of routine chest roentgenography after thoracentesis. Ann Intern Med. 1996;124:816–20.
40. Jones PW, Moyers JP, Rogers JT, Rodriguez RM, Lee YC, Light RW. Ultrasound-guided thoracentesis: is it a safer method? Chest. 2003;123:418–23.
41. Cervini P, Hesley GK, Thompson RL, Sampathkumar P, Knudsen JM. Incidence of infectious complications after an ultrasound-guided intervention. AJR Am J Roentgenol. 2010;195:846–50.
42. Carney M, Ravin CE. Intercostal artery laceration during thoracocentesis: increased risk in elderly patients. Chest. 1979;75:520–2.
43. Tarver RD, Broderick LS, Conces DJ Jr. Reexpansion pulmonary edema. J Thorac Imaging. 1996;11:198–209.
44. Pavlin J, Cheney FW Jr. Unilateral pulmonary edema in rabbits after reexpansion of collapsed lung. J Appl Physiol Respir Environ Exerc Physiol. 1979;46:31–5.

45. Cantey EP, Walter JM, Corbridge T, Barsuk JH. Complications of thoracentesis: incidence, risk factors, and strategies for prevention. Curr Opin Pulm Med. 2016;22:378–85.
46. Christopoulou-Aletra H, Papavramidou N. "Empyemas" of the thoracic cavity in the Hippocratic corpus. Ann Thorac Surg. 2008;85:1132–4.
47. Hewett FC. Thoracentesis: the plan of continuous aspiration. Br Med J. 1876;1:317.
48. Light RW, Lee YCG. Textbook of pleural diseases. London: Arnold; 2003.
49. Gayer G, Rozenman J, Hoffmann C, Apter S, Simansky DA, Yellin A, Itzchak Y. CT diagnosis of malpositioned chest tubes. Br J Radiol. 2000;73:786–90.
50. Millikan JS, Moore EE, Steiner E, Aragon GE, Van Way CW 3rd. Complications of tube thoracostomy for acute trauma. Am J Surg. 1980;140:738–41.
51. Tang AT, Velissaris TJ, Weeden DF. An evidence-based approach to drainage of the pleural cavity: evaluation of best practice. J Eval Clin Pract. 2002;8:333–40.
52. Mahmood K, Wahidi MM. Straightening out chest tubes: what size, what type, and when. Clin Chest Med. 2013;34:63–71.
53. Mayo PH, Goltz HR, Tafreshi M, Doelken P. Safety of ultrasound-guided thoracentesis in patients receiving mechanical ventilation. Chest. 2004;125:1059–62.
54. Moulton JS. Image-guided management of complicated pleural fluid collections. Radiol Clin North Am. 2000;38:345–74.
55. Silverman SG, Mueller PR, Saini S, Hahn PF, Simeone JF, Forman BH, Steiner E, Ferrucci JT. Thoracic empyema: management with image-guided catheter drainage. Radiology. 1988;169:5–9.
56. vanSonnenberg E, Nakamoto SK, Mueller PR, Casola G, Neff CC, Friedman PJ, Ferrucci JT Jr, Simeone JF. CT- and ultrasound-guided catheter drainage of empyemas after chest-tube failure. Radiology. 1984;151:349–53.
57. Kwiatt M, Tarbox A, Seamon MJ, Swaroop M, Cipolla J, Allen C, Hallenbeck S, Davido HT, Lindsey DE, Doraiswamy VA, Galwankar S, Tulman D, Latchana N, Papadimos TJ, Cook CH, Stawicki SP. Thoracostomy tubes: a comprehensive review of complications and related topics. Int J Crit Illn Inj Sci. 2014;4:143–55.
58. Cooke DT, David EA. Large-bore and small-bore chest tubes: types, function, and placement. Thorac Surg Clin. 2013;23:17–24, v.
59. Baumann MH, Patel PB, Roney CW, Petrini MF. Comparison of function of commercially available pleural drainage units and catheters. Chest. 2003;123:1878–86.
60. Cafarotti S, Dall'Armi V, Cusumano G, Margaritora S, Meacci E, Lococo F, Vita ML, Porziella V, Bonassi S, Cesario A, Granone P. Small-bore wire-guided chest drains: safety, tolerability, and effectiveness in pneumothorax, malignant effusions, and pleural empyema. J Thorac Cardiovasc Surg. 2011;141:683–7.
61. Rahman NM, Maskell NA, West A, Teoh R, Arnold A, Mackinlay C, Peckham D, Davies CW, Ali N, Kinnear W, Bentley A, Kahan BC, Wrightson JM, Davies HE, Hooper CE, Lee YC, Hedley EL, Crosthwaite N, Choo L, Helm EJ, Gleeson FV, Nunn AJ, Davies RJ. Intrapleural use of tissue plasminogen activator and DNase in pleural infection. N Engl J Med. 2011;365:518–26.
62. Light RW. Pleural controversy: optimal chest tube size for drainage. Respirology. 2011;16:244–8.
63. Fysh ET, Tan SK, Read CA, Lee F, McKenzie K, Olsen N, Weerasena I, Threlfall T, de Klerk N, Musk AW, Lee YC. Pleurodesis outcome in malignant pleural mesothelioma. Thorax. 2013;68:594–6.
64. Lui MM, Thomas R, Lee YC. Complications of indwelling pleural catheter use and their management. BMJ Open Respir Res. 2016;3:e000123.
65. Herlihy JP, Loyalka P, Gnananandh J, Gregoric ID, Dahlberg CG, Kar B, Delgado RM 3rd. PleurX catheter for the management of refractory pleural effusions in congestive heart failure. Tex Heart Inst J. 2009;36:38–43.
66. Fysh ET, Tremblay A, Feller-Kopman D, Mishra EK, Slade M, Garske L, Clive AO, Lamb C, Boshuizen R, Ng BJ, Rosenstengel AW, Yarmus L, Rahman NM, Maskell NA, Lee YC. Clinical outcomes of indwelling pleural catheter-related pleural infections: an international multicenter study. Chest. 2013;144:1597–602.
67. Mahmood K, Bower C. Treatment of infection associated with tunneled pleural catheters. J Bronchology Interv Pulmonol. 2010;17:69–72.
68. Chandrasekhar AJ, Reynes CJ, Churchill RJ. Ultrasonically guided percutaneous biopsy of peripheral pulmonary masses. Chest. 1976;70:627–30.
69. Yang PC, Chang DB, Yu CJ, Lee YC, Wu HD, Kuo SH, Luh KT. Ultrasound-guided core biopsy of thoracic tumors. Am Rev Respir Dis. 1992;146:763–7.
70. Targhetta R, Bourgeois JM, Marty-Double C, Coste E, Proust A, Balmes P, Pourcelot L. Peripheral pulmonary lesions: ultrasonic features and ultrasonically guided fine needle aspiration biopsy. J Ultrasound Med. 1993;12:369–74.
71. Hsu WH, Chiang CD, Hsu JY, Kwan PC, Chen CL, Chen CY. Ultrasound-guided fine-needle aspiration biopsy of lung cancers. J Clin Ultrasound. 1996;24:225–33.
72. Chen CC, Hsu WH, Huang CM, Hsu JY, Chiang CD. Ultrasound-guided fine needle aspiration biopsy of small pulmonary nodules abutting to the chest wall. Zhonghua Yi Xue Za Zhi (Taipei). 1996;57:106–11.
73. Chen CC, Hsu WH, Huang CM, Chen CY, Kwan PC, Chiang CD. Ultrasound-guided fine-needle aspiration biopsy of solitary pulmonary nodules. J Clin Ultrasound. 1995;23:531–6.
74. Knudsen DU, Nielsen SM, Hariri J, Christensen J, Kristensen S. Ultrasonographically guided fine-needle aspiration biopsy of intrathoracic tumors. Acta Radiol. 1996;37:327–31.
75. Sheth S, Hamper UM, Stanley DB, Wheeler JH, Smith PA. US guidance for thoracic biopsy: a valuable alternative to CT. Radiology. 1999;210:721–6.
76. Yang PC. Ultrasound-guided transthoracic biopsy of peripheral lung, pleural, and chest-wall lesions. J Thorac Imaging. 1997;12:272–84.

77. Yang PC. Ultrasound-guided transthoracic biopsy of the chest. Radiol Clin North Am. 2000;38:323–43.
78. Rivera MP, Mehta AC, Wahidi MM. Establishing the diagnosis of lung cancer: diagnosis and management of lung cancer, 3rd ed: American College of Chest Physicians evidence-based clinical practice guidelines. Chest. 2013;143:e142S–65S.
79. Jarmakani M, Duguay S, Rust K, Conner K, Wagner JM. Ultrasound versus computed tomographic guidance for percutaneous biopsy of chest lesions. J Ultrasound Med. 2016;35:1865–72.
80. Liao WY, Chen MZ, Chang YL, Wu HD, Yu CJ, Kuo PH, Yang PC. US-guided transthoracic cutting biopsy for peripheral thoracic lesions less than 3 cm in diameter. Radiology. 2000;217:685–91.
81. Middleton WD, Teefey SA, Dahiya N. Ultrasound-guided chest biopsies. Ultrasound Q. 2006;22:241–52.
82. Andersson T, Lindgren PG, Elvin A. Ultrasound guided tumour biopsy in the anterior mediastinum. An alternative to thoracotomy and mediastinoscopy. Acta Radiol. 1992;33:423–6.
83. Gupta S, Gulati M, Rajwanshi A, Gupta D, Suri S. Sonographically guided fine-needle aspiration biopsy of superior mediastinal lesions by the suprasternal route. AJR Am J Roentgenol. 1998;171:1303–6.
84. Heilo A. Tumors in the mediastinum: US-guided histologic core-needle biopsy. Radiology. 1993;189:143–6.
85. Sawhney S, Jain R, Berry M. Tru-cut biopsy of mediastinal masses guided by real-time sonography. Clin Radiol. 1991;44:16–9.
86. Wernecke K, Vassallo P, Peters PE, von Bassewitz DB. Mediastinal tumors: biopsy under US guidance. Radiology. 1989;172:473–6.
87. Marchetti GP, Pinelli V, Tassi GF. 100 years of thoracoscopy: historical notes. Respiration. 2011;82:187–92.
88. Macha HN, Reichle G, von Zwehl D, Kemmer HP, Bas R, Morgan JA. The role of ultrasound assisted thoracoscopy in the diagnosis of pleural disease. Clinical experience in 687 cases. Eur J Cardiothorac Surg. 1993;7:19–22.
89. Hersh CP, Feller-Kopman D, Wahidi M, Garland R, Herth F, Ernst A. Ultrasound guidance for medical thoracoscopy: a novel approach. Respiration. 2003;70:299–301.
90. Marchetti G, Valsecchi A, Indellicati D, Arondi S, Trigiani M, Pinelli V. Ultrasound-guided medical thoracoscopy in the absence of pleural effusion. Chest. 2015;147:1008–12.
91. Valsecchi A, Arondi S, Marchetti G. Medical thoracoscopy: analysis on diagnostic yield through 30 years of experience. Ann Thorac Med. 2016;11:177–82.
92. Loddenkemper R, Mai J, Scheffler N, Brandt HJ. Prospective individual comparison of blind needle biopsy and of thoracoscopy in the diagnosis and differential diagnosis of tuberculous pleurisy. Scand J Respir Dis Suppl. 1978;102:196–8.
93. Dole SS, Godbole GP, Pophale HS. To study efficacy of medical thoracoscopy in undiagnosed pleural effusions. J Assoc Physicians India. 2016;64:20–3.
94. Kiani A, Abedini A, Karimi M, Samadi K, Sheikhy K, Farzanegan B, Pour Abdollah M, Jamaati H, Jabardarjani HR, Masjedi MR. Diagnostic yield of medical thoracoscopy in undiagnosed pleural effusion. Tanaffos. 2015;14:227–31.
95. Michaud G, Berkowitz DM, Ernst A. Pleuroscopy for diagnosis and therapy for pleural effusions. Chest. 2010;138:1242–6.
96. Cassanelli N, Caroli G, Dolci G, Dell'Amore A, Luciano G, Bini A, Stella F. Accuracy of transthoracic ultrasound for the detection of pleural adhesions. Eur J Cardiothorac Surg. 2012;42:813–8; discussion 818.
97. Viskum K, Enk B. Complications of thoracoscopy. Poumon Coeur. 1981;37:25–8.
98. Viallat JR, Rey F, Astoul P, Boutin C. Thoracoscopic talc poudrage pleurodesis for malignant effusions. A review of 360 cases. Chest. 1996;110:1387–93.
99. de Campos JR, Vargas FS, de Campos Werebe E, Cardoso P, Teixeira LR, Jatene FB, Light RW. Thoracoscopy talc poudrage: a 15-year experience. Chest. 2001;119:801–6.
100. Colt HG. Thoracoscopy. A prospective study of safety and outcome. Chest. 1995;108:324–9.
101. Brims FJ, Arif M, Chauhan AJ. Outcomes and complications following medical thoracoscopy. Clin Respir J. 2012;6:144–9.

Assessment of Diaphragm Function by Ultrasounds

13

Francesco Feletti, Bruna Malta, and Andrea Aliverti

13.1 Introduction

Breathing is a process achieved by the highly coordinated action of the diaphragm with the other respiratory muscles, including the rib cage muscles (intercostals, parasternal, scalene, and neck muscles) and the abdominal muscles. The diaphragm is a wide dome-shaped aponeurotic formation, interposed between the chest and abdomen, and it is considered the primary muscle of ventilation, responsible in healthy subjects of most of the inspiratory work during spontaneous breathing in resting conditions. Its mechanical action, in inspiration, can be grossly simplified with a cylinder-piston model in which, by analogy, the trunk is the cylinder and the diaphragm the piston. In physiological conditions, the inspiratory action of the diaphragm results from the combination of two mechanisms. The first is the reduction of its zone of apposition (ZOA) on the inner surface of the rib cage (i.e., the portion of the muscular fibres extending from their insertion on the ribs to the point where the diaphragm peels away from the rib cage). The second is the cupola flattening. As a result, a protrusion of the abdomen and expansion of lower costal margin takes place, being, in fact, the thorax similar to an expandable cylinder with variable section.

Despite being a skeletal muscle, given its domed shape, the diaphragm combines muscular tension and muscular curvature. Consequently, the pressure which the diaphragm can develop depends on its three-dimensional shape and curvature radius, the extension of the ZOA, the force-length characteristics of the muscle, and the compliance of the abdomen. The latter affects the diaphragm work of compression of the abdominal contents and expansion of the abdominal wall.

The operating conditions of the diaphragm can be altered by simple exogenous factors, such as the posture assumed by the subject under examination which, in particular, affects the geometry of the diaphragm and the compliance of the abdominal cavity, or by several pathological conditions that determine diaphragm dysfunction (Table 13.1).

Diaphragm dysfunction can be classified as paralysis or weakness; the former is a complete

F. Feletti (✉)
Dipartimento di Diagnostica per Immagini, Ausl della Romagna, Ospedale S. Maria delle Croci, Ravenna, Italy

Dipartimento di Elettronica, Informazione e Bioingegneria, Politecnico di Milano, Milan, Italy
e-mail: francesco.feletti@auslromagna.it

B. Malta
Dipartimento di Diagnostica per Immagini, Ausl di Ferrara, Ospedale Universitario di Ferrara, Ferrara, Italy
e-mail: mltbrn@unife.it

A. Aliverti
Dipartimento di Elettronica, Informazione e Bioingegneria, Politecnico di Milano, Milan, Italy
e-mail: andrea.aliverti@polimi.it

F. Feletti et al. (eds.), *Thoracic Ultrasound and Integrated Imaging*,
https://doi.org/10.1007/978-3-319-93055-8_13

Table 13.1 Causes of diaphragm dysfunction

– Isolated phrenic nerve dysfunction (due to traumas, tumours, radiation therapy, compression, surgery)
– Mechanical ventilation (ventilator-induced diaphragm dysfunction, VIDD)
– CNS lesions (such as ALS, SMA, cervical spine tumour)
– Peripheral nervous system lesions (such as herpes zoster, Guillain-Barre syndrome, diabetic neuropathy)
– Neuromuscular junction disorders (such as myasthenia gravis)
– Myopathies (such as muscular dystrophy)

loss of diaphragmatic function while the latter is a partial loss of the ability to generate pressure. Another dysfunction is eventration, a congenital thinning of the diaphragmatic muscle that causes a focal bulge. These dysfunctions are often initially suggested by diaphragmatic elevation at chest radiography. Elevation caused by paralysis or weakness typically involves an entire hemidiaphragm, whereas elevation secondary to eventration involves only a portion of a hemidiaphragm. When interpreting radiographs and other imaging studies, it is crucial to bear in mind that in healthy individuals, the right hemidiaphragm is somewhat higher than the left hemidiaphragm. Furthermore, the anterior and medial portions of the diaphragm usually are higher than the posterior and lateral portions. Diaphragmatic weakness or paralysis may be seen in the context of metabolic or inflammatory disorders, after trauma or surgery, during mechanical ventilation, and with mediastinal masses, myopathies, or disease that cause lung hyperinflation. Dysfunctions can be unilateral or, less commonly, bilateral. Patients with unilateral diaphragmatic paralysis are usually asymptomatic but may have dyspnea and limited ability to exercise. Patients with bilateral diaphragmatic paralysis or severe diaphragmatic weakness are more likely to have symptoms and may present dyspnea or recurrent respiratory failure. In contrast to unilateral impairment, bilateral diaphragmatic dysfunction is usually symptomatic and may lead to ventilatory failure. In this situation, the accessory muscles of respiration must assume all the work of breathing.

One of the causes of diaphragmatic weakness is mechanical ventilation (MV). While MV is lifesaving in patients with acute respiratory failure, prolonged mechanical ventilation is associated with numerous potential complications. MV is required for approximately 40% of patients in medical ICUs. Multiple studies have suggested that MV has an unloading effect on the respiratory muscles that leads to diaphragmatic atrophy and dysfunction, a process called ventilator-induced diaphragmatic dysfunction (VIDD). In experimental animals, the ability of the intact diaphragm to generate pressure is reduced by 40–50% within a few days of instituting “controlled” mechanical ventilation, which permits little or no spontaneous diaphragmatic activity. The endurance of the diaphragm also appears to be adversely affected, with a reduced ability to sustain the diaphragmatic force. It has been seen that nervous impulse at the levels of the phrenic nerve and the neuromuscular junction remains normal. Thus the deleterious effects of mechanical ventilation upon diaphragmatic function are primarily the result of changes that occur within the muscle fibres. Beyond decreased diaphragmatic strength, some histological and biochemical changes have been described in the diaphragms of animals with VIDD. These include muscle fibre atrophy, which appears to be the result of decreased protein synthesis as well as increased protein breakdown. In humans, individuals under MV, a postmortem analysis has shown diffuse diaphragmatic muscle fibres atrophy in accordance with animals studies [1].

Diaphragm dysfunction should be promptly recognized in order to address the underlying causes and also because adapted ventilatory support may be necessary. For example, postoperative diaphragm dysfunction may lead to failed extubation or prolonged mechanical ventilation. Therefore, in many clinical situations, there is a need to assess the diaphragm function. However, due to the non-specific presentation of diaphragm paralysis, diaphragm paralysis is underdiagnosed.

Different structural and functional techniques are available for evaluating the diaphragm. Each technique has its strengths and weaknesses. The most widely used imaging technique for diaphragm analysis is radiography (RX) which, in addition to anatomical information, provides information used for evaluating diaphragm position (chest X-ray) and motion (fluoroscopy). Kinematic information about the diaphragm is crucial for detecting various pulmonary diseases. Attenuated diaphragm movement is sometimes evident at an early stage of diseases, which cannot be detected by conventional static radiography. More sophisticated imaging techniques, such as magnetic resonance imaging (MRI) and computed tomography (CT), have been used to evaluate diaphragm function. Both the techniques enable a three-dimensional reconstruction of the in vivo diaphragm, allowing accurate measurements of muscle length, surface area, and shape [2–4]. These techniques are, however, cumbersome; the instrumentation is not easy to transport and could be used only for specific diagnostic purposes but are not suitable for monitoring. Moreover, excluding MRI, they require ionizing radiation, and the dose administered to the patient must remain below limit values.

Non-imaging diagnostic tests such as pulmonary function tests or spirometry have limited accuracy and reproducibility, while measurement of trans-diaphragmatic pressure and diaphragm EMG are invasive and time-consuming.

Thoracic ultrasound (TUS) is a technique that is being more and more commonly used to study the diaphragm. It is a quick, generally available, dynamic method able to provide accurate information both on the anatomy and on the function of the muscle. Being radiation-free, TUS is particularly important in children. Another advantage of TUS is that it focuses mainly on the lateral and posterior parts of the muscle, which are innervated by the phrenic nerve and are the more mobile parts of the muscle. On the contrary, the anterior central tendon, which is typically shown by fluoroscopy, moves 40% less during respiration [5].

13.2 Diaphragm and Thoracic Ultrasounds

The diaphragm is a dome-shaped muscle [6] separating the thoracic cavity and the abdomen. It consists of a central aponeurosis, the "central tendon," embryologically originating from the transverse septum and a peripheral muscle sheet (Fig. 13.1).

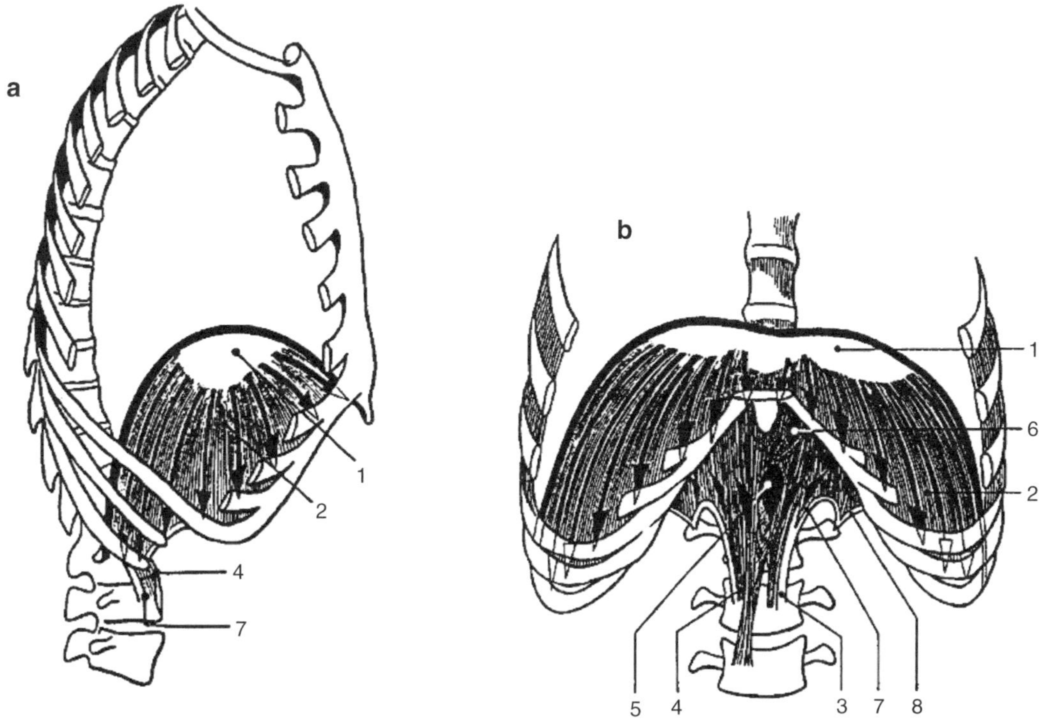

Fig. 13.1 Lateral (**a**) and frontal (**b**) views of the human diaphragm. (1) Central tendon; (2) costal fibres; (3 and 4) crural fibres, right and left pillars; (5) aorta; (6) oesophagus; (7) psoas arches

Muscular fibres originate from the circumference of the thoracic outlet to converge into the central tendon. The muscular part of the diaphragm is conventionally divided into the vertebral and the costal parts. The first one originates from the lumbar spine and the aponeurotic arcuate ligaments, while the second one originates from the lower rib pairs and the xiphoid process of the sternum. The muscular fibres of the costal portion from their insertion on the ribs go in the cranial-dorsal direction, directly apposing to the inner surface of the rib cage; this is the ZOA, representing about the 60% of the total area of the diaphragm. The inner surface covers about 40% of the whole surface of the rib cage [7].

The echographic appearance of the normal diaphragm is that of a hypoechoic layer between two hyperreflective interfaces with the pleura and peritoneum. The internal echotexture is due to hyperechoic fibroadipose septa which separate muscle fibers. The normal diaphragm thickens during inspiration. On the contrary, an atrophic diaphragm appears as a thin strip that does not thicken and move during inspiration. The M-mode provides a mono-dimensional view of the reflectors along a single, chosen ultrasound line, displayed along the time axis. It is used to assess excursion, side-to-side variability, the velocity of movement, and response to phrenic nerve stimulation [5].

13.3 Techniques for Diaphragm Functional Assessment

In order to assess the respiratory movements, TUS examination of the diaphragm is currently carried out during spontaneous respiration, but deep breathing or sniff manoeuvres may also be useful. The supine position offers higher diaphragm excursion, more reproducibility, and less overall and side-to-side variability and is generally preferred. Besides, in the supine position, the inspired volume better correlates with diaphragm movement than in a seated position. Finally, in the supine position, any paradoxical movement is exaggerated, while compensatory action by the anterior abdominal wall is limited. The spleen and the liver windows can be used to visualize the left and the right diaphragm, respectively. The thickness of the diaphragm can be accurately measured using an angle of insonation on the muscular surface close to 90° which maximizes the reflection at the interfaces between muscle and serosas. Excursion measurements require a low-frequency probe, able to provide adequate visualization of the deeper posterior part of the diaphragm. On the other hand, a higher-frequency transducer (7–18 MHz) provides better spatial resolution and allows the correct thickness assessment at the zone of apposition [5] (Fig. 13.2).

13.3.1 Diaphragm Thickness

When diaphragm thickness is evaluated, the ultrasound machine is set in B-mode, and the probe is positioned perpendicularly to the chest wall on the anterior axillary line in the ZOA of the diaphragm to the rib cage, between eighth and ninth or ninth and tenth right ribs in the intercostal space. The right side is chosen because of the presence of the liver, just behind the peritoneal membrane, which is a non-echogenic tissue and makes structures of interest localization easier. Because the costal part of the diaphragm is relatively close to the skin surface, it is possible to use a 7–13 MHz transducer, which has less penetration but enhanced resolution. In a B-mode image, the diaphragm is outlined by two clear, bright parallel lines, corresponding to the pleural and peritoneal membranes. Sometimes between these two lines discontinued less bright lines can be seen which are due to the connective tissue and vessels running between the muscle fibres [7].

Diaphragm thickness is estimated as the distance between the two lines representing the pleural and peritoneal membranes (outer or inner edges or central points) in the zone where they are the most parallel possible (Fig. 13.3). Continuous monitoring of diaphragm thickness is absent in literature. Thickness values are obtained

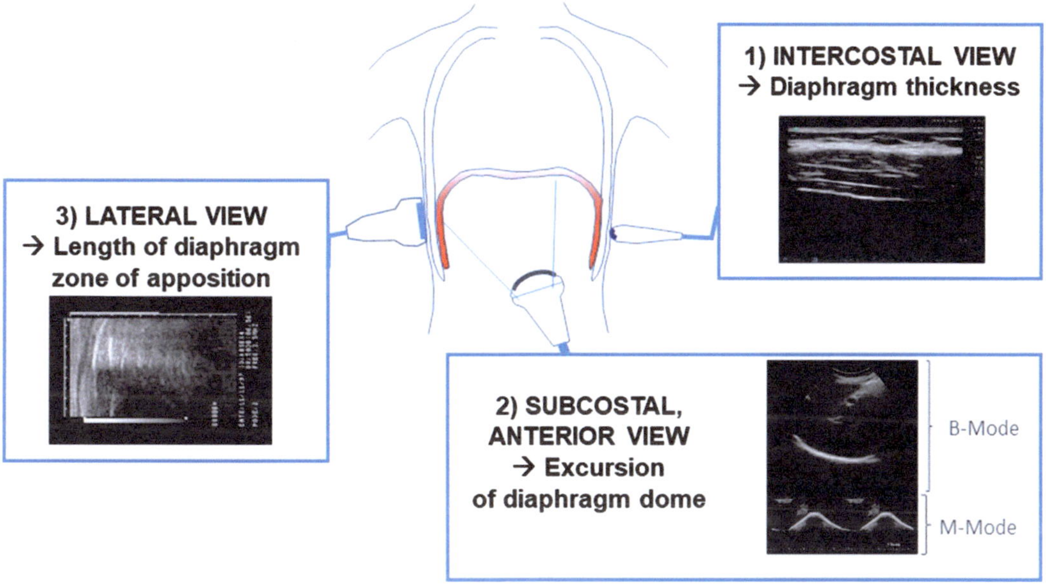

Fig. 13.2 Transducer placement and examples of US images obtained for the three different approaches adopted for diaphragm US analysis. (1) US diaphragm thickness evaluation. A linear transducer (7–18 MHz) is positioned between the eighth and ninth or between the ninth and tenth ribs in the intercostal space (on the anterior axillary line). The obtained US B-mode image visualizes the diaphragm at the zone of apposition. The two bright, echogenic lines represent the pleural and peritoneal membranes. Diaphragm thickness is estimated as the distance between these two lines, where they are mostly parallel. (2) US diaphragm mobility evaluation. A convex transducer (2–6 MHz) is positioned below the costal margin in the midclavicular line (anterior subcostal view). On the B-mode image, the diaphragm silhouette is visible as a thick echogenic line. After having defined a scan line, M-mode allows the visualization of diaphragm motion as a time curve. (3) US diaphragm's zone of apposition (ZOA) evaluation. A large (8–12 cm) linear transducer (7–19 MHz) is positioned vertically against the subject's chest wall just anterior to the right midaxillary line. On B-mode, the bright superficial area corresponds to the lung, whereas the deeper lighter area corresponds to the liver. On the image, the point where the diaphragm separates from the chest wall and the lung interposes can be used to identify the position of the cephalic margin of the zone of apposition, while the costal origin of the diaphragm is identified when the subject breathes in at total lung capacity, where the length of the ZOA approaches zero

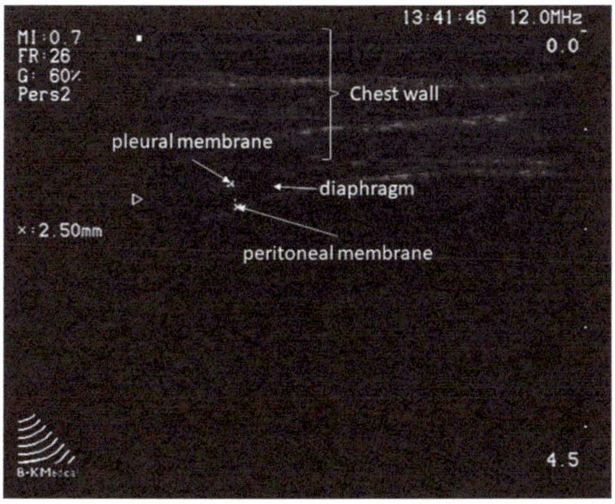

Fig. 13.3 Example of a US image obtained for diaphragm thickness evaluation (see Fig. 13.2-1)

as an average of different images recorded at the end of expiration and at the end of inspiration (Table 13.2).

Average values of the diaphragmatic end-expiratory thickness (T_{EE}) during spontaneous breathing reported in literature are 2.7 ± 1 mm [8], 1.7 ± 2 mm [7], 3.2 ± 1.3 mm [9] in the supine position, and 1.9 ± 0.4 mm in the seated position.

Average values of end-inspiratory thickness (T_{EI}) are 3.7 ± 1.40 and 2.7 ± 0.5 mm, respectively, in the supine and seated positions [9–12].

A diaphragm thickness <2 mm, measured at the end of expiration, has been proposed as the cutoff to define diaphragm atrophy [13, 14]. It is

Table 13.2 Values of diaphragm thickness at functional residual capacity (FRC) and thickening ratio (TR) (from Boon et al. [8])

	N	Age (years)		Thickness (mm)	TR
Men	73	34.7 ± 8.8	Right	3.8 ± 1.5 (1.6–7.6)	1.8 ± 0.5 (1.17–3.9)
			Left	3.7 ± 1.7 (1.2–8.0)	2.0 ± 0.5 (1.1–3.5)
Women	77	34.8 ± 8.5	Right	2.7 ± 1.0 (1.3–5.3)	1.8 ± 0.5 (1.1–3.6)
			Left	3.1 ± 1.9 (1.2–11.8)	1.9 ± 0.5 (1.1–4.2)

essential to define the intercostal space where the thickness of the diaphragm is measured as it varies, with the more inferior portions of the diaphragm being thicker than more superior portions [5]. Discrepancies in mean values may be due to differences in the calculation method and participants' characteristics (age, gender, BMI, smoking status) [8, 12, 15, 16]. Vivier et al. in their study, evaluate diaphragm thickness in patients requiring planned noninvasive ventilation at three levels of pressure support (5, 10, and 15 cm H_2O). They found a decrease in diaphragm thickness at the end of inspiration with increasing pressure support level [10]. Baldwin et al. [11] measured thickness at different lung volumes and compared it to inspiratory capacity. These authors reported that increasing the volume produced an increase in thickness but also a more considerable variability between different subjects. Moreover, at higher volumes lung artefacts are evident.

Thickening. The measurement of thickness alone may miss an acutely paralyzed diaphragm with common thickness and could incorrectly identify atrophy in a low-weight individual with a healthy, yet thin, diaphragm [16]. During inspiration muscle fibres shorten, resulting in diaphragmatic thickening. Therefore, the degree of diaphragm thickening has been proposed to be more sensitive than measurement of thickness alone and represents an indirect measurement of muscle fibre contraction [17]. Diaphragm thickening can be quantified and measured by the diaphragmatic thickening fraction (DTF) calculated as:

$$DTF\left(\%\right) = \frac{T_{EI} - T_{EE}}{T_{EE}} \cdot 100$$

A change in diaphragm thickness of 28–96% has been reported in healthy volunteers, with a change of −35 to 5% in those with a paralyzed diaphragm [5]. Diaphragm thickening of less than 20% is associated with paralysis [5]. A chronically paralyzed diaphragm is thin, atrophic, and does not thicken during inspiration. Diaphragm thinning starts within 48 h after initiation of MV, and diaphragm thickness decreasing rate over time is averaged 6% per day of MV [18]. Ferrari et al. [15] in their study found a good correlation between DTF and maximum inspiratory pressure (MIP) and with tidal volume. These authors proposed, therefore, DTF as a predictor of weaning from the mechanical ventilator after a spontaneous breathing trial, showing that a DFT > 36% is associated with successful weaning. This coefficient has also been used by Summerhill et al. [16] to establish diaphragm paralysis by demonstrating minimal or absent thickening of the hemidiaphragm during inspiration. Diaphragm paralysis is diagnosed with a value of DTF <20%.

Another nondimensional index proposed in the literature is the *thickening ratio* (TR) [19], defined as the ratio between maximal diaphragm thickness (occurring in correspondence of a maximal inspiration, T_{EImax}) and end-expiratory diaphragm thickness (T_{EE}):

$$TR = \frac{T_{EImax}}{T_{EE}}$$

The mean value of typical TR is 1.8 ± 0.5 (ranging between 2 and 3.9) [8, 20]. If at the numerator of the previous formula tidal end-inspiratory thickness is used instead of T_{EImax}, the ratio is lowered to 1.2 ± 0.5 [9].

13.3.2 Diaphragm Mobility

In conditions such as phrenic nerve injury, neuromuscular diseases, after abdominal or cardiac surgery, and critically ill patients under mechanical ventilation, abnormal diaphragmatic motion is observed. M-mode allows evaluation of diaphragm kinematics, motion and excursion, speed of contraction, and duration of the cycle [21]. In order to evaluate diaphragm displacement, continuous monitoring is needed, and the ultrasound machine may be set in M-mode after an initial two-dimensional analysis to select the appropriate exploration line. Typically [22], a convex probe is required with operating frequencies between 2 and 6 MHz to ensure an adequate penetration capacity [5]. The probe is positioned on the upper abdomen and directed toward the dome, the liver or the spleen serving as an acoustic window. Visualization of the left hemidiaphragm may be challenging because of the smaller window provided by the spleen. Through an anterior subcostal view, the diaphragm is seen as a single thick echogenic line, and the movement of the diaphragm as shown by M-mode can be therefore represented on a time curve (Fig. 13.4). The direction of diaphragm movement can be related with the phases of the respiratory cycle: normal inspiratory diaphragmatic movement is caudal since the diaphragm moves toward the probe; typical expiratory trace is cranial, as the diaphragm moves away from the probe. The motion of the diaphragm, moreover, can be related to the phases of the respiratory cycle during mechanical ventilation and therefore potentially used to study patient-ventilator asynchrony (Fig. 13.5). Also, the movement of each hemidiaphragm can be put in correlation with the phases of the respiratory cycle. Whether the diaphragm wanders off from the probe during inspiration, a paradoxical motion shall also be considered. The evaluation of diaphragm excursion with TUS provides values consistent with those obtained using MRI or fluoroscopy [23].

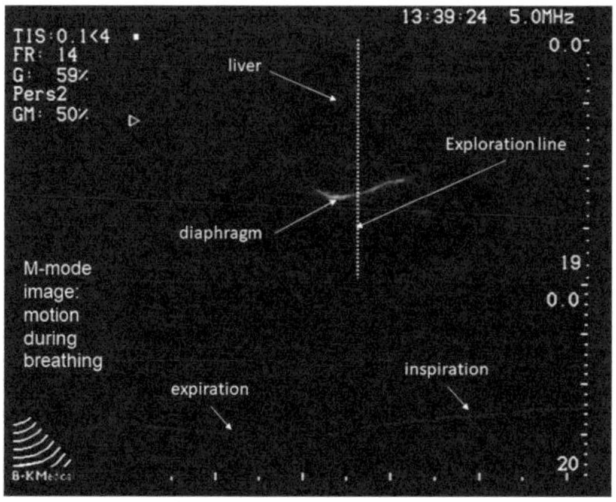

Fig. 13.4 Example of a US image obtained for diaphragm motion evaluation (see Fig. 13.2-2)

Another possibility is to analyze motion through a posterior subcostal view. Nevertheless, this is not commonly used since the patient must be seated, which is not possible in the case of critically ill or mechanically ventilated patients. Similar to the anterior subcostal view, the posterior subcostal view is performed with a low-frequency curvilinear transducer. The probe is placed on a sagittal plane in the posterior subcostal region on either side. The images obtained with this approach are similar to those acquired with the anterior subcostal view and allow measurement of diaphragm excursion. A subxiphoid view with a low-frequency curvilinear transducer (2–6 MHz) oriented upward and dorsally may be used to measure diaphragmatic excursion in children. On an oblique transverse view at the midline, B-mode can be used for a contemporary qualitative evaluation of both sides, while M-mode allows a quantitative measurement of side-to-side variability and excursion amplitude one side at a time [5].

Average values of the diaphragmatic excursion are reported to be in the range of 9–20 mm during quiet spontaneous breathing and 70–100 mm during forced maximal manoeuvres [24]. Boussugues et al. studied M-mode echography diaphragmatic mobility in a group of 210 healthy volunteers in standing position, obtaining the following values of an excursion, for right and left hemidiaphragm, respectively: 18 ± 3 and 18 ± 4 during spontaneous breathing and 66 ± 13 and 73 ± 10 during deep breathing [22]. Similarly, in 2000, Gersovich et al. studied 23 healthy volunteers finding average values of 15 mm (3–21) and 57 mm (17–92), respectively, for calm spontaneous breathing and deep breathing [25]. The same authors found a linear relationship between inspired volumes and diaphragmatic excursion and between BMI and diaphragmatic excursion

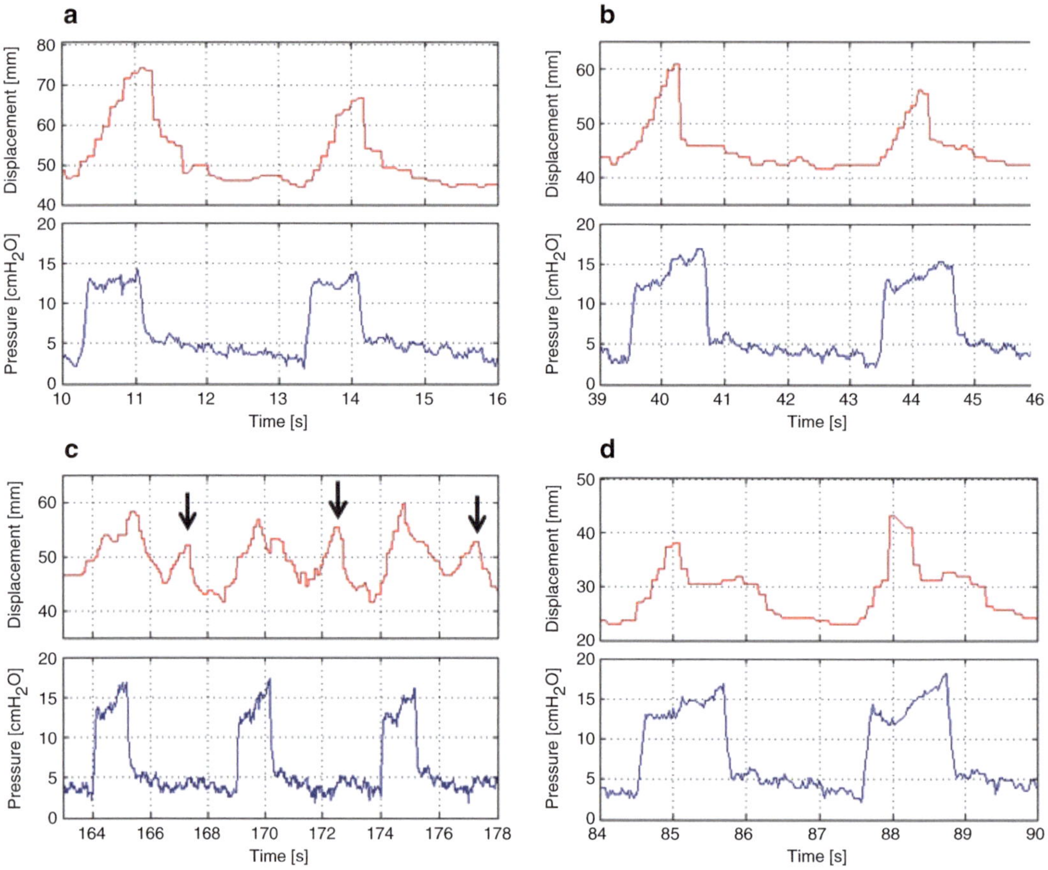

Fig. 13.5 Example of patient-ventilator asynchrony studied on a breath-by-breath basis by US diaphragm motion signal (M-mode) (red curves) synchronized with pressure measured at the airway opening (blue curves) by an acquisition system and software developed at the Politecnico di Milano (unpublished data) in a patient with severe chronic obstructive pulmonary disease (COPD) and myasthenia gravis under pressure support mechanical ventilation (pressure support = 10 cm H_2O, PEEP 5 cm H_2O, inspiratory time 1.2 s) through tracheostomy during acute respiratory failure. (**a**) Breathing showing a good adaptation of the patient to the ventilator, without asynchrony; (**b**) premature diaphragm release, where the diaphragm ends its motion before the support delivered by the ventilator ceases; (**c**) ineffective efforts (indicated by arrows), characterized by patient's inspiratory efforts which fail to trigger the ventilator thus diaphragm displacement increases but the ventilator does not deliver support; (**d**) premature ventilator cycling off, in which ventilator ends insufflation before patient's inspiratory effort ceases

that resulted in being more significant in men [25]. Successively, Kantarci et al. showed that diaphragmatic motion is affected by gender, body mass index (BMI), waist circumference, and age of the individuals [26]. Healthy persons of younger age with a lower BMI and smaller waist circumference may show a decreased amount of diaphragmatic motion. Moreover, in some studies, the relationship between inspired air volume and diaphragm excursion resulted linear in healthy subjects, whereas other studies, regarding patients with lung disease, have reported weak correlation [26]. Yamaguti et al. studied diaphragmatic mobility in lateral decubitus on a limited number of subjects, reporting an excursion of 51 ± 10 and 46 ± 14, for right and left side, respectively [27]. In Table 13.3 the data regarding the typical ranges of motion in healthy adults during quiet breathing (from the resting expiratory position to end inspiration) and deep

Table 13.3 Mean values of diaphragm excursion (data in mm) during spontaneous quiet breathing and deep breathing (aggregated data from [22, 25–27])

	Spontaneous quiet breathing	Deep breathing (from resting expiration to full inspiration)	Voluntary sniff
Men			
Average	18 ± 3	77 ± 11 70 (seated)	–
Lower limit	10	47	18
Women			
Average	16 ± 3	57 ± 10 57 (supine)	–
Lower limit	9	37	16

breathing (from the resting expiratory position to full inspiration) are summarized. In a study comparing pre- and postoperative excursion in adult patients, a diaphragmatic maximal inspiratory amplitude of <24 mm was shown to correlate with a 50% decrease of vital capacity from baseline [28]. An excursion >25 mm in adults has been proposed as a cutoff for excluding severe diaphragm dysfunction [29].

13.3.3 Diaphragm Zone of Apposition

Measurements of diaphragm zone of apposition can be performed by a linear ultrasound probe (80 or 120 mm) placed vertically against the subject's chest wall on the lateral part of the lower rib cage just anterior to the right midaxillary line [30]. This approach allows the visualization of both the ZOA and the point where the diaphragm separates from the chest wall (*costal recess*). The costal origin of the diaphragm is identified when the subject breathes in at total lung capacity, where the length of the ZOA approaches zero. The distance between the costal origin of the diaphragm and its point of separation from the chest wall provides a measure of the ZOA's length at any lung volume or time point. This approach is particularly useful to study patients with chronic obstructive pulmonary disease (COPD) characterized by expiratory flow limitation determining lung hyperinflation which determines, in turn, the shortening of the diaphragm, as well as the other inspiratory muscles, that therefore work at a suboptimal fibre length. In addition, the flattened diaphragm with radially orientated muscle fibres, secondary to hyperinflation, reduces the ZOA and determines the paradoxical inspiratory inward motion of the lower rib cage contributing to dyspnea [31, 32].

13.4 Conclusions and Future Perspectives

Intrarater and interrater reliability of diaphragm US were evaluated and found to be high. For these reasons, there is an increasing interest in the use of ultrasounds as a monitoring tool in diaphragm dysfunctions (Table 13.4). However, this method presents some limitations. The quality of the measurements depends on various factors: localization of the correct intercostal space, perpendicularity of the probe to the diaphragmatic line, stability of the probe itself during the recording time, and lung volume during spontaneous breathing. Another limitation to the spread of ultrasound for diaphragm assessment is a lack of reference values for diaphragm parameters in patients with pulmonary or neuromuscular disease. Only limited studies have evaluated diaphragmatic parameters using ultrasound in patients with lung disease. In conclusion, although imaging protocols are still being fully developed and validated to standardize diaphragm sonography, this technique is already used routinely in some contexts, such as in ICU patients to assess and predict the effects of mechanical ventilation, and has high potential in the evaluation of patients with diaphragm dysfunction due to many causes.

Table 13.4 Clinical usefulness of diaphragm assessment by ultrasounds

Clinical use	Criteria	Cit.
Reveal diaphragm weakness	Less than the normal amplitude of excursion on deep breathing with or without paradoxical motion on sniffing	[33, 34]
Identify diaphragm paralysis and its etiology	– Absence of excursion during quiet/deep breathing – Absence of excursion /paradoxical motion upon sniffing – TF <20%	[17, 33, 35]
Diaphragm muscle weakness assessment in neuromuscular disorders (amyotrophic lateral sclerosis (ALS), Duchenne muscular dystrophy (DMD), Pompe disease, facioscapulohumeral dystrophy (FSHD))		[36–39]
Compare or follow-up movement of the two hemidiaphragms		[40, 41]
Assessment and prediction of extubation failure in weaning from mechanical ventilation	– Diaphragmatic excursions >25 mm increase the likelihood of success of SBT (spontaneous breathing trial) in mechanically ventilated patients – DTF >30–36% during SBT increases the likelihood of success of SBT	[21]
Diagnosis and monitoring of diaphragm function		[42]
Reveal phrenic neuropathy perioperative assessment phrenic nerve injury (causing diaphragm paralysis) in thoracic surgery		[16, 43, 44]
Guidance for needle EMG to enhance accuracy and safety		[45]

References

1. Petrof BJ, Jaber S, Matecki S. Ventilator-induced diaphragmatic dysfunction. Curr Opin Crit Care. 2010;16(1):19–25.
2. Tanaka R, Sanada S, Kobayashi T. Automated analysis for the respiratory kinetics with the screening dynamic chest radiography using a flat-panel detector system. Int Congr Ser. 2003;1256:179–86.
3. Pettiaux N, Cassart M, Paiva M, Estenne M. Three-dimensional reconstruction of human diaphragm with the use of spiral computed tomography. J Appl Physiol. 1997;82(3):998–1002. 122.
4. Cluzel P, Similowski T, Chartrand-lefebvre C, Zelter M, Grenier PA. Technical developments diaphragm and chest wall: assessment of the inspiratory pump with MR imaging—preliminary observations. Radiology. 2000;215(2):27–33.
5. Sarwal A, Walker FO, Cartwright MS. Neuromuscular ultrasound for evaluation of the diaphragm. Muscle Nerve. 2013;47(3):319–29.
6. De Troyer A, Wilson TA. Action of the diaphragm on the rib cage. J Appl Physiol. 2016;121(2):391–40.
7. Ueki J, De Bruin PF, Pride NB. In vivo assessment of diaphragm contraction by ultrasound in normal subjects. Thorax. 1995;50(11):1157–61.
8. Boon AJ, Harper CJ, Ghahfarokhi LS, Strommen JA, Watson JC, Sorenson EJ. Two-dimensional ultrasound imaging of the diaphragm: quantitative values in normal subjects. Muscle Nerve. 2013;47:884–9.
9. Harper CJ, Shahgholi L, Cieslak K, Hellyer NJ, Strommen JA, Boon AJ. Variability in diaphragm motion during normal breathing, assessed with b-mode ultrasound. J Orthop Sports Phys Ther. 2013;43(12):927–31.
10. Vivier E, Mekontso Dessap A, Dimassi S, Vargas F, Lyazidi A, Thille AW, Brochard L. Diaphragm ultrasonography to estimate the work of breathing during non-invasive ventilation. Intensive Care Med. 2012;38(5):796–803.
11. Baldwin CE, Paratz JD, Bersten AD. Diaphragm and peripheral muscle thickness on ultrasound: intra-rater reliability and variability of a methodology using nonstandard recumbent positions. Respirology. 2011;16(7):1136–43.
12. Najwatul N, Rahman A, Lee R. Quantification of diaphragm muscle thickness using ultrasound imaging: a preliminary study. In: Proceedings of the 6th international conference on rehabilitation engineering and assistive technology. 2012; vol. 41, p. 1–3.
13. Chavhan GB, et al. Multimodality imaging of the pediatric diaphragm: anatomy and pathologic conditions. Radiographics. 2010;30:1797–817.

14. McCool FD, et al. Dysfunction of the diaphragm. N Engl J Med. 2012;366(10):932–42.
15. Ferrari G, De Filippi G, Elia F, Panero F, Volpicelli G, Aprà F. Diaphragm ultrasound as a new index of discontinuation from mechanical ventilation. Crit Ultrasound J. 2014;6(1):8.
16. Summerhill EM, El-Sameed YA, Glidden TJ, McCool FD. Monitoring recovery from diaphragm paralysis with ultrasound. Chest. 2008;133(3):737–43.
17. Gottesman E, McCool FD. Ultrasound evaluation of the paralyzed diaphragm. Am J Respir Crit Care Med. 1997;155(5):1570–4.
18. Grosu HB, Lee YI, Lee J, Eden E, Eikermann M, Rose KM. Diaphragm muscle thinning in patients who are mechanically ventilated. Chest. 2012;142(6):1455–60.
19. Sota T, Wada T, Miyagi M, Tamaki A, Osaki M, Hagino H. The relationship of diaphragm thickening ratio and respiratory muscle strength in young healthy adults. Physiotherapy. 2015;101(Suppl 1):e1425–6.
20. Baria MR, Shahgholi L, Sorenson EJ, Harper CJ, Lim KG, Strommen JA, Mottram CD, Boon AJ. B-mode ultrasound assessment of diaphragm structure and function in patients with COPD. Chest. 2014;146(3):680–5.
21. Matamis D, Soilemezi E, Tsagourias M, Akoumianaki E, Dimassi S, Boroli F, Brochard L. Sonographic evaluation of the diaphragm in critically ill patients. Technique and clinical applications. Intensive Care Med. 2013;39(5):801–10.
22. Boussugues A, Gole Y, Blanc P. Diaphragmatic motion studied by m-mode ultrasonography: methods, reproducibility, and normal values. Chest. 2009;135(2):391–400.
23. Ayoub J, et al. Diaphragm kinetics coupled with spirometry. M-mode ultrasonographic and fluoroscopic study; preliminary results. J Radiol. 1997;78(8):563–8.
24. Haji K, Royse A, Green C, Botha J, Canty D, Rosye C. Interpreting diaphragmatic movement with bedside imaging, review article. J Crit Care. 2016;34:56–65.
25. Gersovich EO, Cronan M, McGahan JP, Jain K, Jones CD, McDonald C. Ultrasonographic evaluation of diaphragmatic motion. J Ultrasound Med. 2001;20:597–604.
26. Kantarci F, Mihmanli I, Demirel K, Harmanci K, Akman C, Aydogan F, Mihmanl A, Uysa O. Normal diaphragmatic motion and the effects of body composition, determination with M-mode sonography. J Ultrasound Med. 2004;23:255–60.
27. Yamaguti WP, Paulin E, Shibao S, Kodaira S, Chammas MC, Carvalho CRF. Ultrasound evaluation of diaphragmatic mobility in different postures in healthy subjects. J Bras Pneumol. 2007;33(4):407–13.
28. Kim SH, et al. An evaluation of diaphragmatic movement by M-mode sonography as a predictor of pulmonary dysfunction after upper abdominal surgery. Anesth Analg. 2010;110(5):1349–54.
29. Lerolle N, et al. Ultrasonographic diagnostic criterion for severe diaphragmatic dysfunction after cardiac surgery. Chest. 2009;135(2):401–7.
30. Aliverti A, et al. Chest wall kinematic determinants of diaphragm length by optoelectronic plethysmography and ultrasonography. J Appl Physiol. 2003;94:621–30.
31. Gorman RB, McKenzie DK, Pride NB, Tolman JF, Gandevia SC. Diaphragm length during tidal breathing in patients with chronic obstructive pulmonary disease. Am J Respir Crit Care Med. 2002;166:1461–9.
32. Priori R, Aliverti A, Albuquerque AL, Quaranta M, Albert P, Calverley PM. The effect of posture on asynchronous chest wall movement in COPD. J Appl Physiol. 2013;114:1066–75.
33. Urvoas E, et al. Diaphragmatic paralysis in children: diagnosis by TM-mode ultrasound. Pediatr Radiol. 1994;24(8):564–8.
34. Nason LK, et al. Imaging of the diaphragm: anatomy and function. Radiographics. 2012;32(2):E51–70.
35. Sanchez de Toledo J, et al. Diagnosis of abnormal diaphragm motion after cardiothoracic surgery: ultrasound performed by a cardiac intensivist vs. fluoroscopy. Congenit Heart Dis. 2010;5(6):565–72.
36. Pinto S, Alves P, Pimentel B, Swash M, de Carvalho M. Ultrasound for assessment of diaphragm in ALS. Clin Neurophysiol. 2016;127(1):892–7.
37. De Bruin PF, Ueki J, Bush A, Khan Y, Watson A, Pride NB. Diaphragm thickness and inspiratory strength in patients with Duchenne muscular dystrophy. Thorax. 1997;52(5):472–5.
38. Santos DB, Boussaid G, Stojkovic T, Orlikowski D, Letilly N, Behin A, Butel S, Lofaso F, Prigent H. Respiratory muscle dysfunction in facioscapulohumeral muscular dystrophy. Neuromuscul Disord. 2015;25(8):632–9.
39. Noda Y, Sekiguchi K, Kohara N, Kanda F, Toda T. Ultrasonographic diaphragm thickness correlates with compound muscle action potential amplitude and forced vital capacity. Muscle Nerve. 2016;53(4):522–7.
40. Epelman M, et al. M-mode sonography of diaphragmatic motion: description of technique and experience in 278 pediatric patients. Pediatr Radiol. 2005;35(7):661–7.
41. Kim WY, et al. Diaphragm dysfunction assessed by ultrasonography: influence on weaning from mechanical ventilation. Crit Care Med. 2011;39(12):2627–30.
42. Mier-Jedrzejowicz A, Brophy C, Moxham J, Green M. Assessment of diaphragm weakness. Am Rev Respir Dis. 1988;137(4):877–83.
43. Boon AJ, Sekiguchi H, Harper CJ, Strommen JA, Ghahfarokhi LS, Watson JC, Sorenson EJ. Sensitivity and specificity of diagnostic ultrasound in the diagnosis of phrenic neuropathy. Neurology. 2014;83(14):1264–70.
44. Lerolle N, Guérot E, Dimassi S, Zegdi R, Faisy C, Fagon JY, Diehl JL. Ultrasonographic diagnostic criterion for severe diaphragmatic dysfunction after cardiac surgery. Chest. 2009;135(2):401–7.
45. Chen R, Collins S, Remtulla H, Parkes A, Bolton CF. Phrenic nerve conduction study in normal subjects. Muscle Nerve. 1995;18(3):330–5.

Contrast Medium in Thoracic Ultrasound

14

Christian Görg and Corinna Trenker

14.1 Introduction

The B-mode imaging and color Doppler ultrasound (CDU) techniques are continued by the introduction of contrast-enhanced ultrasound (CEUS) consequently. However, the limitations of this approach do not differ from all other modalities.

Thus, the use of CEUS is restricted to chest wall and pleural lesions, lung lesions with contact to the visceral pleural surface, as well as central lung lesions, in which an atelectasis (AT) or pleural effusion mimics an "acoustic window" (Graph 14.1). In general, the performance of CEUS always necessitates B-mode imaging. To fully understand the principle of CEUS, important basics of lung vascularization, qualitative CDU, and spectral curve analysis are summarized in the present chapter [1, 2].

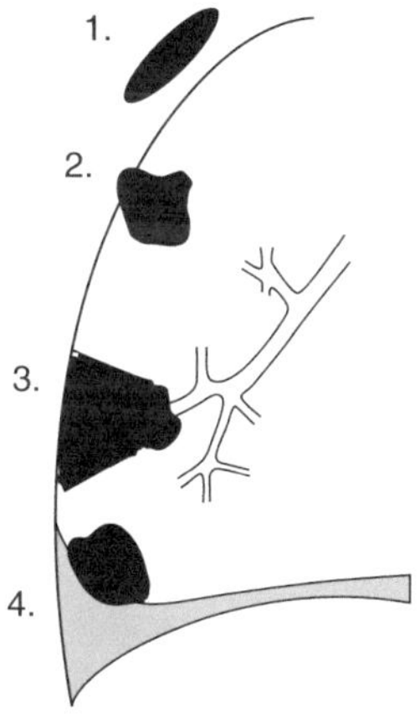

Graph 14.1 Graphic illustration of different localization of tumors which may be examined by ultrasound: (1) thoracic wall lesions, (2) pleural-based lesions, (3) central tumor lesions with atelectasis, and (4) pleural effusion with compressive atelectasis

14.2 Basics of Pulmonary Vascularization

Similar to the liver, the lung is characterized by a dual blood supply. In regard to this, a functional pulmonary vascularization is separated from the nutritive bronchial vascularization. Moreover, an additional intercostal arterial supply for processes originating from the thoracic wall and a tumor-associated neovascularization involving the systemic circulation might be relevant (Fig. 14.1). The pulmonary arteries (PA), which ensure the delivery of deoxygenated blood for

C. Görg (✉)
Interdisciplinary Center of Ultrasound, University Hospital of Giessen and Marburg, Philipps University of Marburg, Marburg, Germany
e-mail: goergc@med.uni-marburg.de

C. Trenker
Department of Hematology, Oncology and Immunology, University Hospital Marburg, Marburg, Germany

F. Feletti et al. (eds.), *Thoracic Ultrasound and Integrated Imaging*,
https://doi.org/10.1007/978-3-319-93055-8_14

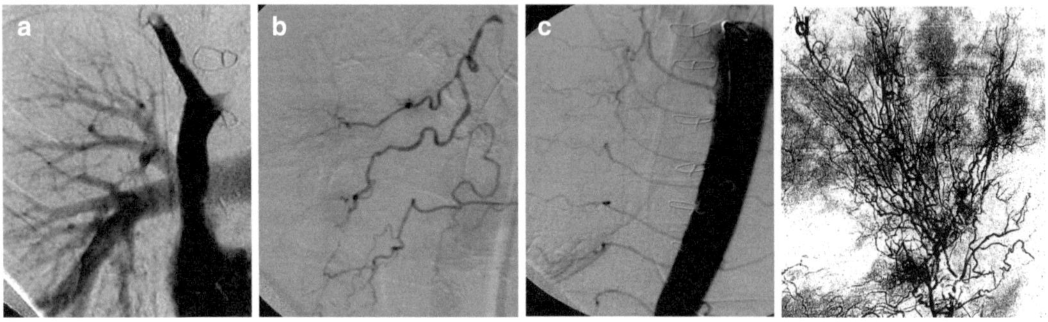

Fig. 14.1 Angiographic images of pulmonary arteries (**a**), bronchial arteries (**b**), intercostal arteries (**c**), and arteries of tumor neoangiogenesis (**d**) [3]

the pulmonary gas exchange, show a branch-like ramification. In contrast to the dilation of systemic arteries due to hypoxic conditions, small PA constrict in the presence of hypoxia to reduce the intrapulmonary shunt flow (Euler-Liljestrand mechanism). Nutritive bronchial arteries (BA) belong to the systemic vascularization. In most individuals, the left BA originate from the aortic arch and from an intercostal artery on the right side, respectively. They form a vascular ring in the area of the lung hilum, from which their branches run parallel to the bronchial branches and pulmonary vessels. The PA and BA vascular systems are frequently connected with anastomoses. However, these vessels are usually closed. Systemic intercostal arteries (ICA) run strictly along the ribs and arise from the aorta. In contrast to PA and BA, ICAs are accessible to visualization by ultrasound examination in healthy volunteers. Essentially, tumor neoangiogenesis (TA) arises from nutritive bronchial arteries [3–5].

14.3 Basics of Color Doppler Ultrasound and Spectral Curve Analysis

In the 1990s fundamental studies about the assessment of vascular supply of pulmonary lesions using CDU were published [6–9]. The performance of spectral curve analysis enabled the derivation of flow curves of BA (Fig. 14.2), PA (Fig. 14.3), ICA (Fig. 14.4), and vessels of tumor neoangiogenesis (Fig. 14.5). Based on this approach multiple patterns of vascularization typical for different pathologies were classified by using CDU [10–12] (Graph 14.2). Pneumonia and atelectasis have a predominant PA vascular supply, whereas in primary malignant lung tumors and metastases, a BA vascularization or systemic neoangiogenetic vessels mainly contribute to the blood supply of these lesions. In subtle derivation of various vessels in a lung consolidation ("mapping"), different flow signals were detected within a lesion indicating a complex tumor vascularization [11, 12] (Fig. 14.6). Qualitative CDU is established in the clinical practice as an exploratory tool, while spectral curve analysis is time-consuming and limited by breath-dependent and pulsatile motion artifacts.

14.4 Basics of CEUS of the Lung

Since the introduction of CEUS to the diagnostic algorithm of liver diseases, its importance has significantly increased over the recent years (especially in the characterization of focal liver lesions) [13]. The currently available second-generation contrast agents enable an enhanced backscattering of the ultrasonic wave by the formation of

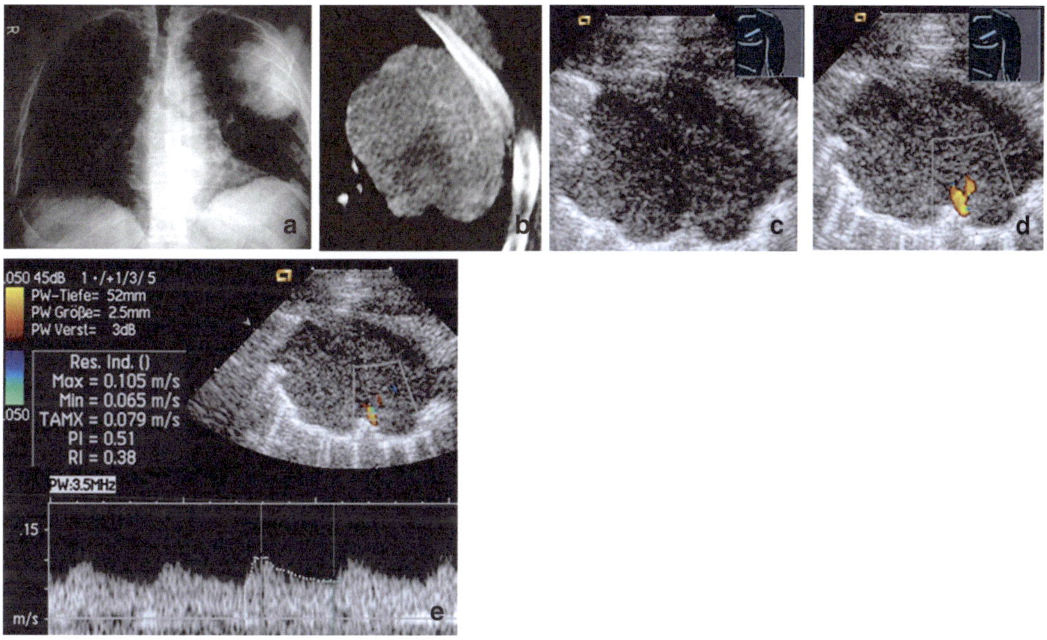

Fig. 14.2 Patient with peripheral lung cancer on X-ray examination (**a**) and CT scan (**b**); B-mode imaging shows a homogeneous echoic lesion (**c**) with reduced flow signal on colour-Doppler ultrasound (CDU) (**d**). Spectral curve analysis shows a low impedant arterial flow signal indicating bronchial arterial supply (**e**)

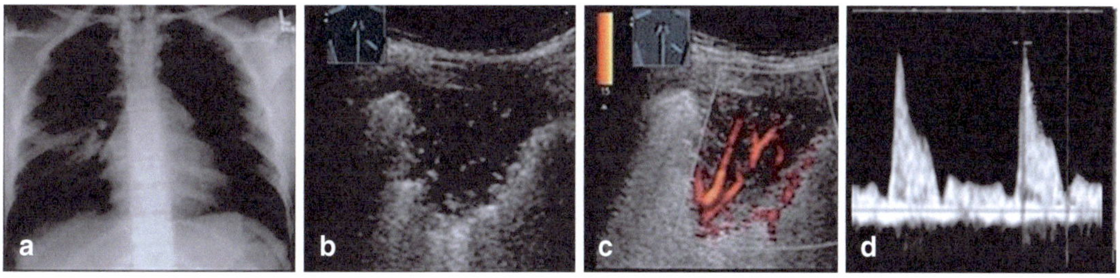

Fig. 14.3 Patient with pneumonia on X-ray examination (**a**); B-mode US presents a homogeneous echoic lesion with air bronchogram (**b**) and with marked flow signal on CDU (**c**). Spectral curve analysis shows a high-impedance arterial flow signal indicating pulmonary arterial supply (**d**)

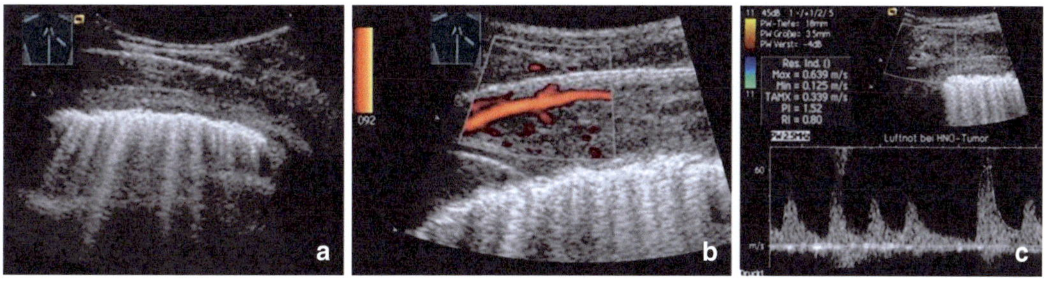

Fig. 14.4 Patient with head and neck cancer and proven pleural metastases; B-mode US presents a homogeneous echoic pleural tumor layer (**a**) with a solitary intercostal vessel on CDU (**b**). Spectral curve analysis shows a high-impedance arterial flow signal indicating intercostal arterial supply in a patient with arrhythmia (**c**)

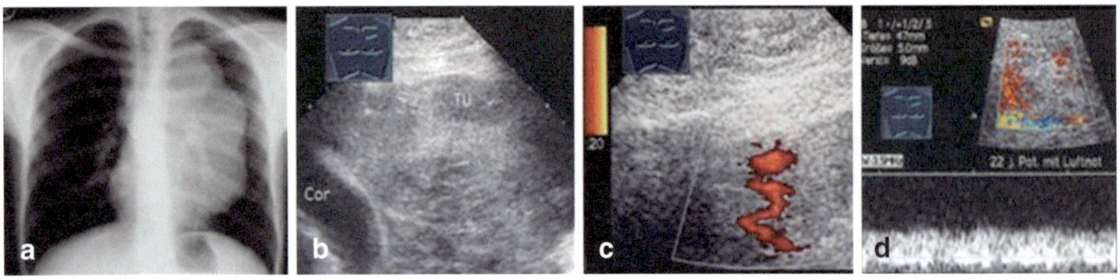

Fig. 14.5 Patient with malignant lymphoma on X-ray examination (**a**); B-mode US presents a homogeneous echoic tumor (TU) (**b**) with reduced flow signal on CDU (**c**). Spectral curve analysis shows a low-impedance arterial flow signal with a nearly constant flow that lacks systolic-diastolic variation indicating vessels of tumor neoangiogenesis (**d**)

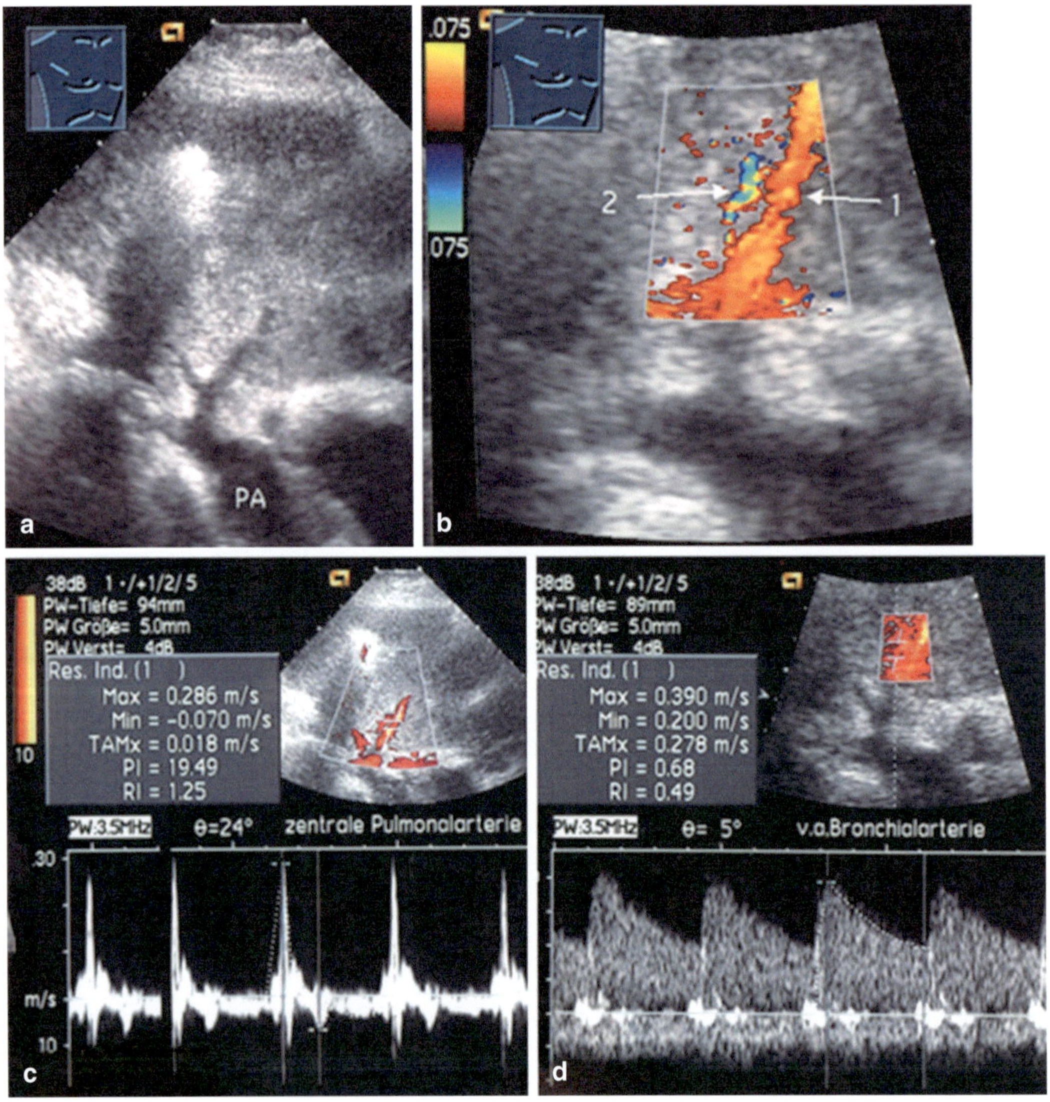

Fig. 14.6 Patient with pneumonia; B-mode imaging presents a homogeneous echoic consolidation of lung tissue (**a**) (PA = pulmonary artery); on CDU two vessels could be differentiated (1 = pulmonary artery, 2 = bronchial artery) (**b**); a high-impedance arterial FS was seen suggesting a pulmonary artery (labelled 1 in **b**) (**c**); a low-impedance monophasic arterial FS directed to the periphery was seen suggesting a bronchial artery (labelled 2 in **b**) (**d**)

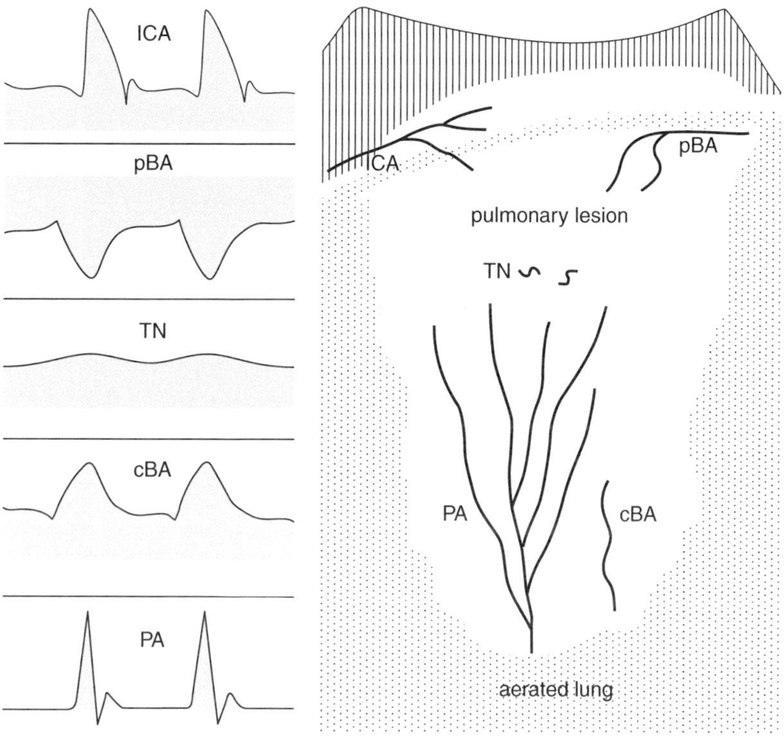

Graph 14.2 Possible arterial supply of pulmonary lesions with corresponding spectral curves. ICA intercostal artery, pBA peripheral bronchial artery, TN tumorneoangiogenesis, cBA central bronchial artery, PA pulmonary artery

microscopic bubbles in the vascular lumen after the application. This leads to an increase in the amplitude of the detected signal finally resulting in a higher contrast of the vascular area compared to CDU. CEUS examination offers the possibility to display even smallest-sized vessels near to the capillary level. Basically, CEUS should be performed according to the guidelines of EFSUMB [13, 14]. Similar to the liver, the lung circulation is characterized by a dual arterial blood supply and thus suitable for CEUS. By using CEUS it is possible to differentiate between an early pulmonary arterial flooding of contrast agent from a delayed systemic flooding of contrast media. Presuming a purely pulmonary vascularization, this moment is marked by an early arterial flooding of the contrast agent (CA) 1–6 s post-intravenous injection. After only a few seconds, the CA can be detected in the right heart by ultrasound examination (Fig. 14.7). The time until any flooding of contrast agent can be revealed ("time to enhancement") depends on the hemodynamic parameters of the patient (heart failure, chronic obstructive pulmonary disease). Contrast enhancement of a pulmonary lesion before contrast medium admission in the chest wall or a parenchymal organ suggests a PA vascularization of the lesion. Flooding of contrast medium coincident with the chest wall or parenchymal organs requires the passing through the lungs and is indicative for a systemic arterial supply. In general the time period is over 7 s but expanded significantly in pathological hemodynamic parameters. Basically, the early arterial phase from the beginning of the PA until the beginning of the BA phase should be always documented by clip, because subtle anomalies of the vascularization can be easily overlooked. The extent of the contrast medium enhancement ("extent of enhancement") depends on the presence or absence of a blood supply, the type of vessel—either PA or BA—and the eventual presence of collaterals or tumor neoangiogenesis. It can be distinguished between an arterial phase (1–30 s) and parenchymal phase (1–5 min). The quantitative assessment of the extent of the contrast media enhancement needs to be adjusted to an intraindividual reference. This offers the opportunity to distinguish between an either reduced or

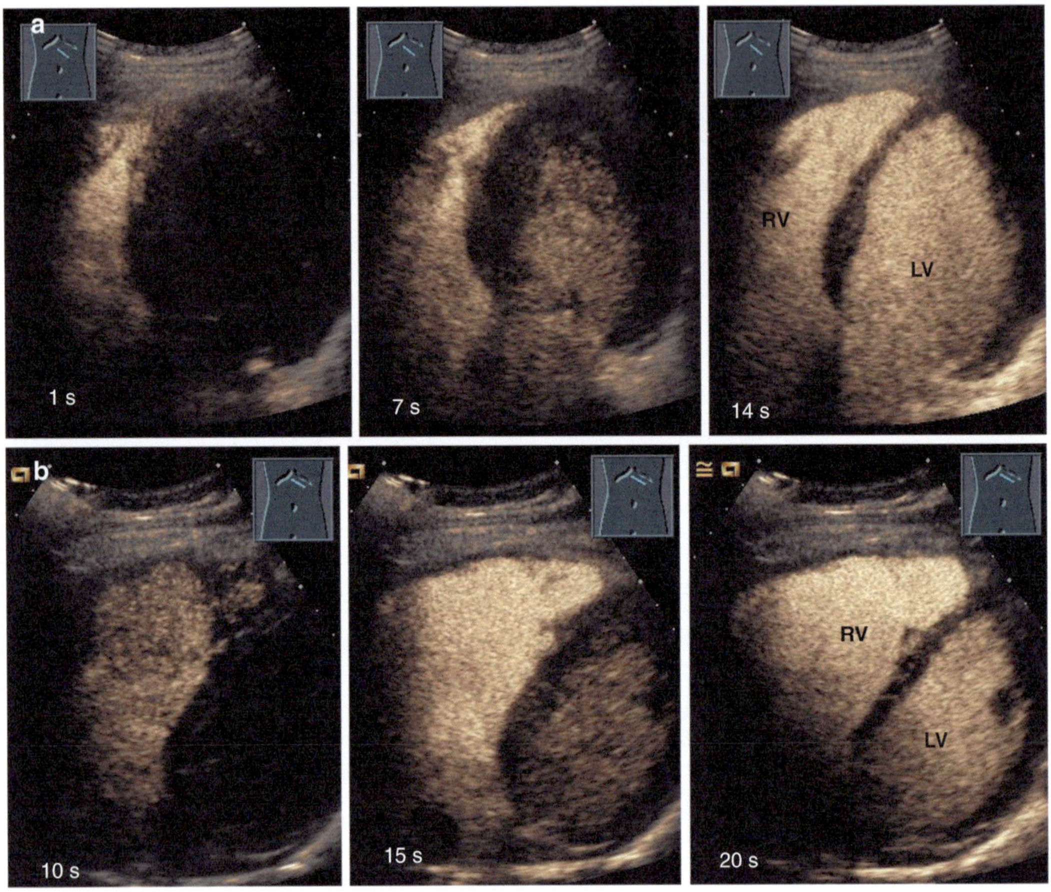

Fig. 14.7 Visualization of the time to contrast enhancement in the subcostal four-chamber view in a healthy proband (series **a**) and a patient with cardiomyopathy (series **b**). Time to enhancement (TE) differs in both series and in the right ventricle (RV) and the left ventricle (LV) indicating influence of varying cardiac output to TE

increased contrast enhancement. Enhancement of parenchymatous organs like spleen and liver leads as in vivo reference. The third criterion may be the differentiation between a homogeneous and inhomogeneous enhancement ("homogeneity of enhancement"). Therefore intraparenchymal lesions were assessed in terms of number, shape (round, wedge-shaped), and location (central, peripheral), whereas the enhancement of the surrounding tissue is considered to be an in vivo reference (Table 14.1). The extravascular administration of the contrast medium provides an additional application modality. It can be administered orally to reveal an esophago-pleural fistula, transcathetrally to control location of a drainage catheter, and intrapleurally to further characterize a polyseptated effusion. For this purpose a few drops of contrast medium are diluted in 20–50 mL normal saline and then applied according to the appropriate indication [15].

Table 14.1 Assessment criteria for contrast-enhanced ultrasound in pleural-based lung lesions

1. Time to contrast enhancement (TE) (differentiation of an early pulmonary arterial vascularization from a delayed bronchial arterial vascularization)
2. Extent of contrast enhancement (EE) (in comparison with the enhancement of parenchymal organs)
3. Homogeneity of contrast enhancement (HE) (enhancement of a lesion in comparison to the enhancement of the surrounding tissue)

However, the indications for thoracic ultrasound especially for CEUS are limited. The clini-

Table 14.2 Potential indications for CEUS in thoracic lesions

1. Clinical condition of visible and palpable tumor of the thoracic wall
2. Clinical condition of localized thoracic pain
3. Complementary investigation of lung consolidations diagnosed by X-ray examination
4. CEUS image guidance for biopsy of thoracic lesions

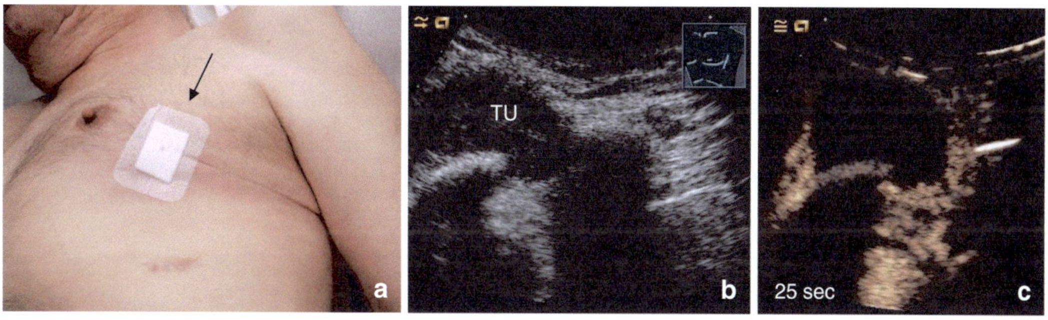

Fig. 14.8 Patient with lung cancer and primary surgery 6 months ago and a palpable tumor (arrow) (**a**); B-mode US shows a homogeneous hypoechoic tumor (TU) (**b**); CEUS shows no enhancement of the lesion suggesting avital tissue (**c**)

cal value of CEUS on the thorax has less evidence [14]. Chest X-ray and computed tomography of the thorax are still irreplaceable and should be (if available) used for interpretation of findings. Due to its high spatial resolution and the possibility to perform a real-time investigation of vascular structures, thoracic ultrasound should in fact not be considered as an independent diagnostic tool but as a valuable extension of the diagnostic procedure limited to particular indication. After B-mode imaging, the use of CEUS should be reserved for particular issues. The following chapter reviews indications of CEUS, and selected keynotes will be discussed (Table 14.2).

14.5 Clinical Keynotes

14.5.1 Symptom-Oriented Examination of a Visible or Palpable Mass of the Chest Wall

The assessment of chest wall lesions represents a domain of conventional B-mode imaging and thus also allows CEUS examination. The indication for the application of contrast agent should just take place in unexplained findings of B-mode imaging. Chest wall lesions are supplied via intercostal arteries, or by tumor angiogenesis; originating from intercostal arteries; therefore a "systemic vascularization" is expected. The essential value of CEUS is the possibility to differentiate between avascular (necrosis, abscess, hematoma, seroma) and vascularized tissue (Figs. 14.8 and 14.9). Whether a vascularized mass is benign or malignant has to be carried out primarily clinically, by B-mode ultrasound and histology. Just in single cases the extension of contrast enhancement provides evidence of the underlying pathology (Fig. 14.10).

14.5.2 Symptom-Oriented Examination in Localized Chest Pain

Chest pain is one of the main symptoms in an emergency area. Conventional B-mode ultrasound is a standard procedure for detecting rib fractures [16] and for the diagnosis of pleurisy [17]. In case of pleural defects in B-mode ultrasound, you should try to clarify whether an infectious pleurisy or an embolic pleurisy is present. Infectious pleurisy shows in CEUS a homogeneous, strong early pulmonary vascularization (Fig. 14.11) [18]. Pleural thickening with marked contrast enhancement

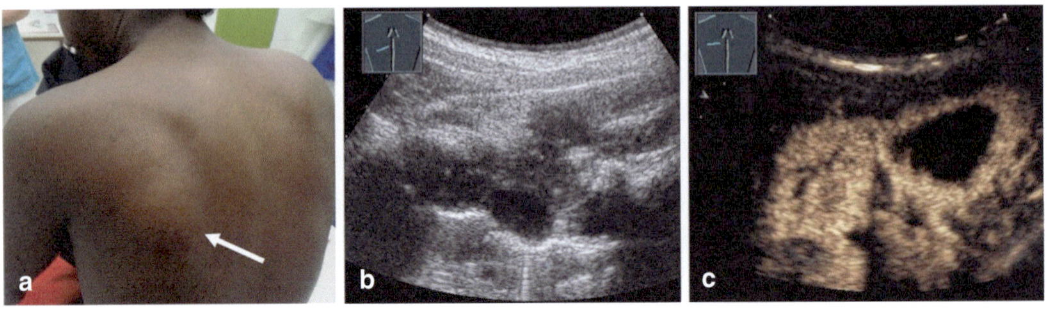

Fig. 14.9 Patient with pain and a visible tumor (arrow) (**a**); B-mode imaging presents an inhomogeneous hypoechoic tumor (TU) (**b**); CEUS shows a complex enhancement of the lesion with areas of no enhancement (**c**). Further investigation confirmed the diagnosis of *tuberculosis*

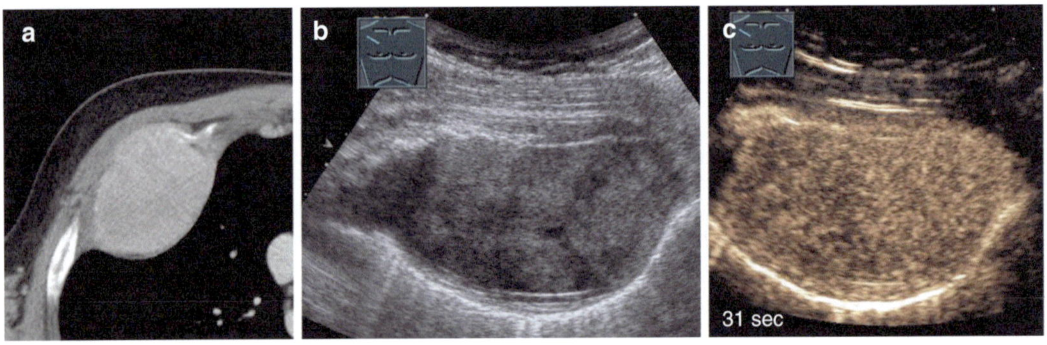

Fig. 14.10 Patient with pain and a palpable tumor (arrow) which was also seen by CT scan (**a**); B-mode imaging shows a homogeneous hypoechoic tumor (**b**); CEUS shows a marked arterial enhancement indicating marked tumor neoangiogenesis (**c**). Further investigation confirmed the diagnosis of *plasmacytoma*

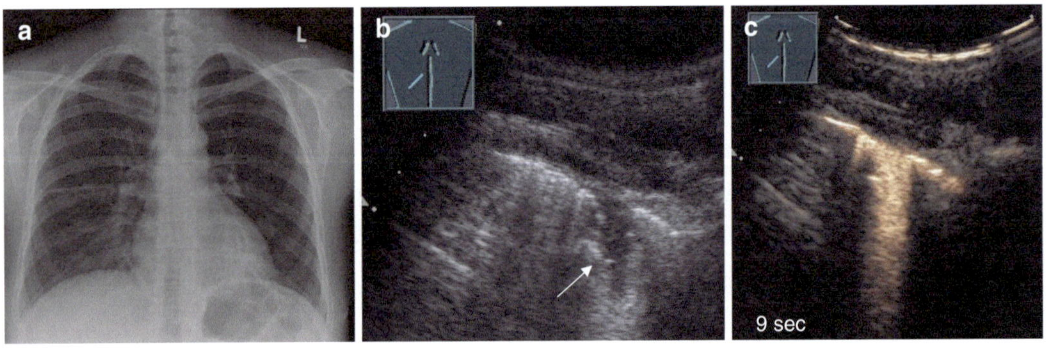

Fig. 14.11 Patient with localized chest pain with a normal thoracic X-ray examination (**a**); B-mode imaging shows a small pleural wedge-shaped lesion (arrow) (**b**); CEUS shows a homogeneous pulmonary arterial enhancement suggesting infectious *pleurisy* (**c**)

can be observed in pleural empyema (Fig. 14.12). Sometimes characteristic CEUS pattern in patients with chronic pleurisy can be observed (Figs. 14.13 and 14.14). A reliable differentiation of chronic pleurisy from a pleural carcinosis is only possible by histological examination. Conventional B-mode ultrasound can be basically used for the diagnosis of embolic pleurisy with underlying pulmonary embolism (PE) [19, 20]. Pathophysiologically the peripheral PE is based on an impaired pulmonary vascularization with formation of a hemorrhage or pulmonary infarction [21]. A first pilot study

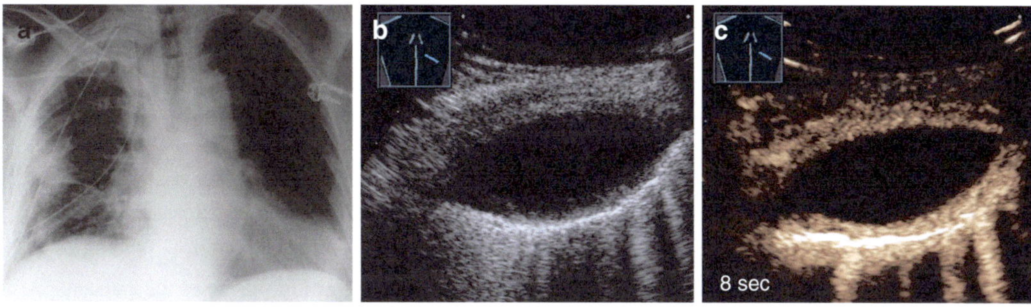

Fig. 14.12 Patient with fever and a right-sided pulmonary consolidation on X-ray examination (**a**); B-mode imaging shows an oval well-demarcated hypoechoic pleural lesion (**b**); on CEUS the lesion shows a marked wall enhancement and no central enhancement (**c**). Further investigation confirmed diagnosis of *pleural empyema*

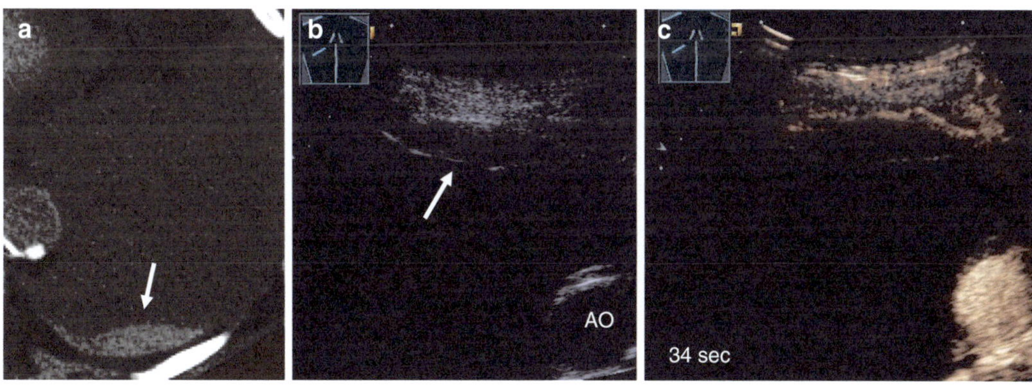

Fig. 14.13 Patient with pleural effusion of unknown cause; CT scan shows hypodense pleural lesion (arrow) (**a**); B-mode imaging shows a hypoechoic pleural lesion (AO = aorta) (arrow) (**b**); CEUS shows nearly no enhancement of the lesion (**c**); US-guided biopsy makes diagnosis of *chronic fibrinous pleuritis*

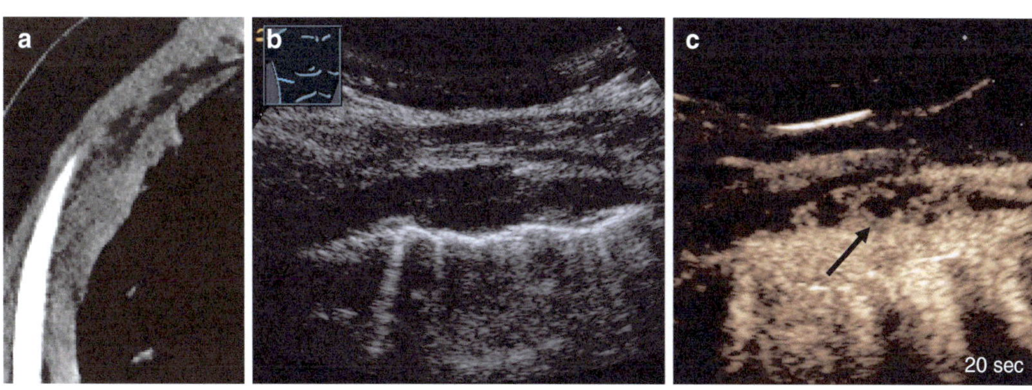

Fig. 14.14 Patient with anamnestic tuberculosis and a marked pleural thickness on CT scan (**a**); B-mode imaging presents a hypoechoic pleural lesion (**b**); CEUS shows a marked enhancement with small areas of no enhancement (arrow) (**c**); US-guided pleural biopsy confirmed diagnosis of *active pleural tuberculosis*

showed that peripheral PE exhibited a defective PA vascularization in CEUS [18, 22]. In this study 80% of the peripheral lung consolidations in patients with pulmonary embolism (PE) diagnosed by computed tomography angiography (CTA) or lung scintigraphy (LS) presented an impaired pulmonary arterial vascularization with peripheral wedge-shaped unenhanced areas in the parenchymal phase of CEUS as a sign of peripheral infarction of the lung (Figs. 14.15 and 14.16) [22].

In cases of a veritable delayed BA vascularization, the impaired PA vascularization can be exclusively observed in a short early arterial time window. A distinct actual infarction is not detectable (Fig. 14.17). The diagnosis of this pathological vascularization requires clip documentation. However, 20% of the secured peripheral embolic pleurisy (EP) presented a homogeneous PA vascularization [22]. This phenomenon may be explained by a fibrinolysis-related revascularization. The detectable vascular changes in peripheral EP in the CEUS can vary in sonographic follow-up. In individual cases of patients with clinical evidence for pulmonary embolism and no evidence in computed tomography regarding PE, CEUS detected pleural defects with impaired pulmonary vascularization (Fig. 14.18) [23]. The role of CEUS in the diagnostic algorithm of embolic pleurisy is still unclear.

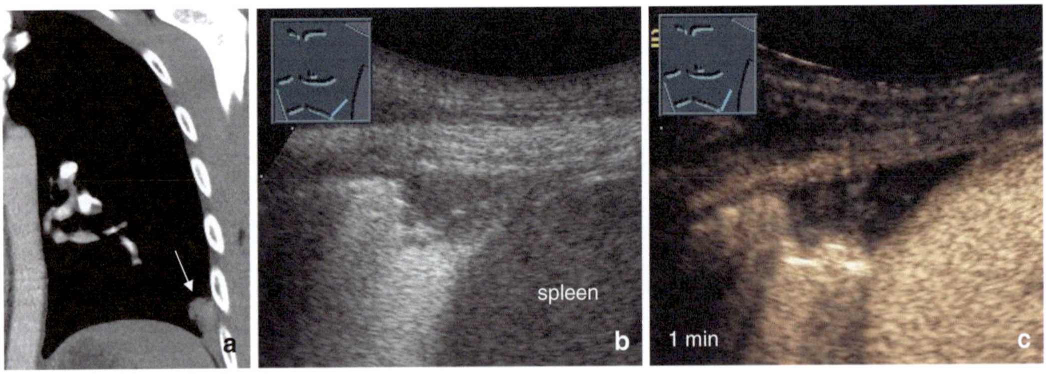

Fig. 14.15 Patient with dyspnea and diagnosis of central pulmonary embolism on CT scan and a small pleural lesion (arrow) (**a**); B-mode imaging presents a wedge-shaped hypoechoic pleural lesion (**b**); CEUS shows no enhancement of the lesion suggesting peripheral *pleural infarction due to pulmonary embolism* (**c**)

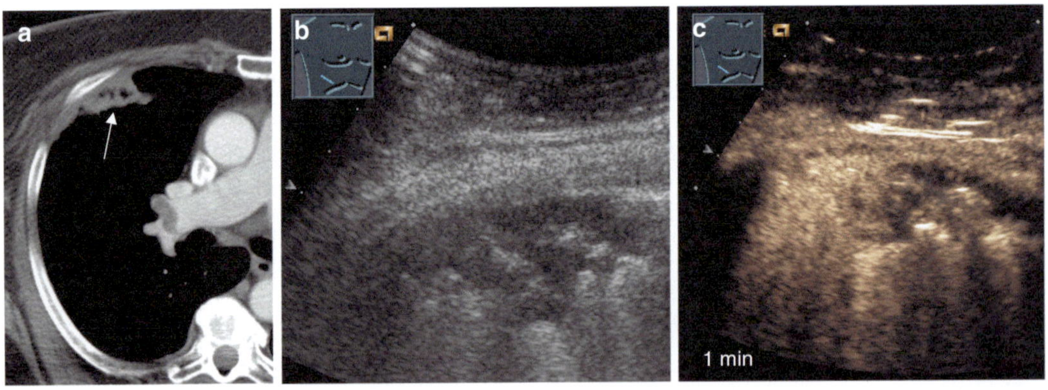

Fig. 14.16 Patient with dyspnea and diagnosis of central pulmonary embolism on CT scan and a small wedge-shaped pleural lesion (arrow) (**a**); B-mode imaging presents a complex hypoechoic pleural lesion with air bronchogram (**b**); CEUS shows a mixed enhancement of the lesion with areas of no enhancement suggesting peripheral *pleural infarction due to pulmonary embolism* (**c**)

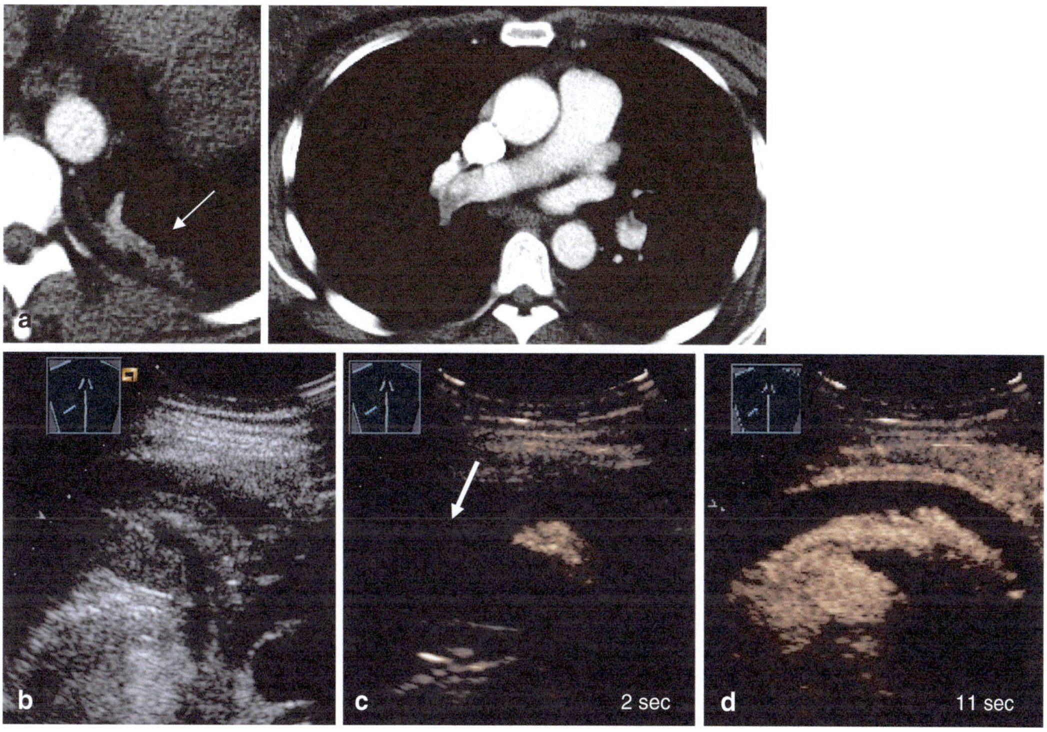

Fig. 14.17 Patient with dyspnea and diagnosis of central pulmonary embolism on CT scan and a small pleural lesion (arrow) (**a**); B-mode imaging presents a small pleural effusion and a consolidated hypoechoic lung tissue (**b**); in the early arterial phase, CEUS shows a consolidated area of no pulmonary arterial enhancement suggesting absence of pulmonary vascularization (**c**); in the later arterial phase, lesion shows a bronchial arterial enhancement of the lesion suggesting peripheral *pleural embolism without signs of infarction* (**d**)

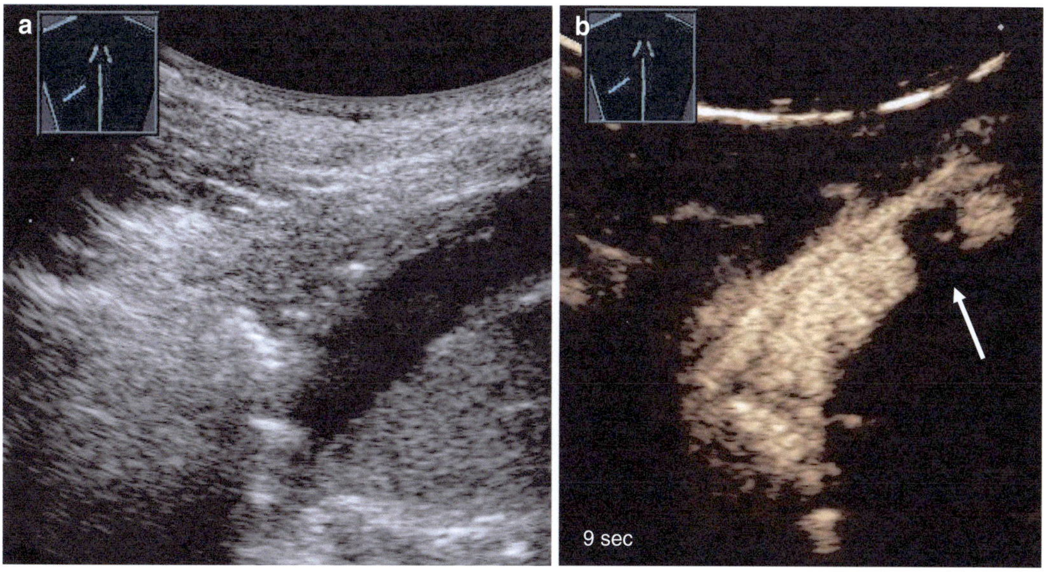

Fig. 14.18 Patient with sudden onset of dyspnea and tachycardia 2 days after appendectomy; deep vein thrombosis was excluded by compression ultrasound, and central pulmonary embolism was excluded by CT scan; B-mode imaging presents a small pleural effusion and a small consolidated hypoechoic lung tissue (**a**); CEUS shows a mixed enhancement with marked pulmonary arterial enhancement but with a small area of no pulmonary enhancement (arrow) suggesting *peripheral embolism* despite negative CT scan for diagnosis of pulmonary embolism (**b**)

14.5.3 Complementary Investigation in Radiological Opacification of the Lung

14.5.3.1 Effusion with Compression Atelectasis

In this clinical constellation the atelectasis, the pleura, and the effusion can be assessed. The compression atelectasis is usually characterized by a homogeneous and clear PA enhancement [24]. However, CEUS should only be used when the etiology of the atelectasis or pleural effusion cannot be assigned safely. CEUS can present nodules (Fig. 14.19), pulmonary infarction (Fig. 14.20), and pulmonary hemorrhage (Fig. 14.21) in atelectatic lung tissue. Pleural metastases are delineated of echogenic effusion by contrast enhancement (Fig. 14.22). In the differential diagnosis of parapneumonic septa in concomitant effusion (Fig. 14.23) and malignant pleural infiltration (Fig. 14.24), CEUS is helpful. Basically, in suspicion of esophageal perforation, the orally administrated contrast medium can be detected in the pleural cavity (Fig. 14.25).

14.5.3.2 Obstructive Atelectasis in Suspected Central Tumor

Obstructive atelectasis can be used as an "acoustic window" for the exploration of central formations behind the atelectasis. CT scan is the standard procedure for diagnosis and staging of central lung tumors. Occasionally, the central tumor cannot be safely separated from the following atelectasis [25, 26]. CEUS represents a possibility of the demarcation of the atelectasis from the central tumor, as atelectasis usually shows a homogeneous PA enhancement, whereas the central tumor is characterized by a generally reduced BA vascularization (Fig. 14.26). So the central tumor can be visualized by using CEUS and potentially also be punctured. In cases of a tumor-induced pulmonary vascular occlusion, mostly in CEUS a reduced BA enhancement of the atelectasis can be observed (Fig. 14.27). In such cases, usually a chronic atelectasis in advanced tumor disease is existent. It is not possible to differentiate this pattern from a tumor-infiltrated atelectasis. In atelectasis due to central lymphoma and lymph node metastasis, the central lesions may show (depending on the extent of their BA tumor neoangiogenesis) an increased contrast enhancement and permit the differential diagnosis of central lung cancer (Fig. 14.28).

14.5.3.3 Pneumonia

In CEUS the uncomplicated pneumonia is characterized by a homogeneous marked PA enhancement [27] (Fig. 14.29). CEUS is merely indicated when there is no or insufficient clinical improvement on therapy. Complications such as necrosis (Fig. 14.30), abscess (Figs. 14.31 and 14.32), infarction (Fig. 14.33), and empyema (Fig. 14.34) can be reliably detected by using the CEUS. Chronic pneumonia with

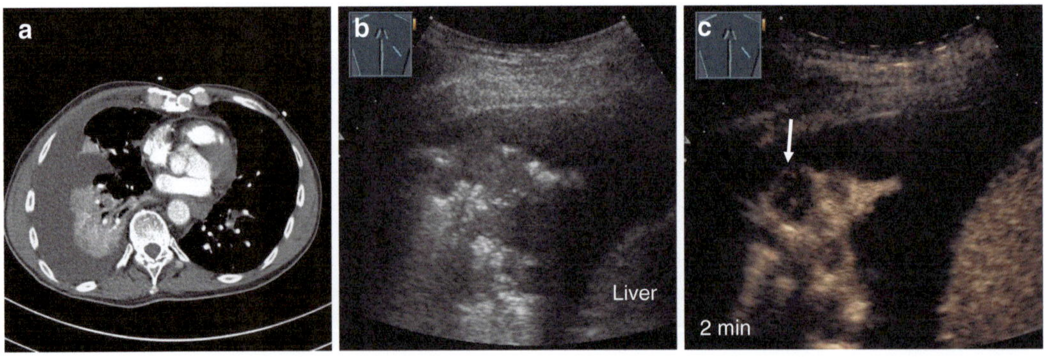

Fig. 14.19 Patient with colorectal cancer and a marked right-sided pleural effusion with compressive atelectasis on CT scan (**a**); B-mode imaging presents pleural effusion with an inhomogeneous air pattern of the lung (**b**); CEUS shows round lesions of reduced enhancement in the consolidated lung suggesting *pulmonary metastasis* (**c**)

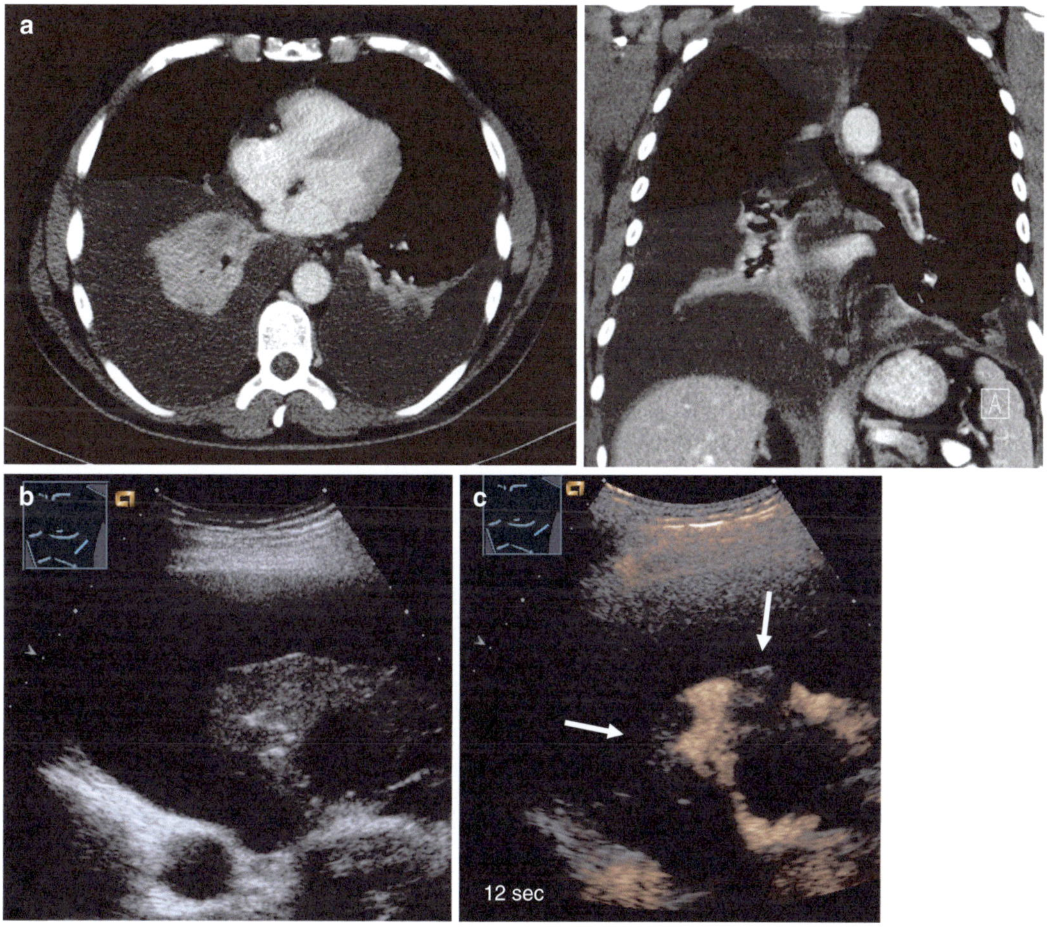

Fig. 14.20 Patient with dyspnea, pulmonary effusion, and confirmed pulmonary embolism by CT scan (**a**); B-mode imaging presents pleural effusion with a homogeneous consolidation of the lung (**b**); CEUS shows wedge-shaped areas of no enhancement in the consolidated lung suggesting *pulmonary infarction due to central pulmonary embolism* (**c**)

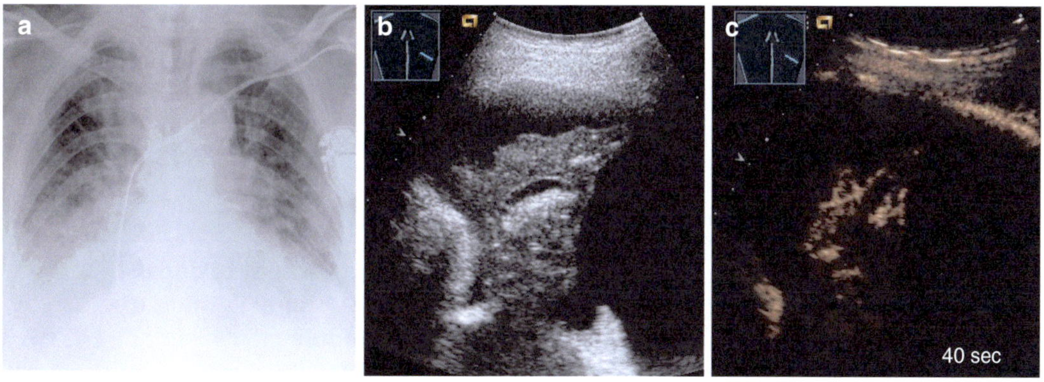

Fig. 14.21 Patient with dyspnea after thoracic trauma; X-ray examination shows pleural effusion (**a**); hemothorax was diagnosed; B-mode imaging presents pleural effusion with a homogeneous consolidation of the lung (**b**); CEUS shows an inhomogeneous enhancement of the lung *suggesting pulmonary hemorrhage* (**c**)

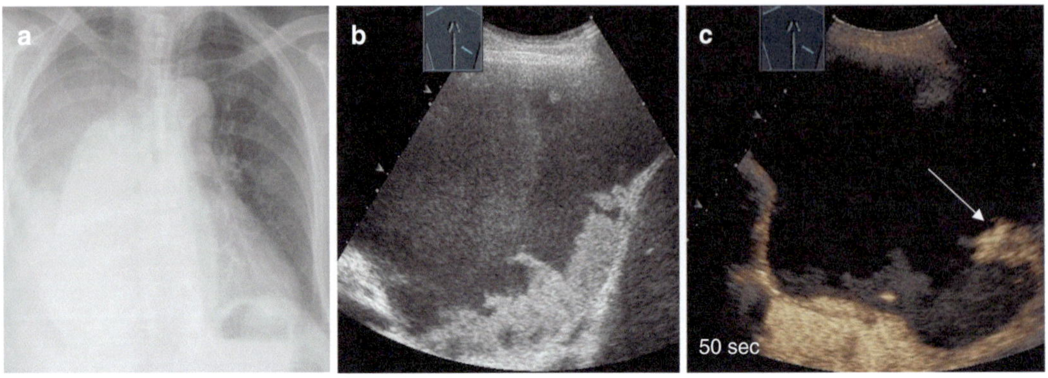

Fig. 14.22 Patient with dyspnea and diagnosis of breast cancer; X-ray examination shows a marked right-sided pleural effusion (**a**), B-mode imaging presents pleural effusion with echoic tissue on the diaphragmal border (**b**); CEUS shows an inhomogeneous enhancement of the echoic tissue suggesting sludge as well as *tumor tissue due to pleural metastases* (arrow) (**c**)

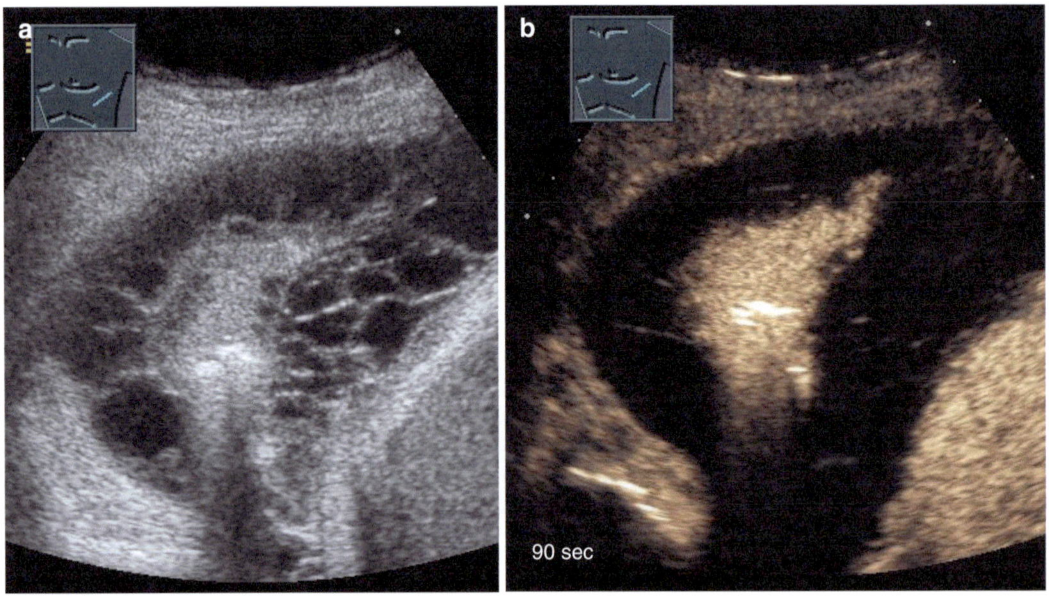

Fig. 14.23 Patient with dyspnea and diagnosis of pneumonia; B-mode imaging presents pleural effusion with marked fibrin strands (**a**); CEUS shows no enhancement of the fibrin strands suggesting parapneumonic *exudative effusion* (**b**)

no regression may reveal a BA enhancement (Fig. 14.35). In these cases the histological analysis of tissue samples remains the diagnostic gold standard. However, the tuberculous pneumonia is also characterized by a BA vascularization. The revealing of a BA vascularization in a patient with the clinically diagnosed pneumonia is always accompanied by a loss of pulmonary vasculature and therefore strongly indicative for a parenchymal pulmonary defect (Figs. 14.36 and 14.37). The CEUS represents no alternative but a complement to the CT scan.

14.5.3.4 The Pleural Lesions/Peripheral Pulmonary Nodule

The diagnosis and assessment of peripheral pulmonary consolidations is the domain of CT scan but in general representable by ultrasound and also by CEUS [29, 30]. One of the key challenges

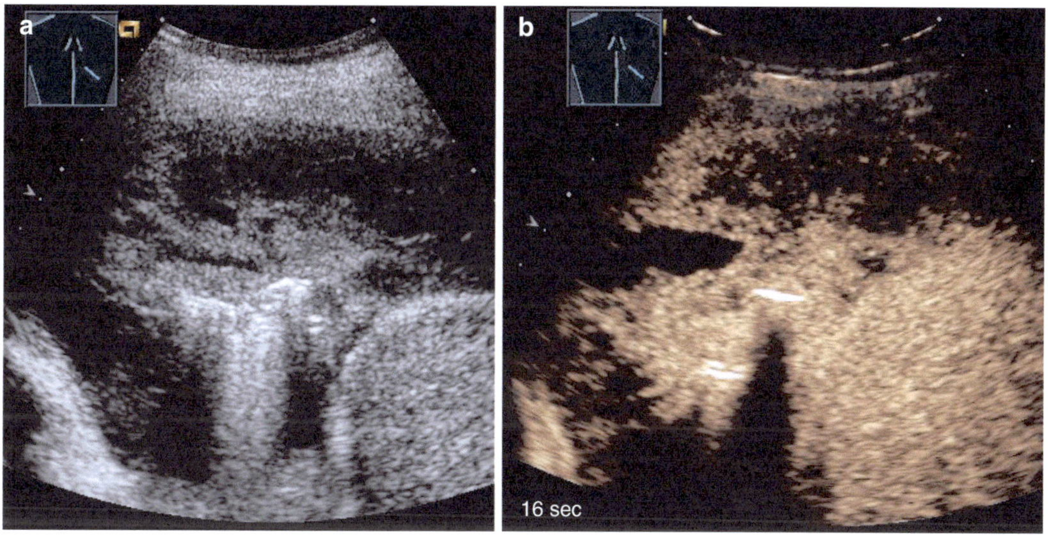

Fig. 14.24 Patient with dyspnea and diagnosis of malignant lymphoma; B-mode imaging presents pleural effusion with marked echoic tissue surrounding the lung (**a**); CEUS shows marked enhancement of the pleural tissue suggesting *pulmonary lymphoma involvement* (**b**)

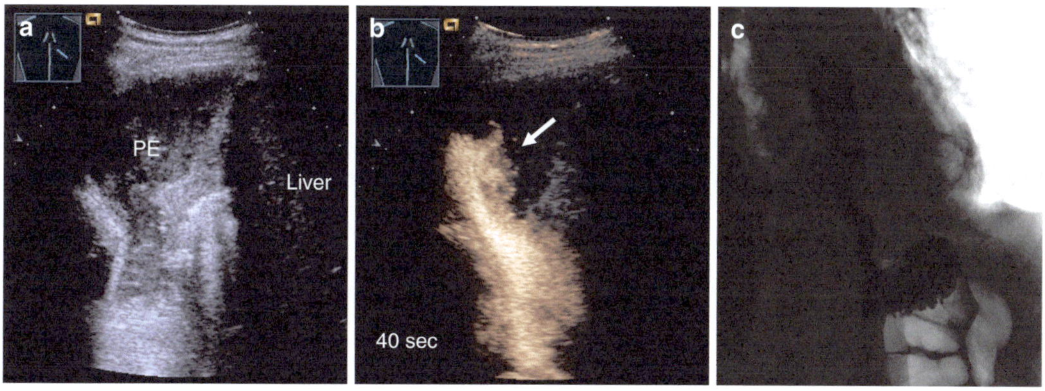

Fig. 14.25 Patient with dyspnea and diagnosis of esophageal cancer; B-mode imaging presents a right-sided echoic pleural effusion (PE) (**a**); CEUS was performed by oral application of contrast medium and shows enhancement of the pleural effusion (arrow) suggesting *esophageal perforation* (**b**); X-ray with esophagography-confirmed diagnosis (**c**)

of routinely used imaging procedure is the evaluation of dignity and the possible histology. Because tumor neoangiogenesis involves predominantly BA, the evaluation of vascularization might be a rational approach in this context [5, 31–33]. The extent of tumor vascularization is variable showing differences in the contrast enhancement in CEUS (Fig. 14.38). Sometimes irregular tumor vessels can be present (Fig. 14.39). Nevertheless, an integrative analysis regarding the clinical context and all additional information is crucial for a correct interpretation of the CEUS imaging results. Subgroups of non-small cell lung cancer can mimic the picture of pneumonia [10] (Fig. 14.40). Pulmonary lymphoma usually also reveals a PA contrast enhancement [34] (Fig. 14.41). Benign pulmonary lesions can be classified by CEUS only in individual cases. A clinical follow-up based on sonography should be performed (Figs. 14.42, 14.43, and 14.44). In the case of therapy relevance, histological confirmation is essential.

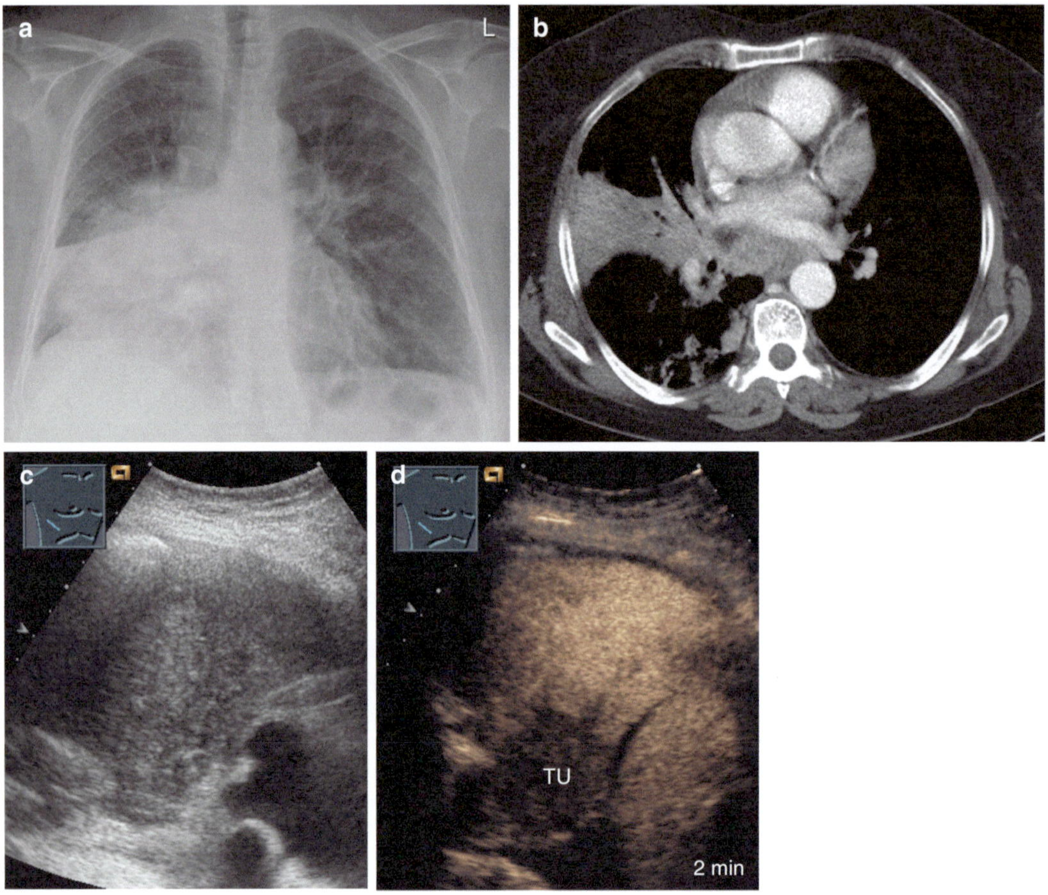

Fig. 14.26 Patient with lung cancer shown on X-ray examination (**a**) and on CT scan (**b**); B-mode imaging presents a homogeneous lung consolidation unable to discriminate between atelectasis and central tumor (**c**); CEUS shows a central hypoechoic tumor lesion (TU) and a hyperechoic atelectatic tissue (**d**)

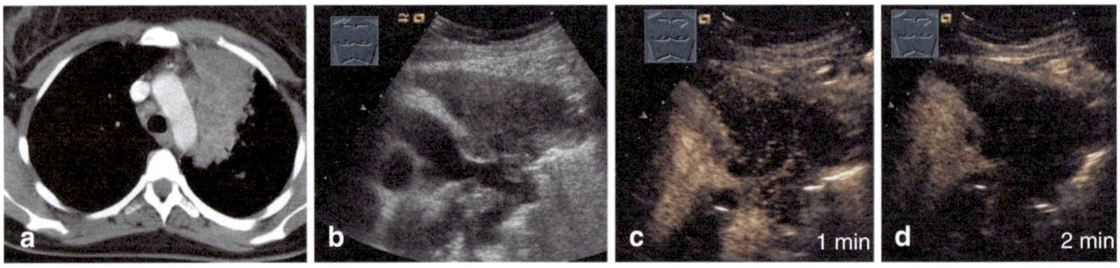

Fig. 14.27 Patient with lung cancer shown on CT scan (**a**); B-mode imaging presents a homogeneous lung consolidation (**b**); CEUS after 1 min (**c**) and 2 min (**d**) shows a reduced contrast enhancement due to bronchial arterial vascularization suggesting occlusion of pulmonary arteries and possible tumor infiltration of the atelectatic tissue

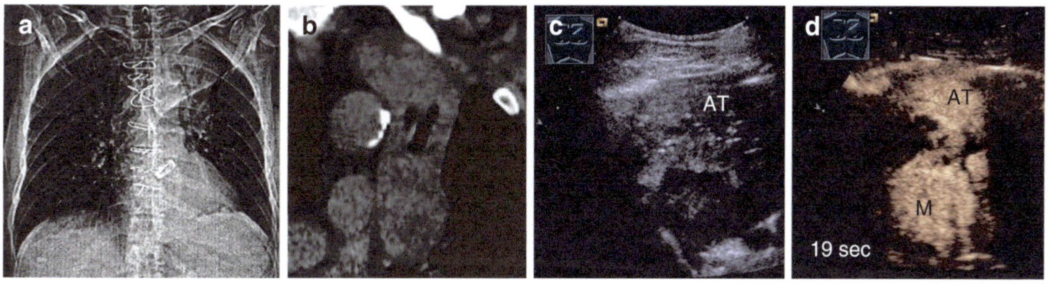

Fig. 14.28 Patient with renal cell cancer (RCC) and evidence of mediastinal tumor and atelectasis of the left upper lobe on X-ray examination (**a**) and on CT scan (**b**); B-mode imaging presents a homogeneous echoic atelectatic tissue (AT) and a central hypoechoic tumor lesion (**c**); CEUS shows a central hyperechoic tumor lesion suggesting *mediastinal metastasis (M) due to RCC* and a hyperechoic atelectatic tissue (**d**)

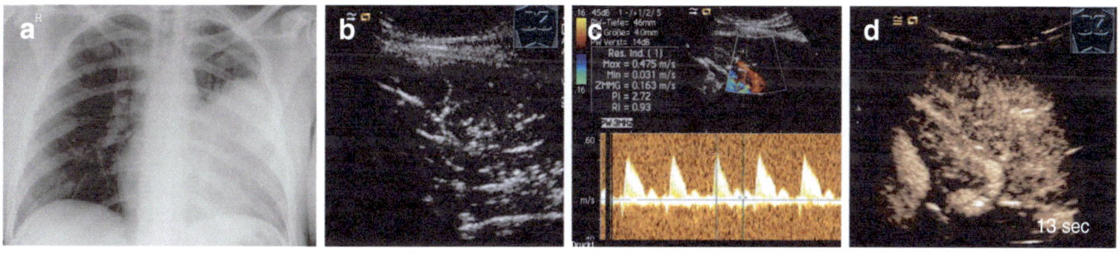

Fig. 14.29 Patient with pneumonia shown on X-ray examination (**a**); B-mode imaging presents a homogeneous lung consolidation with regular air bronchogram (**b**); spectral curve analysis shows a high-impedance flow signal (FS) suggesting pulmonary arterial supply (**c**); CEUS shows a homogeneous pulmonary arterial enhancement characteristic for *pneumonia* (**d**)

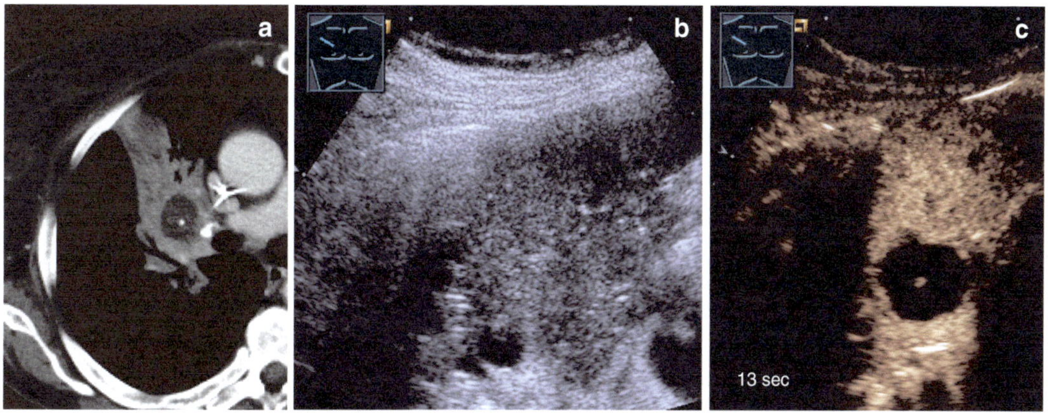

Fig. 14.30 Patient with AML and high-dose chemotherapy and a lung consolidation shown on CT scan (**a**); B-mode imaging presents a homogeneous lung consolidation (**b**); CEUS shows a marked enhancement of the lesion with a round central lesion without contrast enhancement (**c**); further investigation revealed *pulmonary aspergilloma*

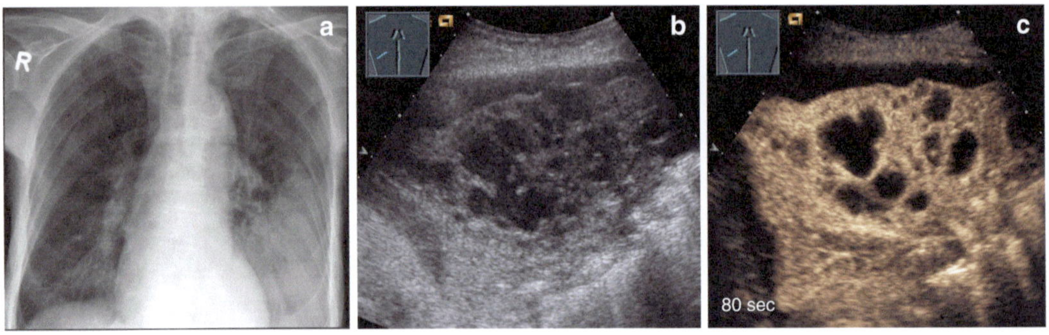

Fig. 14.31 Patient with clinical diagnosis of pneumonia and the corresponding lung infiltration on X-ray examination (**a**): B-mode imaging presents an inhomogeneous lung consolidation with multiple round hypoechoic lesions within the lung tissue (**b**); CEUS shows a marked enhancement of the lesion with multiple non-enhanced round areas suggesting *lung abscesses* (**c**)

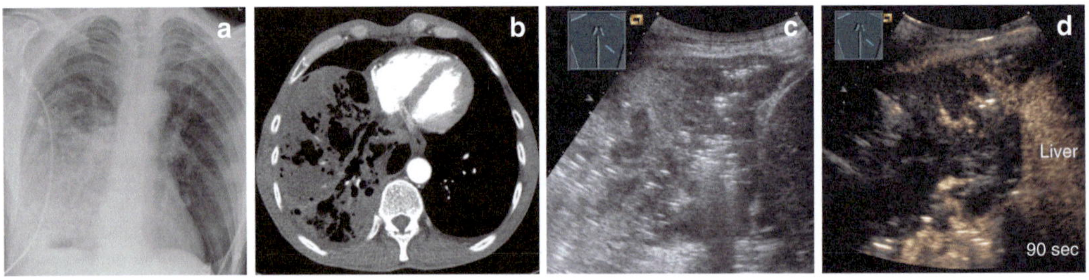

Fig. 14.32 Patient with chronic alcoholic disease and clinical diagnosis of pneumonia; the corresponding lung infiltration is shown on X-ray (**a**) and on CT scan (**b**): B-mode imaging presents an inhomogeneous lung consolidation with irregular air distribution (**c**); CEUS shows a large area of no enhancement suggesting a nearly complete *lobe abscess* (**d**); resection of the right lower lobe was performed

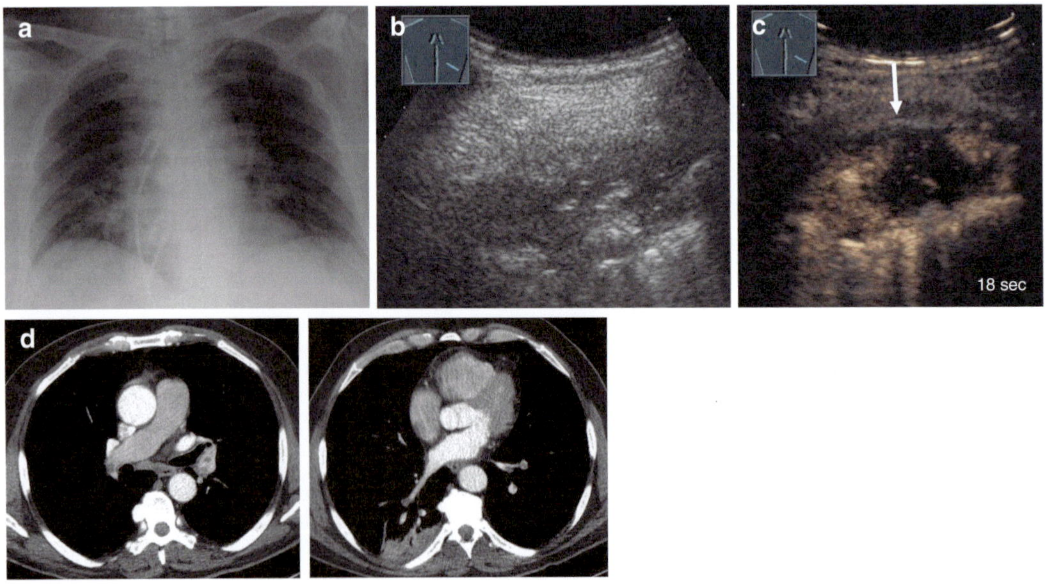

Fig. 14.33 Patient with clinical diagnosis of pneumonia; the corresponding lung infiltration is shown on X-ray examination (**a**); B-mode imaging presents a lung consolidation with air bronchogram (**b**); CEUS shows an inhomogeneous enhancement with a wedge-shaped area of no enhancement suggesting *infarct pneumonia* (**c**); CT scan confirmed diagnosis of central pulmonary embolism (**d**)

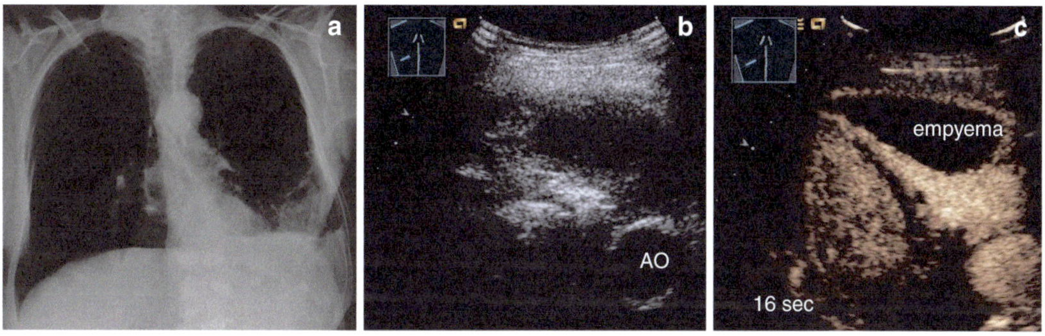

Fig. 14.34 Patient with clinical diagnosis of pneumonia and the corresponding lung infiltration on X-ray examination; B-mode imaging presents an inhomogeneous lung consolidation with a peripheral hypoechoic area and central signs of air bronchogram (**a**); CEUS shows a homogeneous central enhancement with a pleural-based oval well-delineated area of no enhancement (**b**); further investigation confirmed diagnosis of *parapneumonic pleural empyema* (**c**)

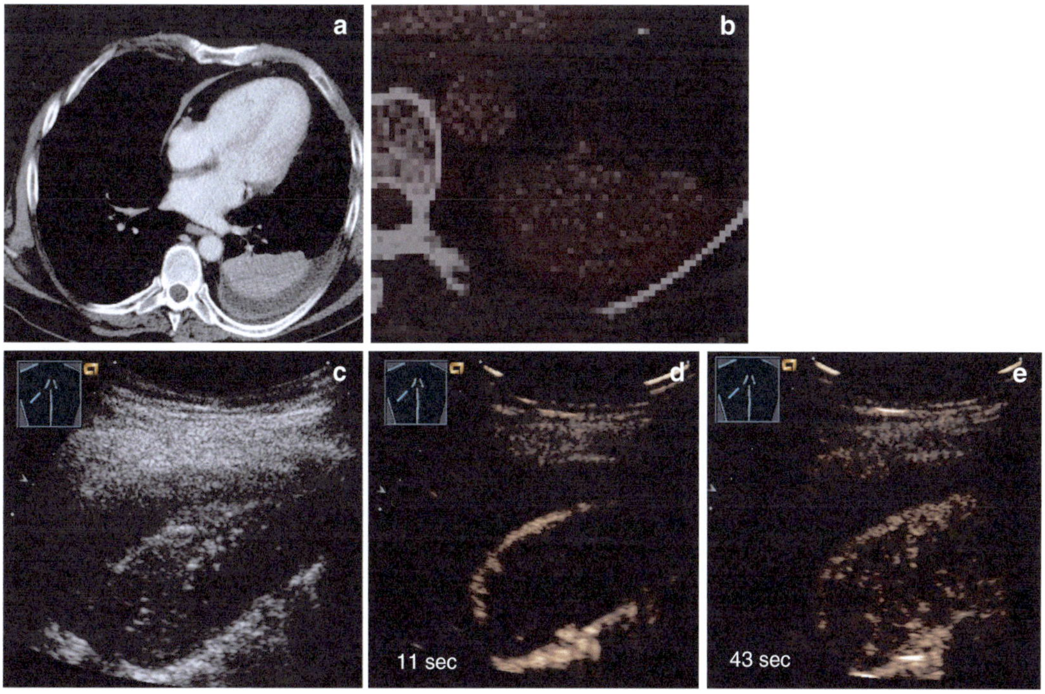

Fig. 14.35 Patient with schizophrenia and clinical diagnosis of pneumonia with a homogeneous infiltration of the lung shown on CT scan (**a, b**); B-mode imaging presents a complete lung consolidation (**c**); CEUS shows after 11 s (**d**) and 43 s (**e**) a reduced contrast enhancement due to bronchial arterial vascularization; US-guided biopsy was performed which excluded malignancy and makes the diagnosis of *chronic pneumonia*. Finally "*rounded atelectasis*" was diagnosed [28]

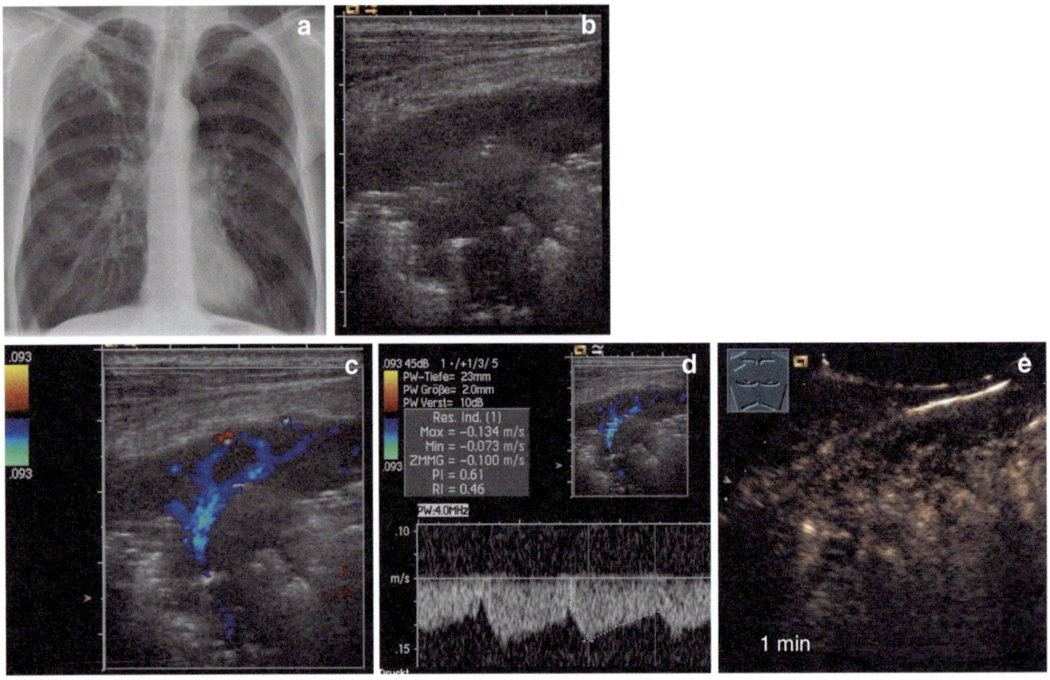

Fig. 14.36 Patient with fever, hemoptoe, and clinical diagnosis of consolidation in the apex of the lung suggesting tuberculosis shown on X-ray examination (**a**); B-mode imaging presents a complex lung consolidation with air bronchogram (**b**); CDU shows a flow directed to the hilus suggesting bronchial arterial supply (**c**); spectral curve analysis shows a low-impedance flow signal indicating bronchial arteries (**d**); CEUS shows a reduced inhomogeneous enhancement (**e**); US-guided biopsy was performed which excluded tuberculosis with the diagnosis of *chronic pneumonia*

14.5.3.5 Imaging-Guided Intervention

The ultrasound-guided intervention is an essential part of thoracic ultrasound. CEUS allows the differentiation of liquid and solid tissue and increases the procedural safety of puncturing and/or draining of abscesses of the thoracic wall, pleural empyema (Fig. 14.45), and lung abscess (Fig. 14.46) [35]. CEUS helps to differentiate between not vascularized tumor and vascularized tumor tissue. The CEUS-guided biopsy should be limited to areas with contrast enhancement (Figs. 14.47 and 14.48). By using CEUS tissue samples of central tumors with concomitant atelectasis can be taken transthoracically (Fig. 14.49). To control the correct position of a pleural catheter, an extravascular administration of contrast medium is necessary (Fig. 14.50). Complications after intervention, like an active bleeding, can be detected by CEUS (Figs. 14.51 and 14.52).

14.5.3.6 Summary

Different arterial supply of intercostal arteries, bronchial arteries, pulmonary arteries, and arteries of tumor neoangiogenesis may play a role in thoracic tumor vascularization. CEUS of the chest is limited to pleural-based lesion. CEUS in peripheral lesions and lesions of the thoracic wall will be evaluated by time to enhancement (TE),

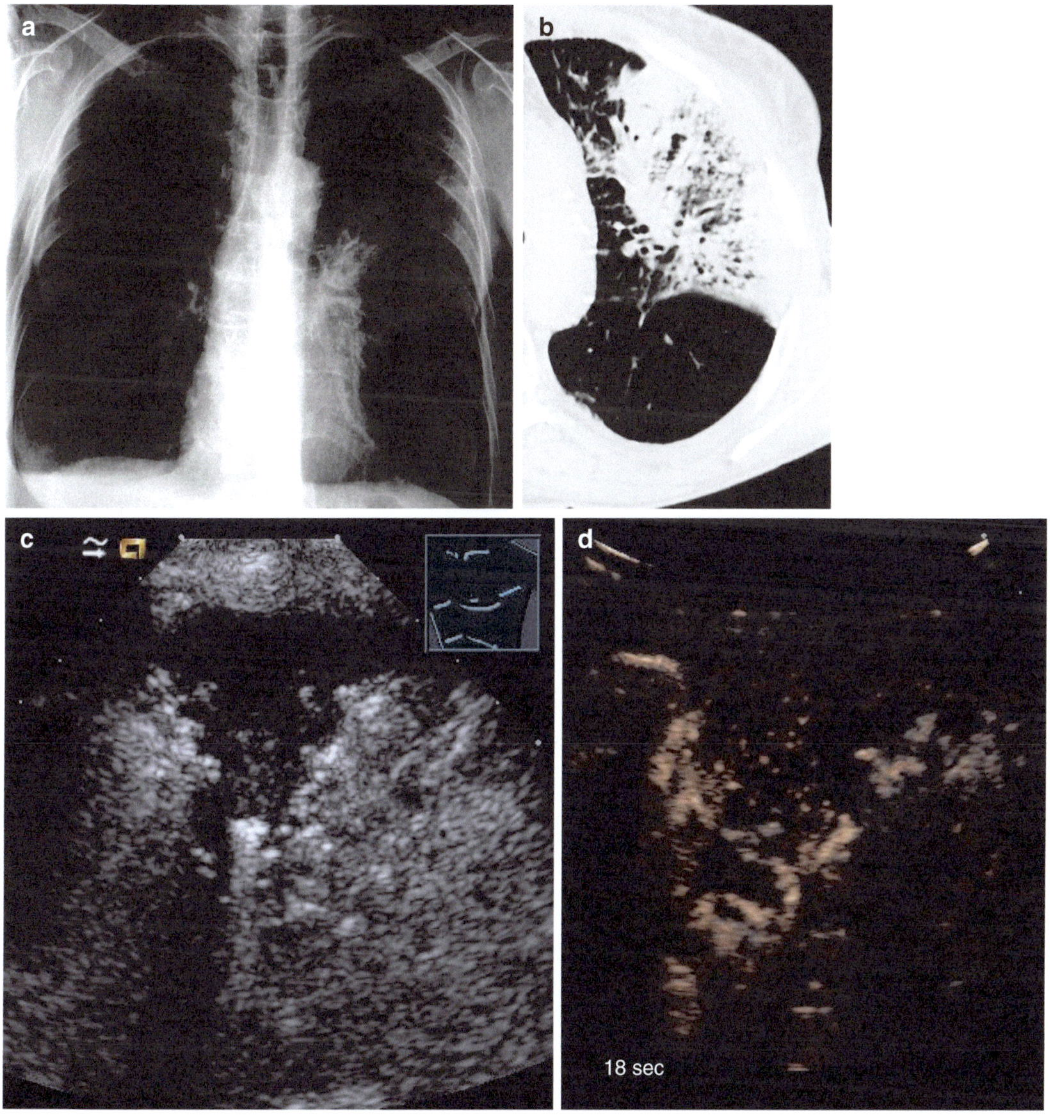

Fig. 14.37 Patient with lung cancer after radiation therapy; a wedge-shaped lung infiltration was found on X-ray examination (**a**) and on CT scan (**b**) suggesting *radiation pneumonia*; B-mode imaging presents an inhomogeneous lung consolidation with diminished air distribution (**c**); CEUS shows a reduced enhancement suggesting bronchial arterial supply indicating chronic injury of lung tissue (**d**)

extent of enhancement (EE), and homogeneity of enhancement (HE). CEUS enables to distinguish PA supply from BA supply by TE. Various peripheral lesions have characteristic CEUS patterns regarding TE, EE, and HE. There are clinical conditions which may reveal diagnostic advantages of CEUS in comparison to B-mode US and additional information to computed tomography. CEUS may be helpful (1) to characterize tumors of the chest wall, especially for differentiation of non-vital and vital tissue; (2) to differentiate infectious pleurisy from embolic pleurisy; (3) to

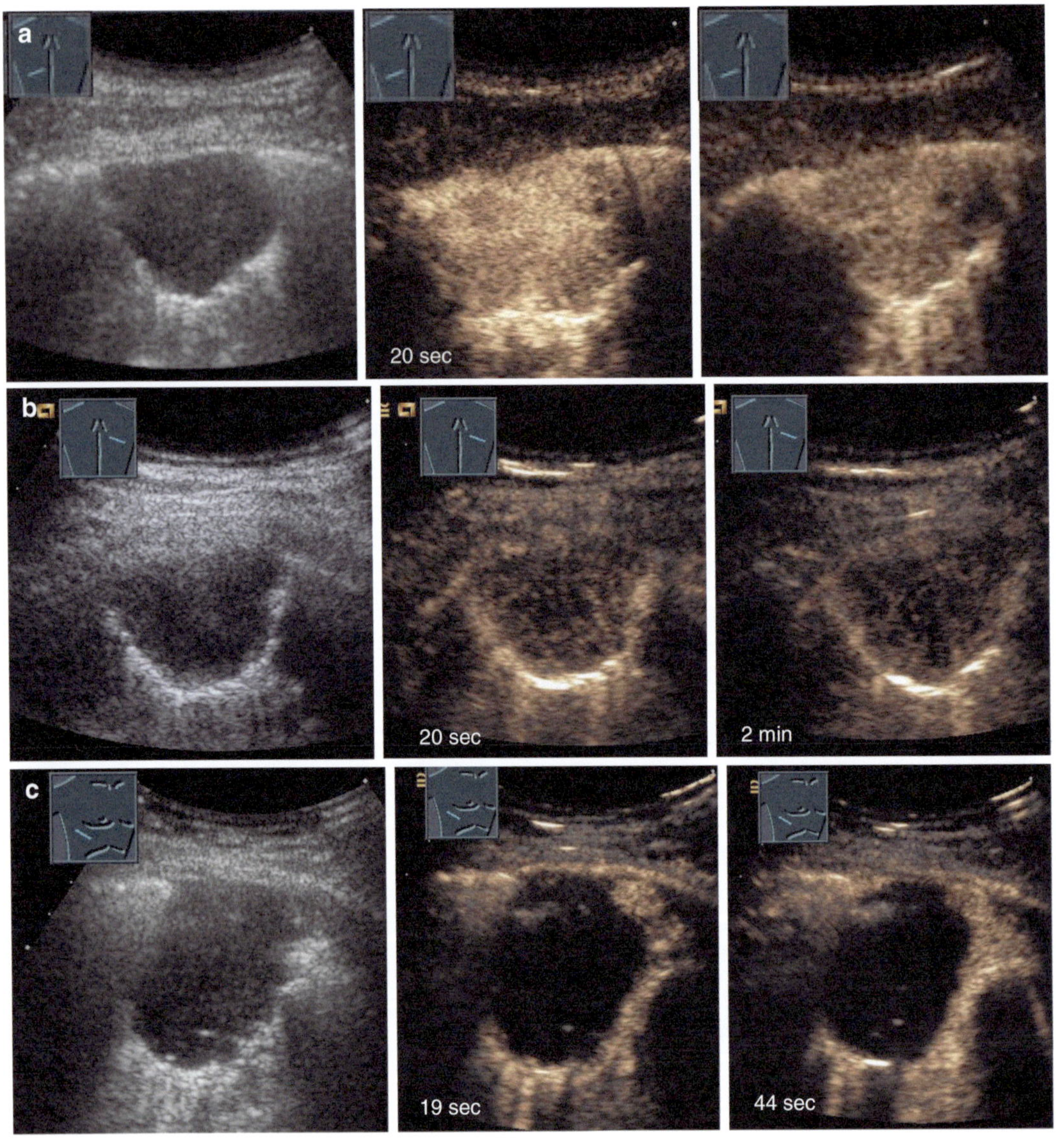

Fig. 14.38 Peripheral malignant lesions with different patterns of bronchial arterial supply indicating different extent of tumor neoangiogenesis: B-mode ultrasound (left) and patterns of marked arterial supply in a patient with renal cell cancer and pulmonary metastasis (**a**1–3); B-mode ultrasound (left) and patterns of reduced arterial supply in a patient with peripheral non-small cell lung cancer (NSCLC) (**b**1–3); B-mode ultrasound (left) and patterns of nearly no arterial supply in a patient with peripheral NSCLC (**c**1–3)

characterize opacification of lung tissue due to compression atelectasis, obstructive atelectasis, pneumonia, and benign and malignant tumors (in these cases CEUS may give relevant additional information in atypical or complicated courses of disease); and (4) to assist in interventional procedures and detect interventional associated complications.

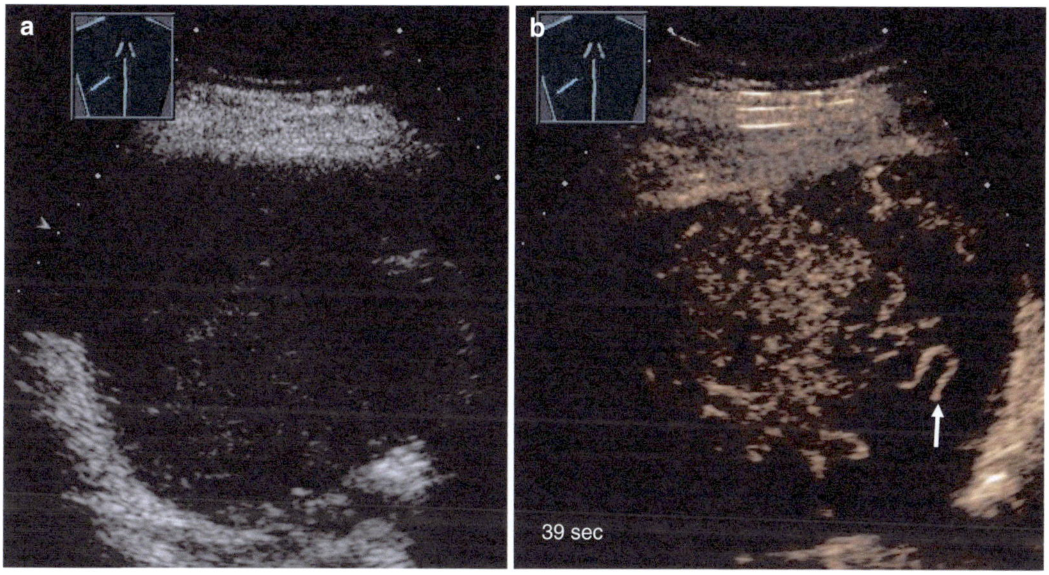

Fig. 14.39 Patient with sarcoma; B-mode imaging presents a large left sided homogeneous echoic round pulmonary tumor (**a**); CEUS shows a chaotic vascularization with tortuous vessels indicating *tumor neoangiogenesis* (arrow) (**b**)

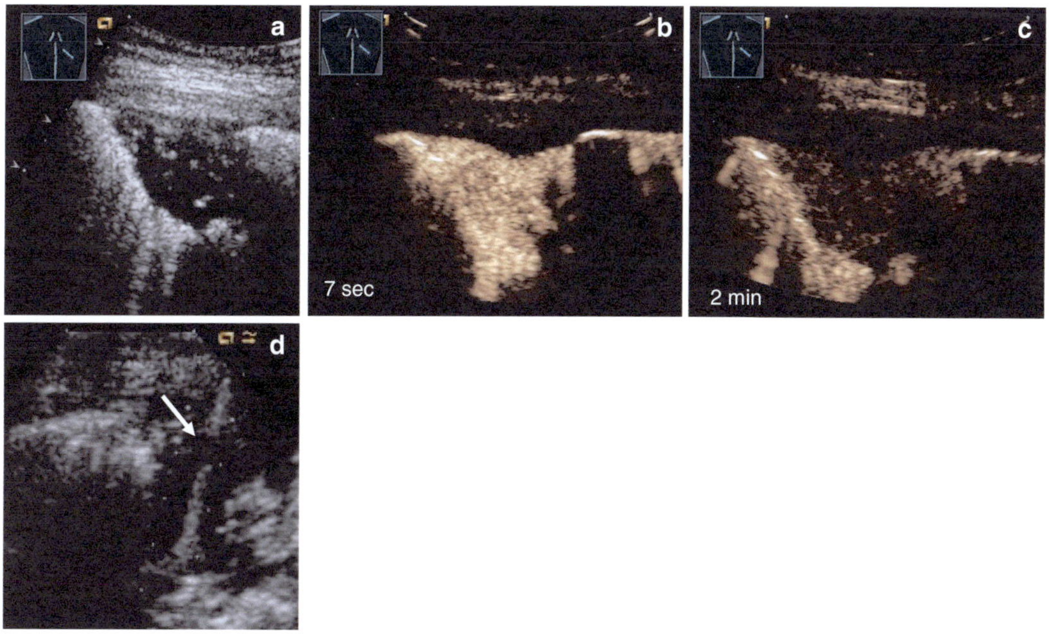

Fig. 14.40 Patient with lung consolidation and clinical suspected pneumonia; B-mode imaging presents a well-delineated hypoechoic area with air bronchogram convenient for pneumonia (**a**); CEUS after 7 s shows a marked pulmonary arterial enhancement (**b**); convenient for pneumonia with a reduced enhancement in the parenchymal phase (**c**); US-guided biopsy revealed diagnosis of *bronchioloalveolar carcinoma* (**d**)

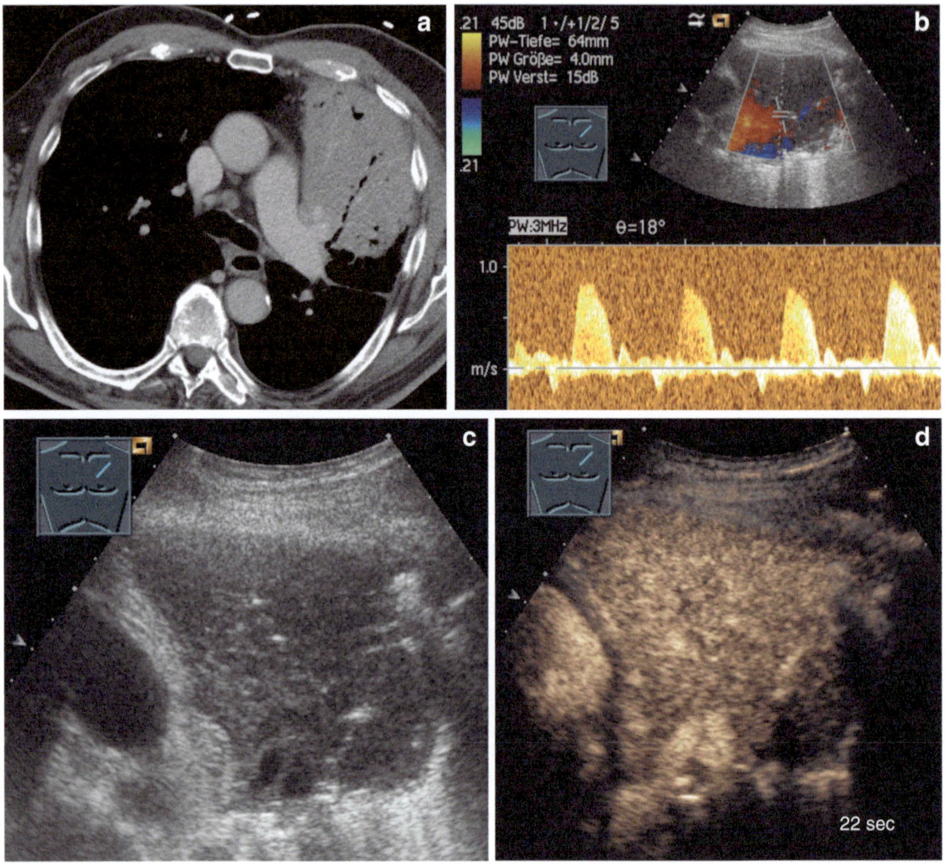

Fig. 14.41 Patient with lung consolidation and clinical suspicion of pneumonia shown on CT scan (**a**); spectral curve analysis shows a high-impedance flow signal indicating pulmonary arterial supply (**b**); B-mode imaging presents a well-delineated hypoechoic area with reduced air bronchogram convenient for pneumonia (**c**); CEUS after 22 s shows a marked pulmonary arterial enhancement convenient for pneumonia (**d**); US-guided biopsy revealed diagnosis of *primary lymphoma of the lung*

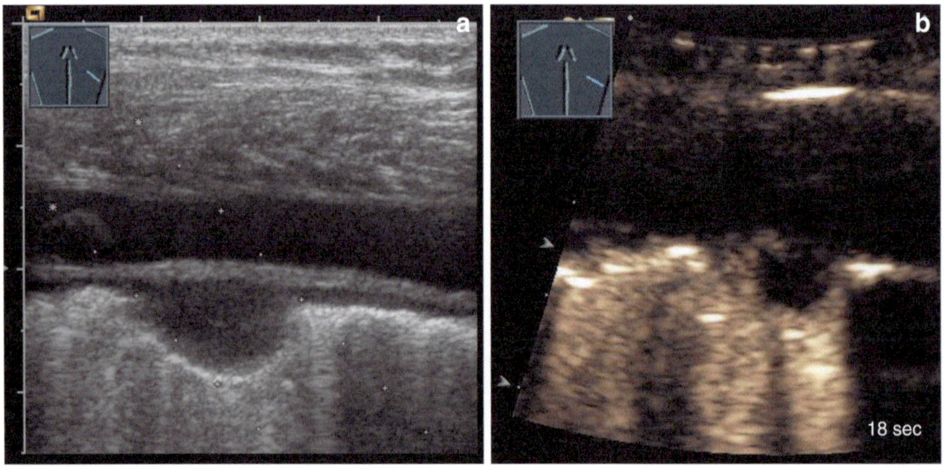

Fig. 14.42 Patient with suspected tuberculosis and evidence of pleural-based nodules in B-mode US (**a**); CEUS shows a border enhancement with central no enhancement (**b**); US-guided biopsy confirmed diagnosis of *active tuberculosis*

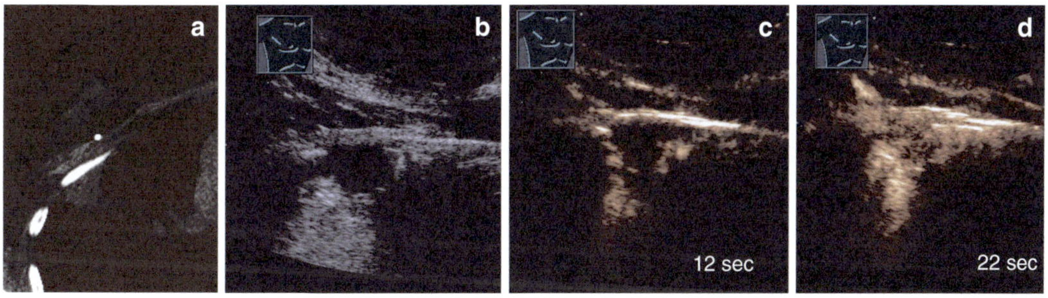

Fig. 14.43 Patient with anamnestic breast cancer and systemic sarcoidosis; CT scan shows pleural-based lesion (**a**); B-mode imaging presents a hypoechoic pleural-based round lesion; (**b**); CEUS shows a time to enhancement after 12 s indicating bronchial arterial supply (**c**) with a marked extent of enhancement after 22 s (**d**); US-guided biopsy revealed *sarcoid granuloma*

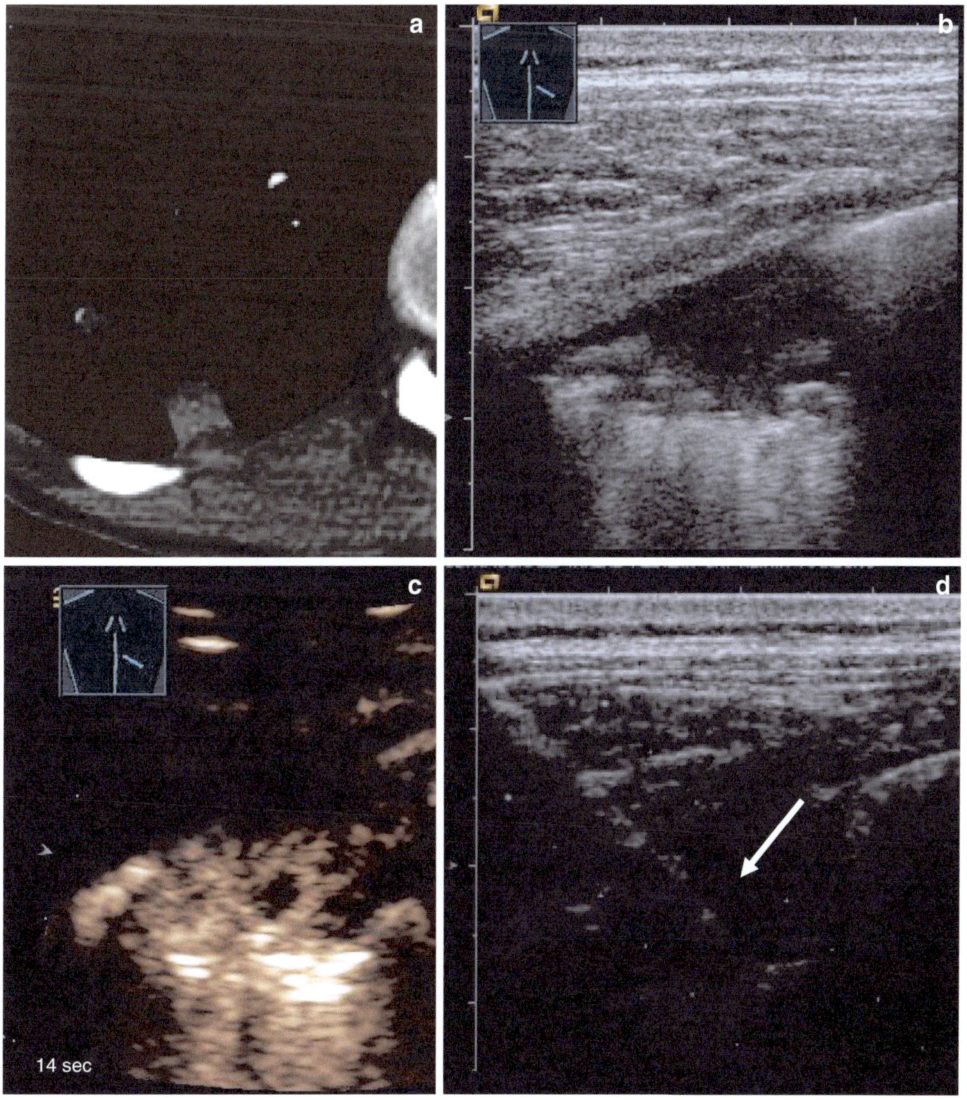

Fig. 14.44 Patient with focal pleural lesion of unknown cause shown on CT scan (**a**); B-mode imaging presents an irregular delineated lesion with air bronchogram (**b**); CEUS shows a time to enhancement before chest wall enhancement indicating pulmonary arterial supply (**c**); US-guided biopsy (arrow) revealed *pneumonia* (**d**)

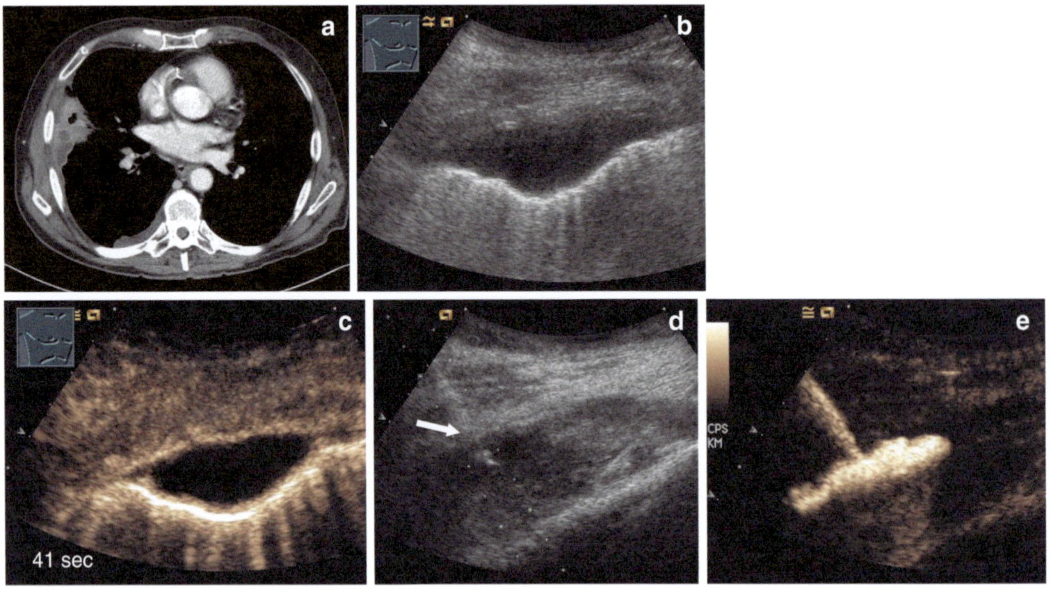

Fig. 14.45 Patient with suspected pleural empyema on CT scan (**a**); B-mode imaging presents a pleural-based oval lesion (**b**); CEUS shows a strong border enhancement with central no enhancement characteristic for *pleural empyema* (**c**); US-guided catheter drainage was performed (arrow) (**d**), and correct position was confirmed by extravasal transcathetral application of contrast medium (**e**)

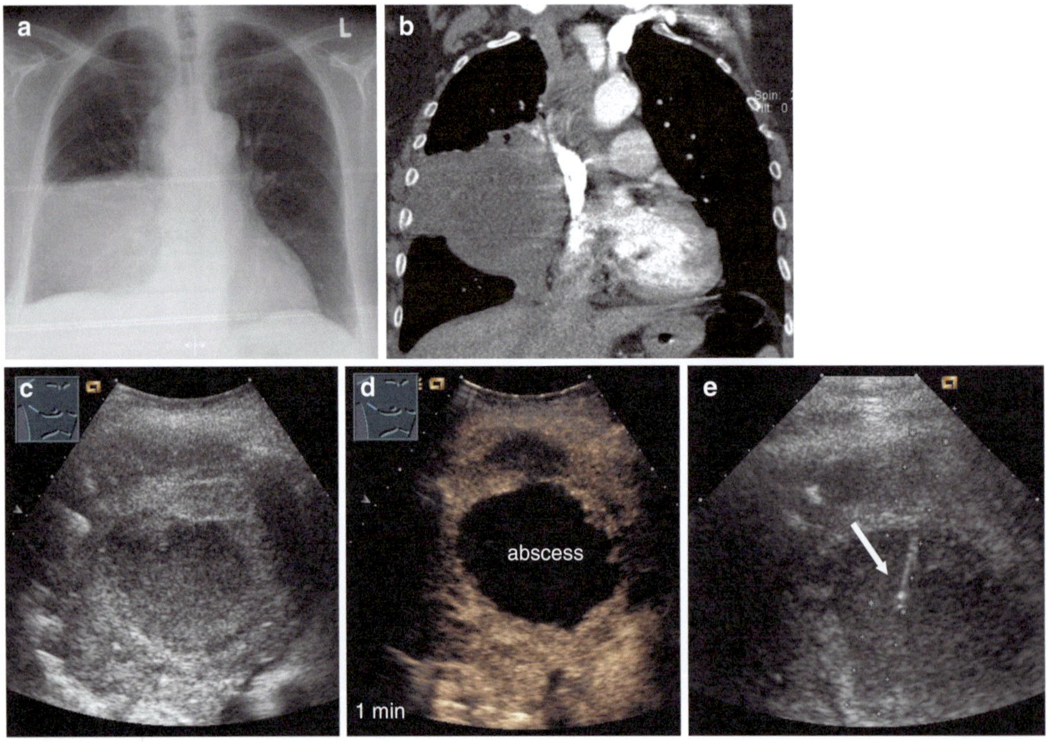

Fig. 14.46 Patient with obstructive atelectasis and pulmonal abscess found on X-ray examination (**a**) and CT scan (**b**); B-mode imaging presents a consolidation with a central well-delineated hypoechoic area (**c**); CEUS shows no enhancement of the central area indicating pulmonary abscess/liquidification (**d**); US-guided drainage (arrow) confirmed diagnosis of *pulmonary abscess* (**e**)

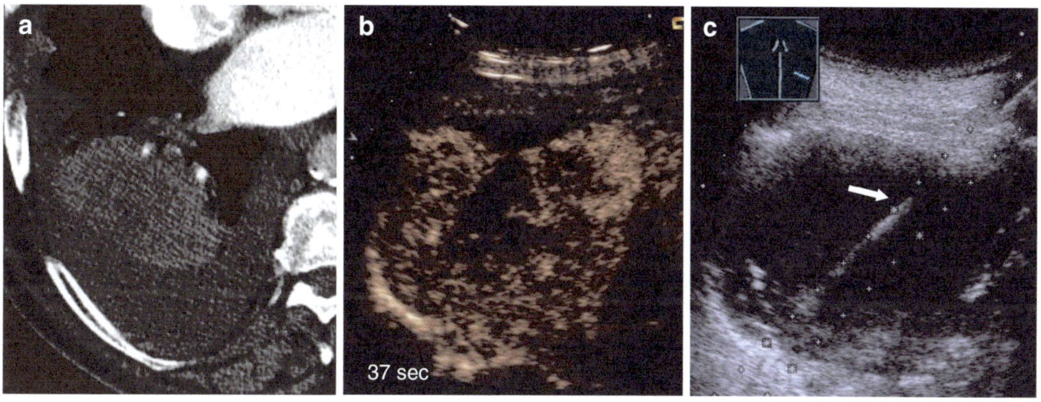

Fig. 14.47 Patient with suspected lung cancer on CT scan (**a**); B-mode imaging presents an inhomogeneous bronchial arterial enhancement (**b**); US-guided biopsy (arrow) revealed adenocarcinoma (**c**)

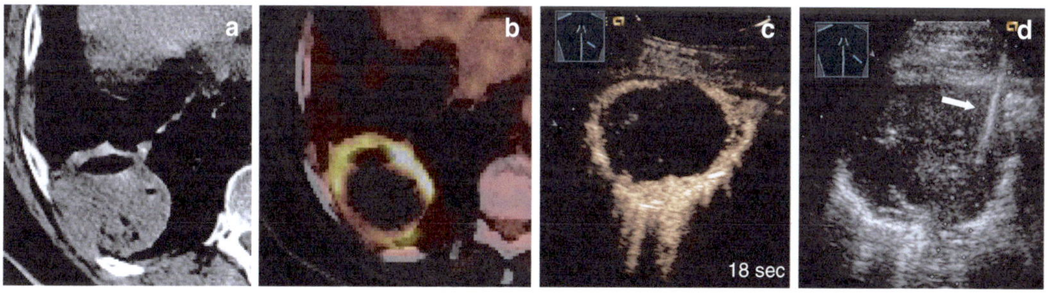

Fig. 14.48 Patient with suspected lung cancer on CT scan (**a**) and PET-CT (**b**); CEUS shows border enhancement and central no enhancement (**c**); US-guided biopsy (arrow) revealed lung cancer (**d**)

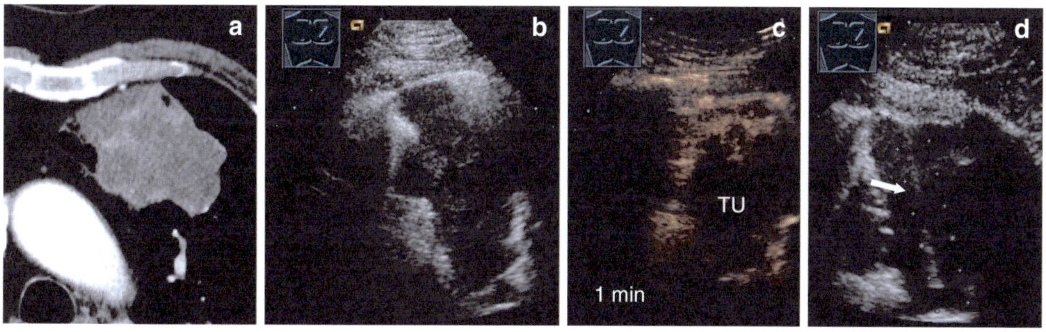

Fig. 14.49 Patient with suspected lung cancer on CT scan (**a**); B-mode imaging presents a complex consolidation (**b**); CEUS shows a marked border enhancement of suspected atelectatic tissue with a central hypoenhancement of suspected tumor tissue (TU) (**c**); US-guided biopsy (arrow) revealed lung cancer (**d**)

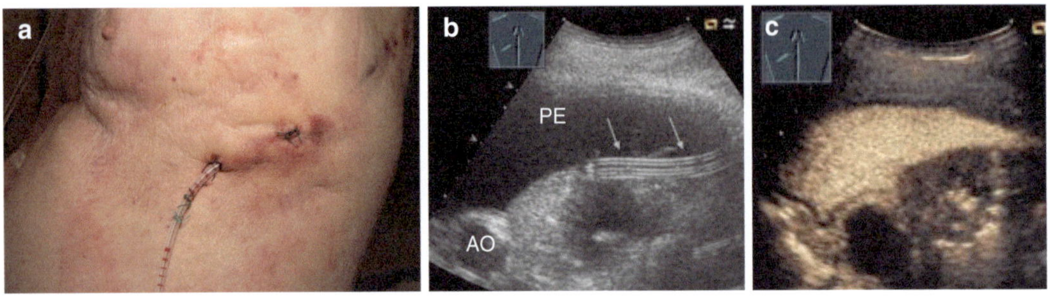

Fig. 14.50 Patient with malignant pleural effusion and an US-guided implantation of a permanent intracutaneous tunnelled pleural catheter (arrow) (AO = aorta) (**a**); B-mode imaging shows the catheter within the pleural cavity (arrow) (**b**); correct position of the catheter was confirmed by extravasal transcathetral application of contrast medium (**c**)

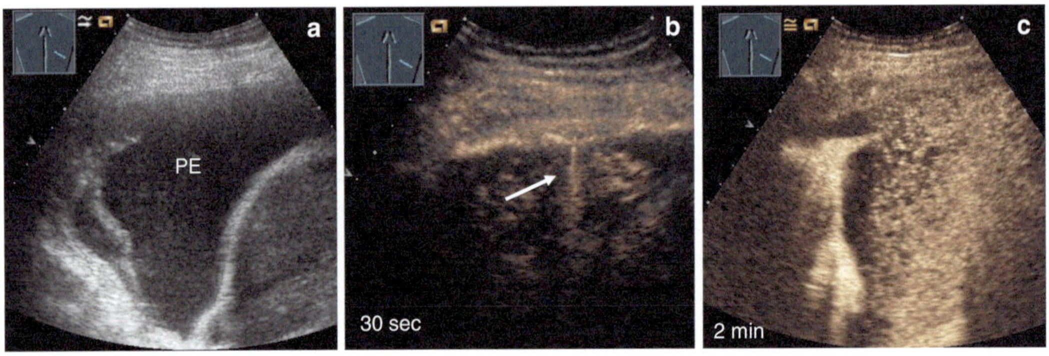

Fig. 14.51 Patient with right-sided pleural effusion (PE) shown on B-mode US (**a**); after function of the PE, an active bleeding was suspected and confirmed by detection of a contrast jet with CEUS (arrow) (**b**); after 2 min multiple bubbles were seen in the pleural cavity (**c**)

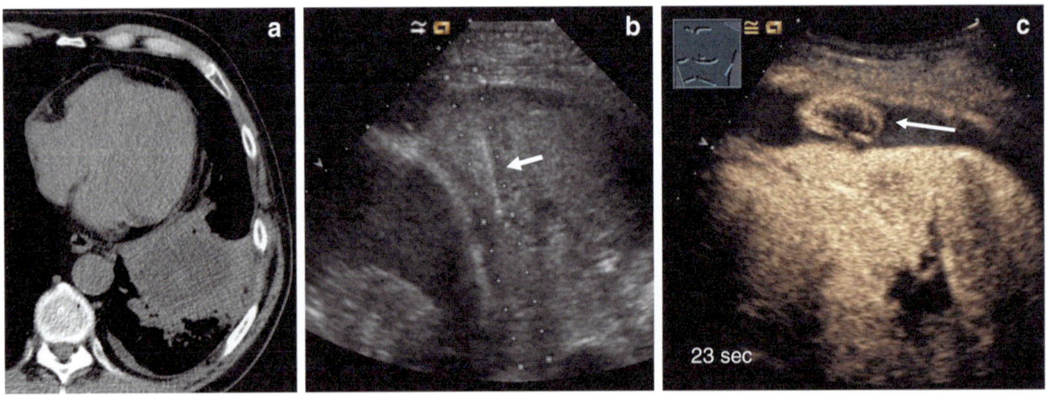

Fig. 14.52 Patient with suspected lung cancer on CT scan (**a**); US-guided biopsy confirmed diagnosis (arrow) (**b**); after biopsy active bleeding was suspected and confirmed by detection of a contrast medium cloud (arrow) with CEUS (**c**)

References

1. Görg C, Bert T. Trancutaneous colour Doppler sonography of lung consolidations: review and pictorial essay. Part 1: pathophysiologic and CDS basics of pulmonary vascularity. Ultraschall Med. 2004;25:221–6.
2. Görg C, Bert T. Trancutaneous colour Doppler sonography of lung consolidations: review and pictorial essay. Part 2: CDS patterns of pulmonary consolidations. Ultraschall Med. 2004;25:285–91.
3. Müller KM, Meyer-Schwickerath M. Bronchial arteries in various stages of bronchogenic carcinoma. Pathol Res Pract. 1978;163:34–46.
4. Hsu WH, Ikezoe J, Chen CY, Kwan PC, Hsu CP, et al. Color Doppler ultrasound signals of thoracic lesions: correlation with resected histologic specimens. Am J Respir Crit Care Med. 1996;153:1938–51.
5. Babo HV, Müller KMG, Huzky A, Bosnjakovic-Buscher S. Die Bronchialarteriographie bei Erkrankungen der Lunge. Radiologe. 1979;19:506–13.
6. Civardi G, Fornari F, Cavanna L, Di Stasi M, Sbolli G, et al. Vascular signals from pleural-based lung lesions studied with pulsed Doppler ultrasonography. J Clin Ultrasound. 1993;21:617–22.
7. Hsu WH, Chiang CD, Chen CY, Kwan PC, Hsu JY, et al. Color Doppler ultrasound pulsatile flow signals of thoracic lesions: comparison of lung cancer and benign lesions. Ultrasound Med Biol. 1998;24:1087–95.
8. Yuan A, Chang DB, Yu CJ, Kuo SM, Luh KT, Yang PC. Color Doppler sonography of benign and malignant pulmonary masses. Am J Roentgenol. 1994;163:545–9.
9. Yuan A, Yang PC, Lee L, Wu DH, Kuo SH, et al. Reactive pulmonary artery vasoconstriction in pulmonary consolidation by color Doppler ultrasonography. Ultrasound Med Biol. 2000;26:49–56.
10. Görg C, Seifart U, Holzinger I, Wolf M, Zugmaier G. Bronchiolo-alveolar carcinoma: sonographic pattern of "pneumonia". Eur J Ultrasound. 2002;15:109–17.
11. Görg C, Seifart U, Görg K, et al. Color Doppler sonographic mapping of pulmonary lesions: evidence of dual arterial supply by spectral analysis. JUM. 2003;22:1033–9.
12. Görg C, Bert T, Görg K, Heinzel-Gutenbrunner M. Color Doppler sonographic mapping of chest wall lesions. Br J Radiol. 2005;78:303–7.
13. Claudon M, Dietrich CF, Choi BI, et al. Guidelines and good clinical practice recommendations for contrast enhanced ultrasound (CEUS) in the liver—update 2012: a WFUMB-EFSUMB initiative in cooperation with representatives of AFSUMB, AIUM, ASUM, FLAUS and ICUS. Ultrasound Med Biol. 2013;39:187–210.
14. Piscaglia F, Nolsoe C, Dietrich CF, et al. The EFSUMB guidelines and recommendations on the clinical practice of contrast enhanced ultrasound (CEUS): update 2011 on non-hepatic applications. Ultraschall Med. 2012;33:33–59.
15. Ignee A, et al. Der endocavitäre Kontrastmittelultraschall-Verschiedene Anwendungen, eine Übersicht über die Literatur und zukünftige Perspektiven. Ultraschall Med. 2013;34:504–28.
16. Bitschnau R, Gehmacher O, Kopf A, Schreier M, Mathis G. Ultrasound diagnosis of rib and sternum fractures. Ultraschall Med. 1997;18:158–61.
17. Gehmacher O, Kopf A, Scheier M, et al. Can pleurisy be detected with ultrasound? Ultraschall Med. 1997;18:214–9.
18. Görg C, Bert T, Görg K. Contrast enhanced sonography for differential diagnosis of pleurisy and focal pleural lesions of unknown cause. Chest. 2005;128:3894–9.
19. Mathis G, Blank W, Reisig A, Lechleitner P, Schuler A, Beckh S. Thoracic ultrasound for diagnosing pulmonary embolism: a prospective multicenter study of 352 patients. Chest. 2005;28:1531–8.
20. Nazerian P, Simone Vanni S, Volpicelli G, et al. Accuracy of point-of-care multiorgan ultrasonography for the diagnosis of pulmonary embolism. Chest. 2014;145:950–7.
21. Mathis G, Dirschmid K. Pulmonary infarction: sonographic appearance with pathologic correlation. Eur J Radiol. 1993;17:170–4.
22. Bartelt S, Trencer C, Görg C, Neesse A. Contrast-enhanced ultrasound of embolic consolidations in patients with pulmonary embolism: a pilot study. J Clin Ultrasound. 2016;44(3):129–35. https://doi.org/10.1002/jcu.22313.
23. Trenker C, Neesse A, Pastor S, Bartelt S, Görg C. Hinweis auf embolische Pleuraläsionen in der CEUS bei klinischem Verdacht einer Lungenarterienembolie und fehlenden Nachweis einer zentralen LAE in der. CT Ultraschall Medizin Suppl. 2015;1(36):S4–122.
24. Görg C, Bert T, Kring R. Contrast enhanced sonography of the lung for differential diagnosis of atelectasis. JUM. 2006;25:35–9.
25. Görg C. Transcutaneous contrast-enhanced sonography of pleural-based pulmonary lesions. Eur J Radiol. 2007;64:213–21.
26. Holland A, Brinkmann C, Görg C. B-Bild-Sonographie und kontrastmittelunterstützte Sonographie (KUS) bei obstruktionsbedingten Lungenatelektasen. Ultraschall Med. 2007;28(Suppl 1):12_4.
27. Linde H-N, Holland A, Greene BH, Görg C. Kontrastunterstützte Sonographie (CEUS) bei Pneumonie: Darstellungsmuster und prognostische Bedeutung- eine retrospektive Studie bei n=50. Patienten Ultraschall Med. 2012;33:146–51.
28. Stathopoulos GT, Karamessini MT, Sotiriadi AE, Pastromas VG. Rounded atelectasis of the lung. Respir Med. 2005;99:615–23.
29. Görg C, Bert T. Transcutaneous contrast enhanced sonography of peripheral lung lesions: review and pictorial essay. Am J Roentgenol. 2006;187:420–9.

30. Görg C, Bert T, Kring R, Dempfle A. Transcutaneous contrast enhanced sonography of the chest for evaluation of pleural based pulmonary lesions. Ultraschall Med. 2006;27:437–44.
31. Kolin A, Koutllakis T. Role of arterial occlusion in pulmonary scar cancers. Hum Pathol. 1988;19:1161–70.
32. Caremani M, Benci A, Lapini L, et al. Contrast enhanced ultrasonography (CEUS) in peripheral lung lesions: a study of 60 cases. J Ultrasound. 2008;11:89–96.
33. Sartori S, Postorivo S, Di Vece F, et al. Contrast-enhanced ultrasonography in peripheral lung consolidations: what's its actual role? World J Radiol. 2013;5(10):372–80.
34. Trenker C, Wilhelm M, Rexin P, Görg C. Kontrastmittelverhalten von Lungenlymphomen in der CEUS-eine retrospektive Studie. Ultraschall Medizin Suppl. 2015;1(36):S5–125.
35. Sperandeo M, Sperandeo G, Varriale A, et al. Contrast-enhanced ultrasound (CEUS) for the study of peripheral lung lesions: a preliminary study. Ultrasound Med Biol. 2006;32:1467–72.

Chest Sonography to Assess Lung Recruitment in Patients with Acute Respiratory Distress Syndrome

15

Lorenzo Ball, Noemi Baretta, Simone Bazurro, and Paolo Pelosi

15.1 Introduction

Many studies investigated the role of lung recruitment in the management of acute respiratory distress syndrome (ARDS), a serious disease that leads to death in 40–60% of cases [1]. Recruitment can refer either to the maintenance of lung aeration through specific ventilator settings, in particular positive end-expiratory pressure (PEEP), or to a transient increase of transpulmonary pressure obtained with the ventilator, aimed at restoring aeration in non-aerated regions, referred to as *recruitment manoeuvre* [2].

ARDS patients typically require invasive mechanical ventilation and the application of PEEP and end-expiratory lung de-recruitment while improving the lung aeration and oxygenation [3], and its use has been often proposed in conjunction with recruitment manoeuvres. Nonetheless, the role of both higher levels of PEEP [4] and recruitment manoeuvres [5] is still controversial and challenged by the findings of recent trials [6]. Prone positioning can improve gas exchange and survival in early severe ARDS patients, with a mechanism likely mediated by lung recruitment and improvement of the ventilation-perfusion matching [7]. The bedside assessment of lung recruitment could be useful to assess the effectiveness of a recruitment manoeuvre, of a change of PEEP level or their impact on hemodynamic, potentially leading to a patient-tailored ventilator setting [1, 8].

Several methods were proposed to evaluate the effectiveness of recruitment. Chest radiography played an historical role, as it was the first tool used to assess patients with ARDS, and the presence of bilateral alveolar infiltrates was part of the first definition of the syndrome [9]; nowadays its use is slowly but steadily decreasing in favour of other bedside techniques such as lung ultrasound (LUS), as it shows low sensitivity and specificity and exposes patients and intensive care unit (ICU) staff to ionizing radiations [10]. Computed tomography (CT) provides information about the presence of symmetric or asymmetric densities and gravity-dependent atelectasis [11]: its high resolution and the possibility to perform quantitative analysis of the lung tissue aeration make it a gold standard for the assessment of ARDS [12]; however it is associated with an elevated radiation exposure and requires transporting the patient outside the ICU as well as time-consuming post-acquisition analysis of data in order to derive quantitative data [13]. For all these reasons, lung CT has an undoubted clinical value, but its quantitative analysis is limited to the research setting. At the bedside, a method based on the analysis of static pressure-volume (PV) curve has been proposed and validated

L. Ball · N. Baretta · S. Bazurro · P. Pelosi (✉)
Dipartimento di Scienze Diagnostiche e Chirurgiche Integrate, Università degli Studi di Genova e Ospedale Policlinico San Martino, IRCCS per l'Oncologia, Genova, Italy
e-mail: simone.morganti@unipv.it

F. Feletti et al. (eds.), *Thoracic Ultrasound and Integrated Imaging*,
https://doi.org/10.1007/978-3-319-93055-8_15

against CT [14]; but also this method has pitfalls, including the need for deep sedation and neuromuscular blockade, limiting its application to patients in controlled ventilation modes. Moreover, this method has limits in discriminating recruitment from hyperinflation.

Lung ultrasound (LUS) has an increasingly relevant role in the bedside assessment of critically ill patients, including for the assessment of lung recruitment, first reported one decade ago [1]. Transthoracic LUS can provide information concerning lung aeration through scores or morphological evaluation and can be conveniently integrated by echocardiography, for hemodynamic monitoring. It is reasonable to assume that a change in lung aeration resulting from any therapy changes LUS patterns [15, 16]. Moreover, positive pressure ventilation and higher PEEP levels can negatively influence cardiac performances and lead to haemodynamic impairment. Pulmonary hypertension is an often neglected aspect of ARDS, and an increase in pulmonary vascular resistance and mild to severe right ventricle dysfunction have been reported in up to 30% of ARDS patients [10]. The end stage of such dysfunction is cor pulmonale, whose hallmarks are represented by right ventricle dilatation and septal dyskinesia resulting from volume and pressure overload. Therefore, a comprehensive examination comprising lung and heart ultrasound could help in defining a compromise ventilation strategy able to improve gas exchange while avoiding overdistension and detrimental heart-lung interaction.

15.2 LUS Re-aeration Assessment

15.2.1 Based on Scoring Systems

LUS is unable to visualize healthy lungs, but artefactual B-lines arise in the presence of alveolo-interstitial syndrome, while in case of complete loss of aeration, the consolidated lung can be directly seen. Several scoring systems have been developed to estimate lung aeration, based on the visual assessment of LUS patterns in specific lung regions bilaterally. As PEEP can influence lung aeration in ARDS patients, changes in LUS following a PEEP change could reflect the changes in lung aeration. This hypothesis was tested by Bouhemad and colleagues in 2011 [17]. The authors performed LUS at 0 and 15 cm H_2O PEEP level, assigning a LUS score based on the worst image obtained examining all the intercostal spaces in six chest regions bilaterally, classifying the pattern into four previously described patterns, described below:

- Normal (N) pattern: characterized by the presence of lung sliding sign and less than two B-lines
- Moderate loss of aeration (B1 pattern): distinct B-lines with well-defined spacing
- Severe loss of lung aeration (B2 pattern): multiple coalescent B-lines, resulting from partial filling of alveolar spaces by pulmonary oedema or confluent bronchopneumonia foci
- Complete loss of lung aeration (C pattern), appearing as a tissue image with dynamic air bronchograms

Starting from this classification, Bouhemad developed a re-aeration/loss of aeration scoring system, based on the comparison of the pattern in the corresponding chest region before and after PEEP changes, as illustrated in Table 15.1. This score was validated against the pressure-volume curve method, showing a good agreement and therefore demonstrating that LUS can track PEEP-induced aeration changes. This method has several advantages and pitfalls. First, it can

Table 15.1 Ultrasound re-aeration score on 12 bilateral chest fields (6 per hemithorax)

Re-aeration score			Loss of aeration score		
From pattern	To pattern	Points	From pattern	To pattern	Points
B1	N	1	N	B1	2
B2	B1	1		B2	3
	N	3		C	5
C	B2	1	B1	B2	1
	B1	3		C	3
	N	5	B2	C	1

Adapted by Bouhemad et al. *"Bedside Ultrasound Assessment of Positive End-Expiratory Pressure-induced Lung Recruitment"*

be performed at the bedside, not requiring deep sedation nor neuromuscular blockade, and allows a regional analysis of lung aeration. However, its sensitivity is limited when recruitment is limited in size, and in most patients the changes in aeration scores were due to changes in the anterior and lateral parts of the chest, with most of the posterior consolidated regions remaining unchanged. This should lead to interpret cautiously this scoring system, as it might be unable to distinguish between recruitment and hyperinflation: while the reversal of a lung collapse region clearly corresponds to recruitment, the disappearance of B-lines could be due to either the recruitment of previously collapsed areas or hyperinflation of already aerated respiratory units. The balance between recruitment and hyperinflation is a cornerstone of the respiratory management of ARDS [18]. In addition to scoring systems, researchers have tried to develop computer-based analysis of LUS, but these algorithms have not yet been validated in this setting [19, 20].

15.2.2 Based on Morphological Assessment

Stefanidis et al. in 2011 have enrolled ten patients with ARDS under mechanical ventilation and administered a PEEP titration trial at 5, 10, and 15 cm H_2O. For reproducibility reasons, the authors limited the assessment to the dependent right lung regions, accessed through a transhepatic acoustic window, and evaluated the effectiveness of LUS in the assessment of the non-aerated areas at different levels of PEEP, investigating also the relationship between the recruitable lung as indicated by LUS and arterial oxygen partial pressure (PaO_2). All patients were examined in semi-recumbent position with the probe positioned longitudinally along the posterior-axillary line, and then the images were measured by two independent radiologists, blinded to PEEP level and blood gas analysis, to measure the sonographic area of non-aerated lung. As expected, patients showed an increase in oxygenation and a reduction in non-aerated lung progressively from PEEP 5 cm H_2O to PEEP 15 cm H_2O. This method shares advantages and limitations with LUS scoring.

15.2.3 Monitoring the Hemodynamic Effects of Recruitment

There is a close interaction between the lung and the right ventricle (RV) function. This implies that airway pressure changes due to PEEP induce a series of alterations in the right ventricle size and in pulmonary circulation that can lead to right heart haemodynamic impairment, from mild to end-stage manifestation, acute cor pulmonale [21]. These alterations are more likely to occur in severe ARDS patients, both because of the underlying cardiac impairment due to systemic inflammation and because these patients usually need higher PEEP levels [22]. In this context, the haemodynamic assessment by transthoracic or transoesophageal cardiac ultrasound can be complementary to LUS [23]. With the constant decrease in the use of pulmonary artery catheterization, ultrasound raised increasing interest, and right heart failure is reported in as much as one fifth of ARDS patients receiving protective mechanical ventilation [24].

Among the approaches to identify such condition, the estimation of systolic pulmonary artery pressure (sPAP) using continuous Doppler on tricuspid regurgitation is relatively easy to perform: velocity 2.8–2.9 m/s corresponds to a sPAP of about 36 mmHg and can be considered as a reasonable cutoff. However, this method is likely to underestimate sPAP because systolic pulmonary artery pressure also depends on right ventricular systolic function [25]. Many ARDS-related factors can influence the pulmonary arterial pressure, including mechanical ventilation either directly or through changes in right ventricle afterload, but also hypercapnia and acidosis that lead to an increase of vascular tone, and then increase in pulmonary vascular resistance [26].

Another parameter used to identify pulmonary vascular alterations is right ventricle dimensions, especially if compared with the left ventricular size: a ratio between right (RVEDA) and left ventricular diastolic area (LVEDA) above 0.6 defines moderate right ventricular dilation, while >1.0 defines severe impairment and corresponds to a right ventricle bigger than the left one [25].

Finally, a qualitative assessment of interventricular septal dyskinesia helps in the diagnosis and is characterized by leftwards interventricular septum displacement at the onset of left ventricular diastole and rightwards rebound when the left ventricle restarts contraction [25].

15.2.4 Evaluation of Lung Aeration and Weaning from Mechanical Ventilation

LUS aeration assessment has also been proposed to estimate the loss of aeration during spontaneous breathing trials and could be used to predict post-extubation respiratory distress [17]. In a study by Soummer and colleagues, at comparable baseline LUS scores, patients that had a reduction of lung aeration at the end of the spontaneous breathing trials were more likely to develop post-extubation respiratory failure [27]. In this study, a commonly used scoring system was used, assessing six regions bilaterally and assigning 0, 1, 2, and 3 points to normal aeration, B1, B2, and C patterns, respectively. With this scoring system, LUS ≤ 12 at the end of breathing trial was predictive of extubation success, while LUS ≥ 17 was associated with post-extubation respiratory failure. Compared to other techniques of weaning success prediction, LUS allows to observe how the de-recruitment is distributed in the lungs.

15.3 Conclusion

The simplicity, the noninvasiveness, and the possibility to be carried directly at the bedside are the strongest LUS advantages and can be considered equivalent to the pressure-volume curve method in assessing quantitatively PEEP-induced lung recruitment allowing a regional assessment of the lung. Despite this, it does not allow an assessment of PEEP-induced hyperinflation and cannot be the sole method for PEEP titration, but it should be part of a comprehensive evaluation including haemodynamic monitoring and gas exchange assessment.

Conflict of Interest Statement The authors have no conflict of interest to disclose.

References

1. Gardelli G, Feletti F, Gamberini E, Bonarelli S, Nanni A, Mughetti M. Using sonography to assess lung recruitment in patients with acute respiratory distress syndrome. Emerg Radiol. 2009;16(3):219–21.
2. Fan E, Wilcox ME, Brower RG, Stewart TE, Mehta S, Lapinsky SE, et al. Recruitment maneuvers for acute lung injury: a systematic review. Am J Respir Crit Care Med. 2008;178(11):1156–63.
3. Stefanidis K, Dimopoulos S, Tripodaki E-S, Vitzilaios K, Politis P, Piperopoulos P, et al. Lung sonography and recruitment in patients with early acute respiratory distress syndrome: a pilot study. Crit Care. 2011;15(4):R185.
4. Santa Cruz R, Rojas JI, Nervi R, Heredia R, Ciapponi A. High versus low positive end-expiratory pressure (PEEP) levels for mechanically ventilated adult patients with acute lung injury and acute respiratory distress syndrome. Cochrane Database Syst Rev. 2013;(6):CD009098.
5. Hodgson C, Goligher EC, Young ME, Keating JL, Holland AE, Romero L, et al. Recruitment manoeuvres for adults with acute respiratory distress syndrome receiving mechanical ventilation. Cochrane Database Syst Rev. 2016;11:CD006667.
6. Writing Group for the Alveolar Recruitment for Acute Respiratory Distress Syndrome Trial (ART) Investigators, Cavalcanti AB, Suzumura ÉA, Laranjeira LN, Paisani D de M, Damiani LP, et al. Effect of lung recruitment and titrated positive end-expiratory pressure (PEEP) vs low PEEP on mortality in patients with acute respiratory distress syndrome: a randomized clinical trial. JAMA. 2017;318(14):1335–45.
7. Guérin C, Reignier J, Richard J-C, Beuret P, Gacouin A, Boulain T, et al. Prone positioning in severe acute respiratory distress syndrome. N Engl J Med. 2013;368(23):2159–68.
8. Luecke T, Corradi F, Pelosi P. Lung imaging for titration of mechanical ventilation. Curr Opin Anaesthesiol. 2012;25(2):131–40.
9. Ashbaugh DG, Bigelow DB, Petty TL, Levine BE. Acute respiratory distress in adults. Lancet Lond Engl. 1967;2(7511):319–23.
10. Corradi F, Brusasco C, Pelosi P. Chest ultrasound in acute respiratory distress syndrome. Curr Opin Crit Care. 2014;20(1):98–103.

11. Gattinoni L, Caironi P, Pelosi P, Goodman LR. What has computed tomography taught us about the acute respiratory distress syndrome? Am J Respir Crit Care Med. 2001;164(9):1701–11.
12. Ball L, Vercesi V, Costantino F, Chandrapatham K, Pelosi P. Lung imaging: how to get better look inside the lung. Ann Transl Med. 2017;5(14):294.
13. Ball L, Braune A, Corradi F, Brusasco C, Garlaschi A, Kiss T, et al. Ultra-low-dose sequential computed tomography for quantitative lung aeration assessment-a translational study. Intensive Care Med Exp. 2017;5(1):19.
14. Lu Q, Constantin J-M, Nieszkowska A, Elman M, Vieira S, Rouby J-J. Measurement of alveolar derecruitment in patients with acute lung injury: computerized tomography versus pressure-volume curve. Crit Care Lond Engl. 2006;10(3):R95.
15. Du J, Tan J, Yu K, Wang R. Lung recruitment maneuvers using direct ultrasound guidance: a case study. Respir Care. 2015;60(5):e93–6.
16. Tusman G, Acosta CM, Costantini M. Ultrasonography for the assessment of lung recruitment maneuvers. Crit Ultrasound J. 2016;8(1):8.
17. Bouhemad B, Brisson H, Le-Guen M, Arbelot C, Lu Q, Rouby J-J. Bedside ultrasound assessment of positive end-expiratory pressure–induced lung recruitment. Am J Respir Crit Care Med. 2011;183(3):341–7.
18. Güldner A, Braune A, Ball L, Silva PL, Samary C, Insorsi A, et al. Comparative effects of volutrauma and atelectrauma on lung inflammation in experimental acute respiratory distress syndrome. Crit Care Med. 2016;44(9):e854–65.
19. Corradi F, Ball L, Brusasco C, Riccio AM, Baroffio M, Bovio G, et al. Assessment of extravascular lung water by quantitative ultrasound and CT in isolated bovine lung. Respir Physiol Neurobiol. 2013;187(3):244–9.
20. Corradi F, Brusasco C, Vezzani A, Santori G, Manca T, Ball L, et al. Computer-aided quantitative ultrasonography for detection of pulmonary edema in mechanically ventilated cardiac surgery patients. Chest. 2016;150(3):640–51.
21. Au S-M, Vieillard-Baron A. Bedside echocardiography in critically ill patients: a true hemodynamic monitoring tool. J Clin Monit Comput. 2012;26(5):355–60.
22. Bellani G, Laffey JG, Pham T, Fan E, Brochard L, Esteban A, et al. Epidemiology, patterns of care, and mortality for patients with acute respiratory distress syndrome in intensive care units in 50 countries. JAMA. 2016;315(8):788–800.
23. Lazzeri C, Cianchi G, Bonizzoli M, Batacchi S, Peris A, Gensini GF. The potential role and limitations of echocardiography in acute respiratory distress syndrome. Ther Adv Respir Dis. 2016;10(2):136–48.
24. Mekontso Dessap A, Boissier F, Charron C, Bégot E, Repessé X, Legras A, et al. Acute cor pulmonale during protective ventilation for acute respiratory distress syndrome: prevalence, predictors, and clinical impact. Intensive Care Med. 2016;42(5):862–70.
25. Rudski LG, Lai WW, Afilalo J, Hua L, Handschumacher MD, Chandrasekaran K, et al. Guidelines for the echocardiographic assessment of the right heart in adults: a report from the American Society of Echocardiography. J Am Soc Echocardiogr. 2010;23(7):685–713.
26. Mekontso Dessap A, Charron C, Devaquet J, Aboab J, Jardin F, Brochard L, et al. Impact of acute hypercapnia and augmented positive end-expiratory pressure on right ventricle function in severe acute respiratory distress syndrome. Intensive Care Med. 2009;35(11):1850–8.
27. Soummer A, Perbet S, Brisson H, Arbelot C, Constantin J-M, Lu Q, et al. Ultrasound assessment of lung aeration loss during a successful weaning trial predicts postextubation distress. Crit Care Med. 2012;40(7):2064–72.

Part IV

Clinical and Radiological Correlations

16 Clinical Cases

Francesco Feletti, Bruna Malta, and Andrea Aliverti

16.1 Adult Patient with Chronic Septated Pleural Effusion

In this case, plain radiography (Fig. 16.1a, b) showed the obliteration of the posterior costophrenic sinuses (arrow) together with the scissure near the pleural effusion and the concomitance of pulmonary thickening (arrowhead).

The computed tomography (CT) (Fig. 16.1c) made it possible to distinguish, in a manner superior to traditional radiology, the effusion (arrow) from the atelectasic lung (arrowhead).

The thoracic ultrasound (TUS) (Fig. 16.1d) also allowed the effusion (C) to be distinguished from the atelectatic lung (A).

The latter showed an echogenic aspect similar to that of the hepatic parenchyma; peripherally, on the other hand, the partially ventilated zones of the parenchyma showed numerous B lines (B).

The TUS demonstrates the presence of septations (Fig. 16.1e), an aspect not assessable using CT, suggesting its chronic nature and thus indicating the need for subsequent treatment.

In fact, in the case of a highly organized effusion, chest drain insertion risks being unsuccessful and possibly inadvisable (Fig. 16.1f).

If thoracentesis is proposed for diagnostic purposes, TUS may allow the collection of quantitatively adequate samples by directing drainage to larger loculations (Fig. 16.1g).

16.2 Diagnosis and Follow-Up of Pneumonia in a Pediatric Patient

Physical examination and laboratory tests of the 3-year-old patient suggested an infection of the lower respiratory tract.

The X-ray was acquired through a single anteroposterior projection for radiation protection reasons and showed nodular retrocardiac thickening (Fig. 16.2a; A).

The TUS (Fig. 16.2b) showed pulmonary consolidation in contact with the posterior thoracic wall. The consolidated lung appeared echogenic and the aerial bronchogram scarce. The colour

F. Feletti (✉)
Dipartimento di Diagnostica per Immagini, Ausl della Romagna, Ospedale S. Maria delle Croci, Ravenna, Italy

Dipartimento di Elettronica, Informazione e Bioingegneria, Politecnico di Milano, Milan, Italy
e-mail: francesco.feletti@auslromagna.it

B. Malta
Dipartimento di Diagnostica per Immagini, Ausl di Ferrara, Ospedale Universitario di Ferrara, Ferrara, Italy
e-mail: mltbrn@unife.it

A. Aliverti
Dipartimento di Elettronica, Informazione e Bioingegneria, Politecnico di Milano, Milan, Italy
e-mail: andrea.aliverti@polimi.it

F. Feletti et al. (eds.), *Thoracic Ultrasound and Integrated Imaging*,
https://doi.org/10.1007/978-3-319-93055-8_16

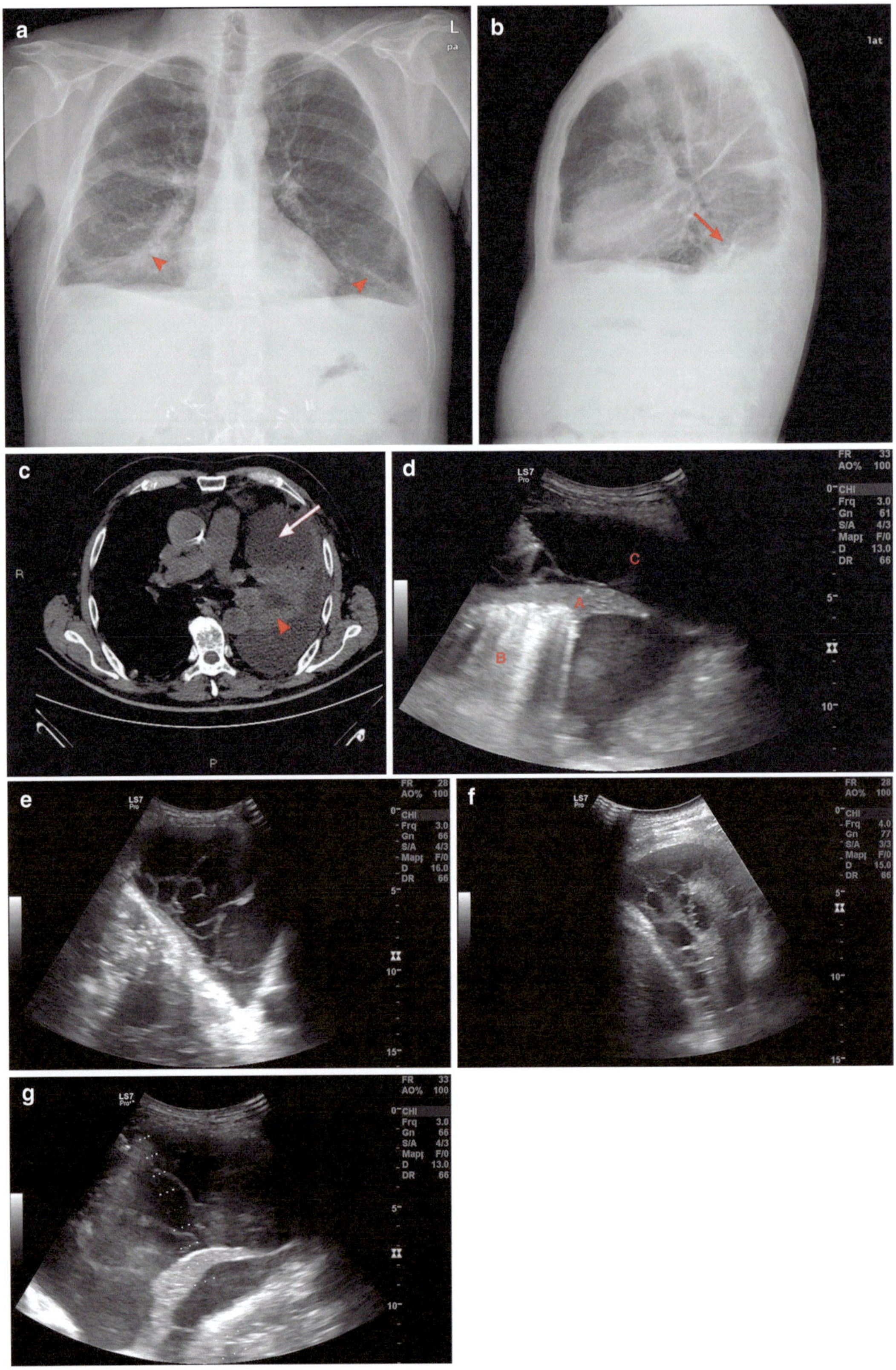

Fig. 16.1 (**a**, **b**) plain radiography; (**c**, **d**) CT; (**d–g**) TUS

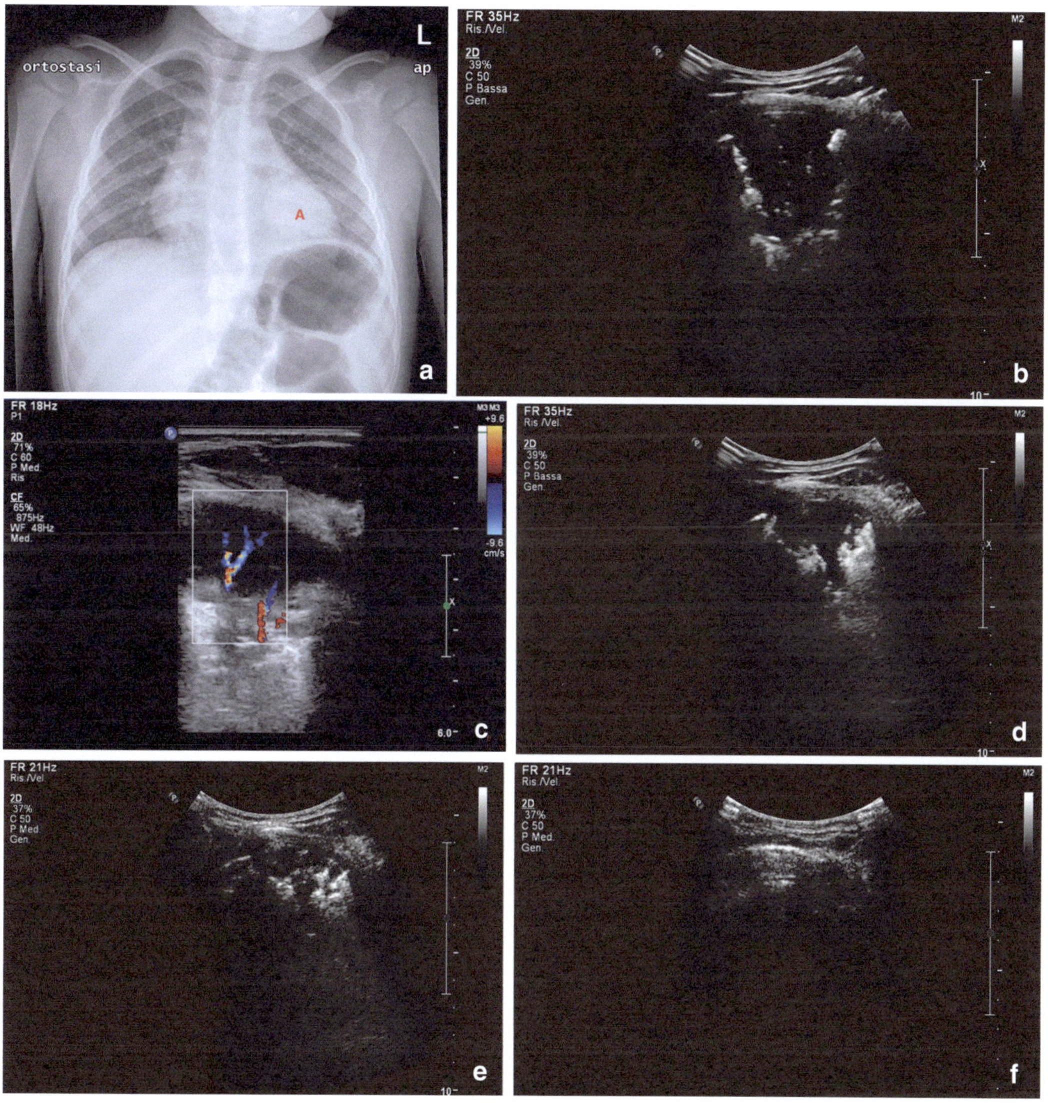

Fig. 16.2 (**a**) plain radiography; (**b–f**) TUS

Doppler demonstrated the natural arboriform disposition of the vascular signals (Fig. 16.2c), testifying that the lung maintained normal vascularization and that pulmonary volume was not reduced.

Based on these aspects, together with the clinical exams, TUS allowed for a differential diagnosis excluding heteroplastic lesions and atelectasis.

The TUS also allowed monitoring of the dimensional reduction of the consolidation over time (Fig. 16.2d, e) and continued after the resolution of the clinical diagnosis until its complete disappearance (Fig. 16.2f), thus avoiding the use of further radiological examinations.

16.3 Metastases in the Soft Tissues of the Thoracic Wall

The adult patient showed palpable swelling corresponding to the sternal manubrium.

TUS identified a newly formed tissue, iso-hypoechogenic in respect to the muscular structures and richly vascularized (Fig. 16.3a, b).

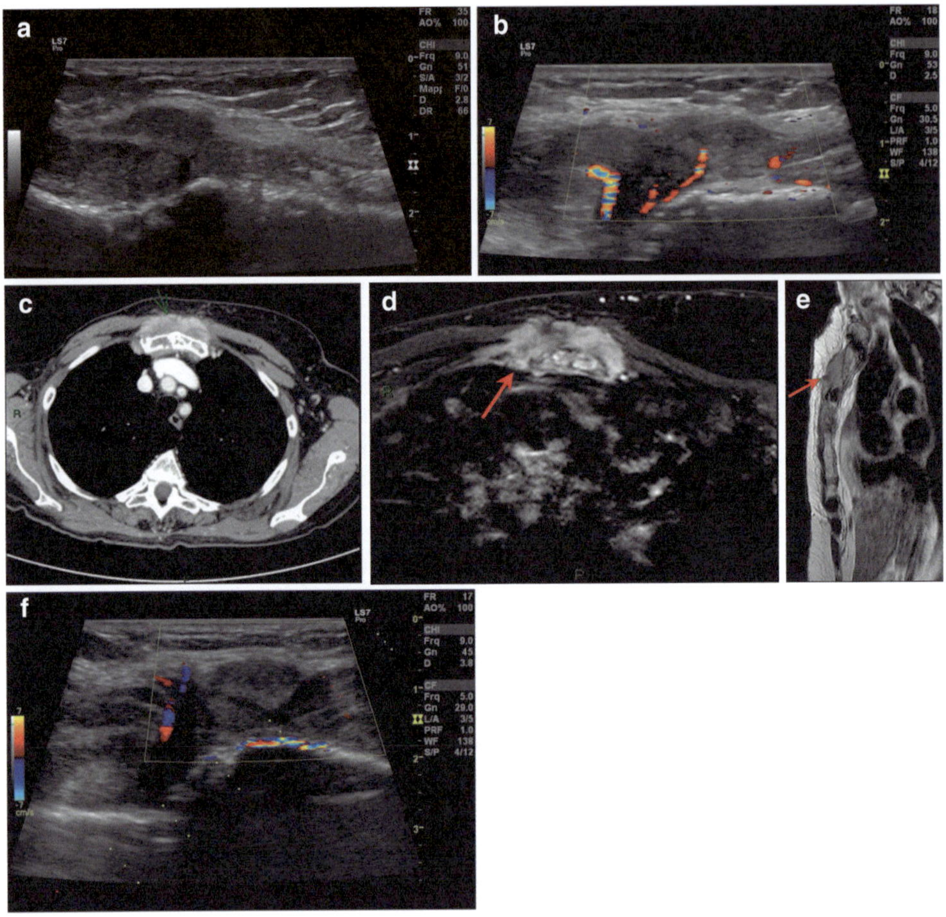

Fig. 16.3 (**a**, **b**) TUS; (**c**) CT; (**d**, **e**) MRI; (**f**) colour-Doppler

The lesion was inseparable from the pectoral muscles, while the underlying sternal bone surface appeared slightly irregular.

The CT (Fig. 16.3c) and magnetic resonance imaging (MRI) (Fig. 16.3d, e) more comprehensively revealed the extent of the lesion and the anatomical relationships of the lesion with the surrounding anatomical structures, in particular with the sternum and the pectoral muscles.

Lastly, the TUS (Fig. 16.3f) provided a guide for biopsy sampling, avoiding larger neoformed vessels. TUS can be used as a first-line imaging method for investigating the soft tissue and bony lesions of the chest wall. It has a high degree of resolution and accuracy, and is useful for safe guidance of percutaneous diagnostic procedures [1].

16.4 Heart Failure

Thoracic ultrasound is more sensitive than plain radiography in the diagnosis of pulmonary edema in acute decompensated heart failure. Therefore, TUS should be used as an adjunct imaging method in patients with dyspnea at risk of acute decompensated heart failure [2]. The TUS showed an abundant bilateral anechogenic pleural effusion (Fig. 16.4a; A).

In the ventilated lung, several B-lines were present, demonstrating thickening of the imbibed pulmonary interstice (Fig. 16.4a; B).

Lastly, the suprahepatic veins were dilated, testifying to the initial stages of liver stasis (Fig. 16.4b; V).

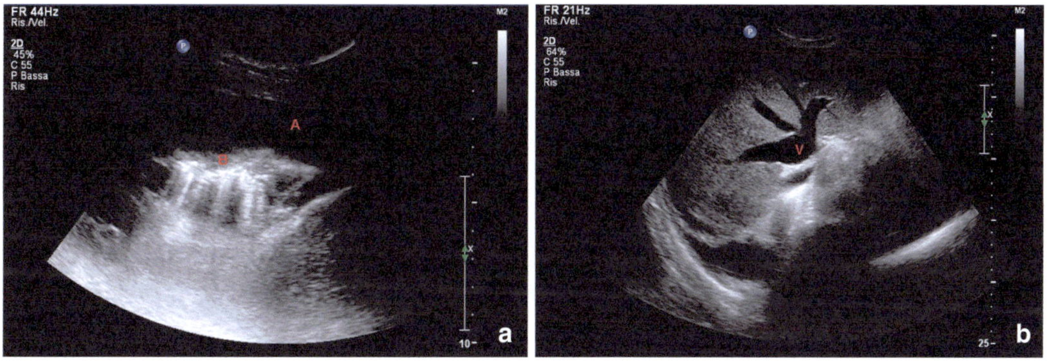

Fig. 16.4 (**a**, **b**): TUS

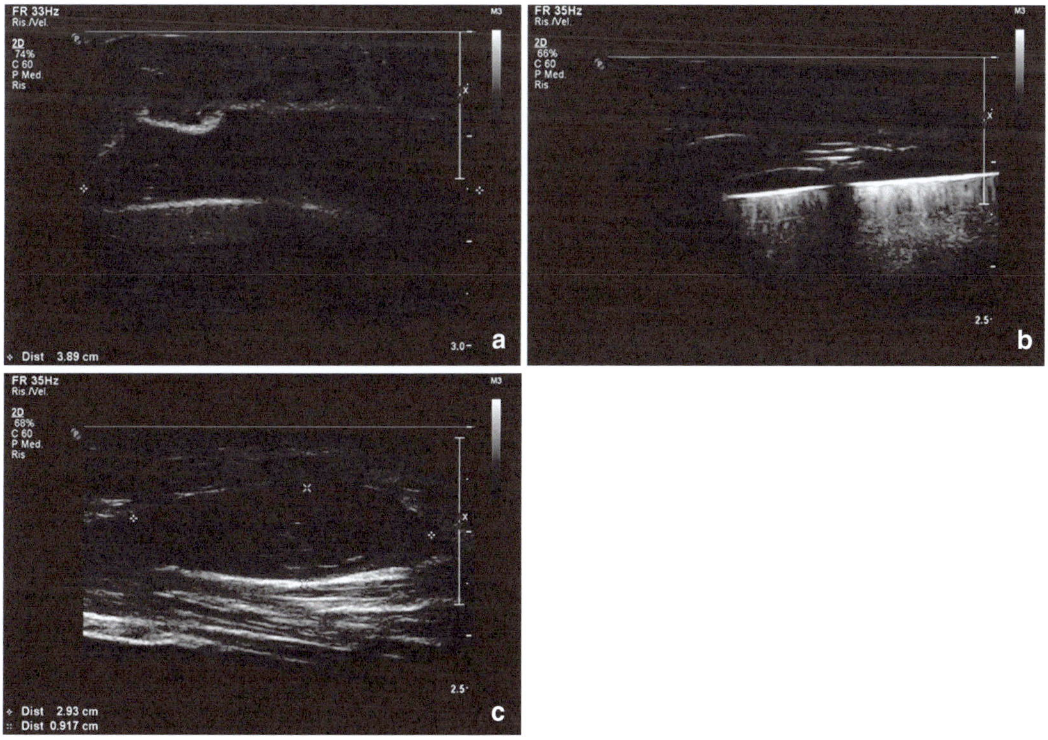

Fig. 16.5 (**a–c**) TUS

16.5 Infection of a Newly Implanted Pacemaker Pocket

Corresponding to the pacemaker pocket, the TUS showed the presence of a hypoechogenic collection with irregular contours (Fig. 16.5a), in the context of which the stimulating electrode was visible (Fig. 16.5b).

The surrounding subcutaneous adipose tissue was hyperechogenic, moderately thickened, and with lymphatic ectasia, as a result of inflammation. However, there were no gas bubbles that would have testified to the involvement of gas-producing bacteria in the infectious process.

A check-up 15 days after pacemaker removal showed the presence of hematoma in the pacemaker pocket (Fig. 16.5c).

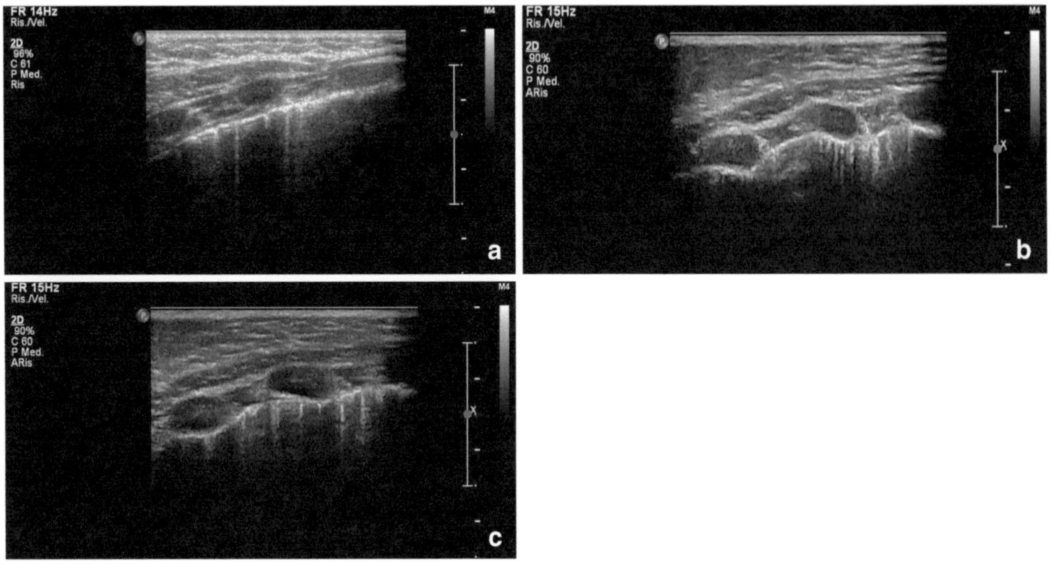

Fig. 16.6 (**a**–**c**) TUS with liear probe

16.6 Infant Trauma

The three-month-old infant was the victim of a road accident with suspected chest trauma.

The TUS identified several B-lines corresponding to the hemiclavear line, an expression of slight lung contusions (Fig. 16.6a–c). It was possible to monitor these lesions with TUS and avoid recourse to radiology.

16.7 Bronchopneumonia in Pediatric Patient

Five-year-old patient with clinical exams suggesting bronchopneumonia and extended pulmonary consolidation in the lower-left pulmonary field (Fig. 16.7a).

TUS showed pulmonary consolidation with a typical arboriform distribution of the aerial bronchogram and vessels (Fig. 16.7–d).

16.8 Pulmonary Neoplasia

In this case, standard radiography (Fig. 16.8a, b) suggested a neoplastic lesion of the pulmonary apex: an extensive consolidation with infiltrative aspects and distortion of the surrounding parenchyma.

The TUS allowed only a partial visualization of the lesion; however, the appearance of the solid lesion was clearly different from the phlogistic (see previous case) or atelectasis, due to the absence of recognizable bronchial or vascular structures and the presence of vascular signals with a different distribution from that of atelectasis (Fig. 16.8c, d).

16.9 White Hemithorax Examination and Bronchial Calcifications

In the case of the left white hemithorax (Fig. 16.9a), TUS permitted the identification of extensive pulmonary consolidations with a tissue-like pattern. In this context, multiple hyperreflective point or linear images, without posterior shadows, may be interpreted as aerial bronchograms (Fig. 16.9b, c).

The presence of aerial bronchograms allows distinction between pneumonia and consolidations of a different kind, such as atelectasis, infarct, and neoplasia.

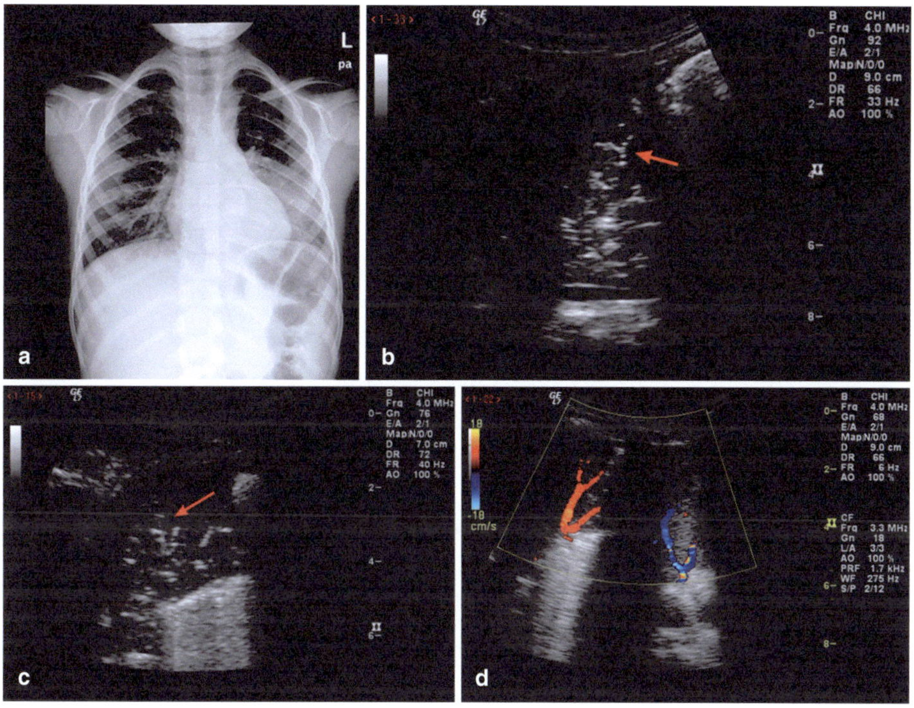

Fig. 16.7 (**a**) plain radiography; (**b–d**) TUS

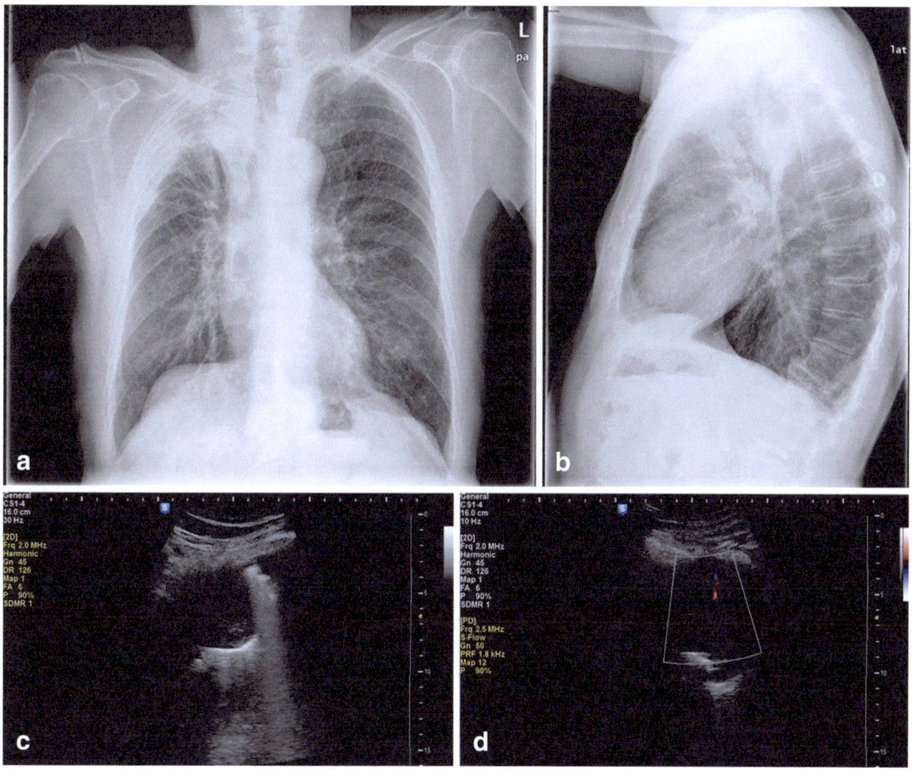

Fig. 16.8 (**a**, **b**) plain radiography; (**c**, **d**) TUS

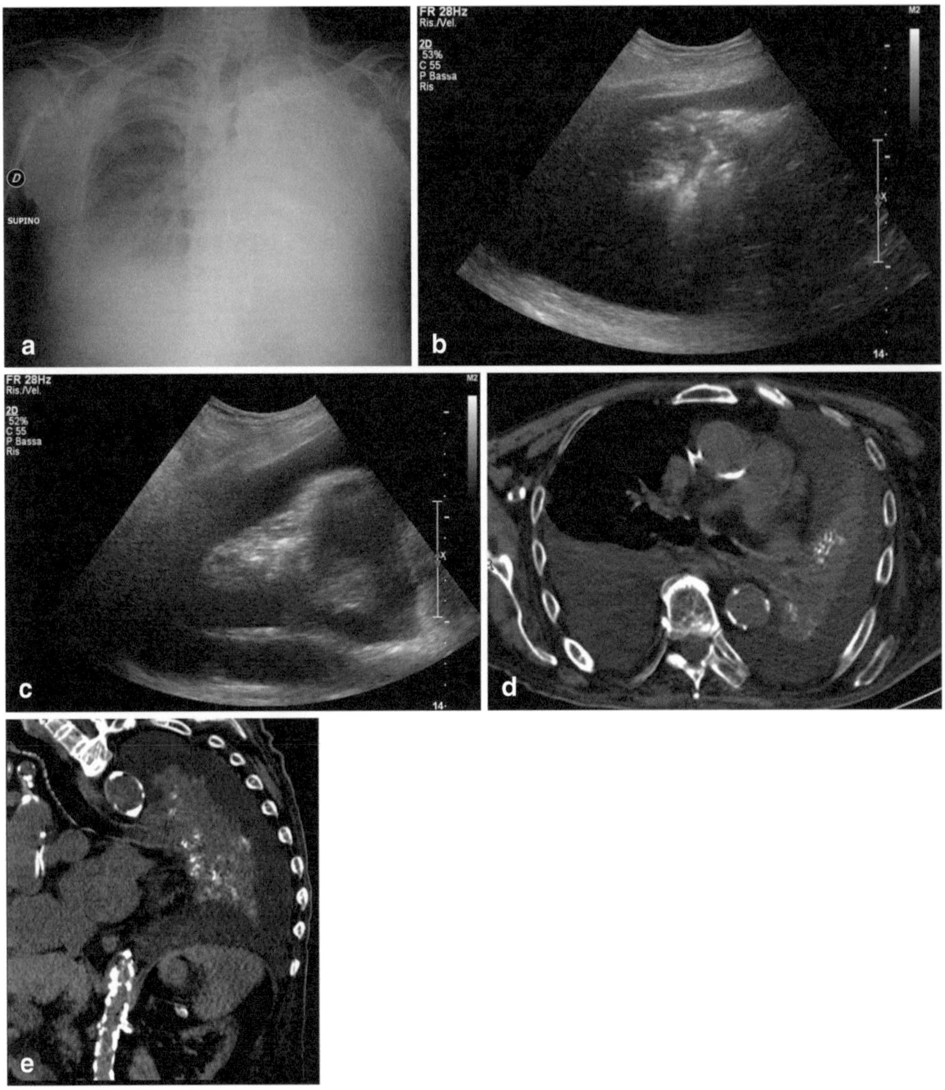

Fig. 16.9 (**a**) plain radiography; (**b**, **c**) TUS; (**d**) CT, axial view; (**e**) CT with curve multi-planar reconstruction

CT (Fig. 16.9d), with the help of curve reconstructions (Fig. 16.9e), allowed the hyper-reflective images to be attributed to the calcifications of bronchial cartilages, excluding the presence of aerial bronchograms.

The possibility that bronchial calcifications simulate air bronchograms has not been described so far. However, bronchial calcifications may be present in numerous conditions, even in pediatric age (Table 16.1), where TUS is widely used.

Further studies of further cases and independent evaluation by multiple ultrasound investigators are necessary to verify that bronchial calcifications are truly indistinguishable from air bronchograms.

Table 16.1 Calcification of bronchial cartilage in childhood

Conditions associated with calcification of bronchial cartilage in childhood
Congenital mitral valvular diseases
Keutel syndrome [3]
Warfarin sodium therapy [4]
Chondrodysplasia punctata [5]
Warfarin embryopathy
Tracheobronchopathia osteochondroplastica [6]
Relapsing polychondritis [7]
Idiopathically [8]

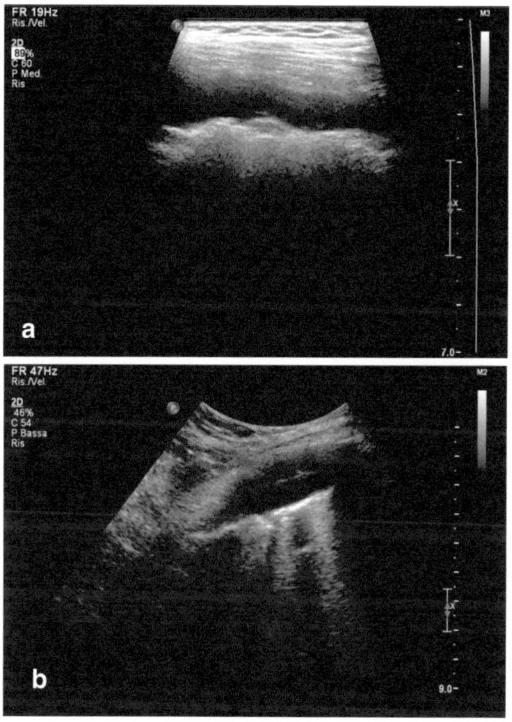

Fig. 16.10 (**a**, **b**) TUS

16.10 Asbestos-Related Disease

In asbestosis, the TUS shows B lines prevalent at the basal zone [9] (Videoclip 1).

Although isolated pleural plaques may be found as a result of trauma, tuberculosis, and hemothorax, multiple pleural plaques are generally associated with asbestos exposure [10] and represent a marker of past exposure [11].

On chest radiograms, deposits of subpleural fat, old costal fractures, and even healthy *serratus posterior superior muscle* and *serratus anterior muscle* can simulate the presence of pleural plaques [12, 13]. On the contrary, ultrasound detection of pleural plaques is optimal and not complicated by possible misinterpretations.

Pleural plaques appear as hypoechogenic thickenings of the parietal pleura on which the visceral pleura normally slides (Fig. 16.10a, b).

TUS has been proposed as a tool to follow up pleural plaques, lung peripheral interstitial thickening, and peripheral pulmonary consolidations identified by CT in workers exposed to asbestos [14].

16.11 Pericardial Effusion

In this case, the chest X-ray showed an evident dimensional increase in the cardiac image (Fig. 16.11a, b). The TUS, however, allowed demonstration of the presence of abundant pericardial effusion, with a thickness of about 4 cm. The heart was compressed and hypokinetic (Fig. 16.11c, d).

The examination can be easily performed also by non-cardiologists and should always be conducted in the event of trauma, even in remote and adverse environments [15].

16.12 Pulmonary Sequestration

A young girl with a positive history of pneumonia recurrent to the right lung base, documented radiologically.

The TUS allowed the identification of an anomalous, ectatic vase, originating from the thoracic aorta in the context of a supradiaphragmatic pulmonary consolidation (Fig. 16.12a, b).

Diagnosis is confirmed by CT-angiography (Fig. 16.12c) and confirmed in surgery (Fig. 16.12d, e).

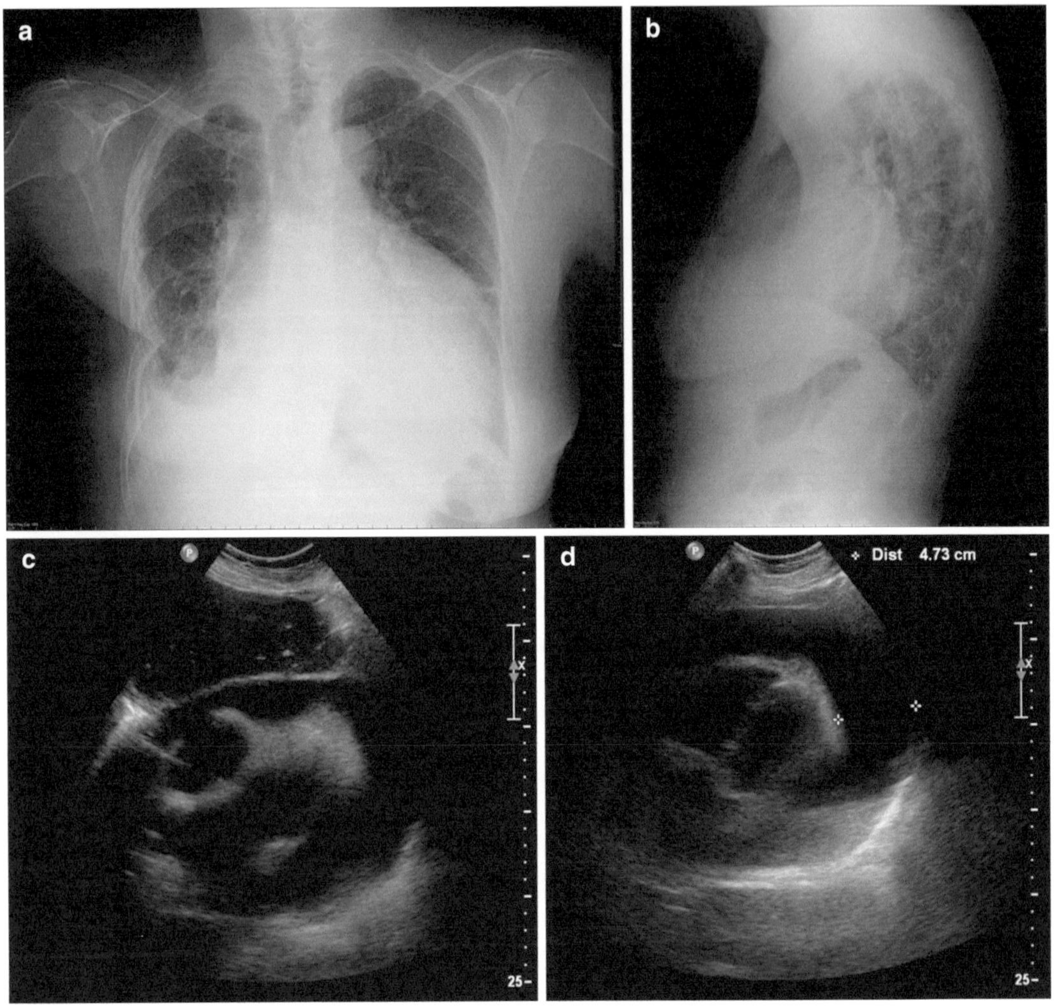

Fig. 16.11 (**a**, **b**) plain radiography; (**c**, **d**) TUS

16.13 Hydrops Fetalis in Premature Infants

Preterm birth at 32 weeks with hydrops fetalis, a condition characterized by severe oedema in soft tissues, bilateral pleural effusion (Fig. 16.13a), as well as peritoneal effusion.

The TUS allowed for quantification of the pleural effusion (Fig. 16.13b), excluding the pericardial effusion (Fig. 16.13c), provided guidance for the man oeuvre of evacuative thoracentesis, allowed for the estimation of the expansion of the atelectatic lung during the thoracentesis and excluded the presence of pneumothorax at the end of thoracentesis. Lastly, the TUS was repeated twice per day for the next ten days in order to monitor pleural effusion and ventilation status of the pulmonary parenchyma.

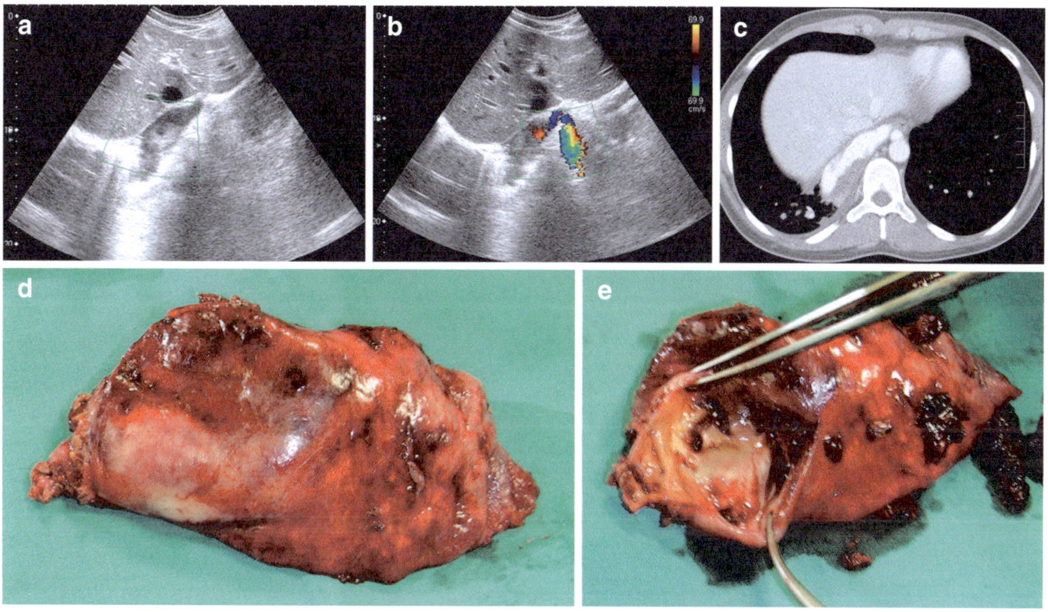

Fig. 16.12 (**a**, **b**) TUS; (**c**) CT; (**d**, **e**) surgical piece. (Reprinted with permission from Feletti et al. [16])

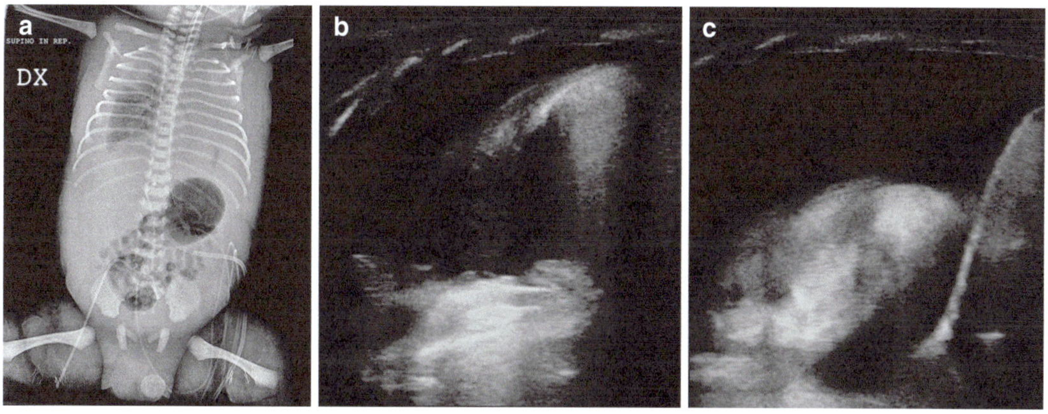

Fig. 16.13 (**a**) plain radiograpy; (**b**, **c**) TUS (Reprinted with permission from Feletti et al. [16])

16.14 Post-traumatic Hemato-Pneumatocele

An 11-year-old boy suffered blunt thoracic trauma as a consequence of a high energy road accident. Chest and computed tomography (CT) revealed multiple subpleural contusions, some coastal fractures, and a subpleural post-traumatic hemato-pneumatocele of the upper segment of the right lower lobe (Fig. 16.14a–d). TUS was used for the follow-up instead of radiology, allowing minimization of X-ray exposure.

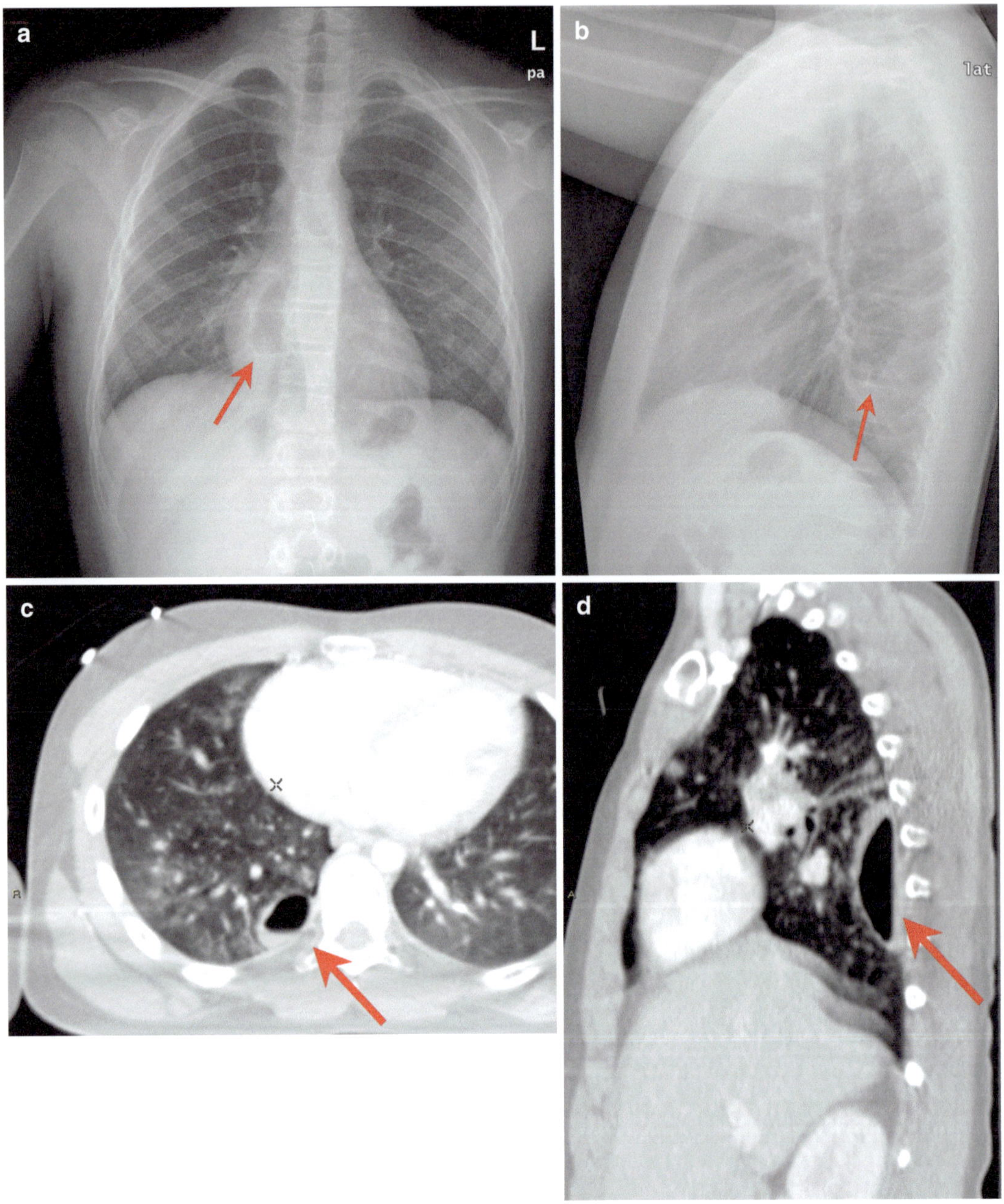

Fig. 16.14 Chest radiography (**a, b**); CT (**c**) axial view; (**d**) sagittal reconstruction; (**e**) B-Mode; (**f**) color doppler

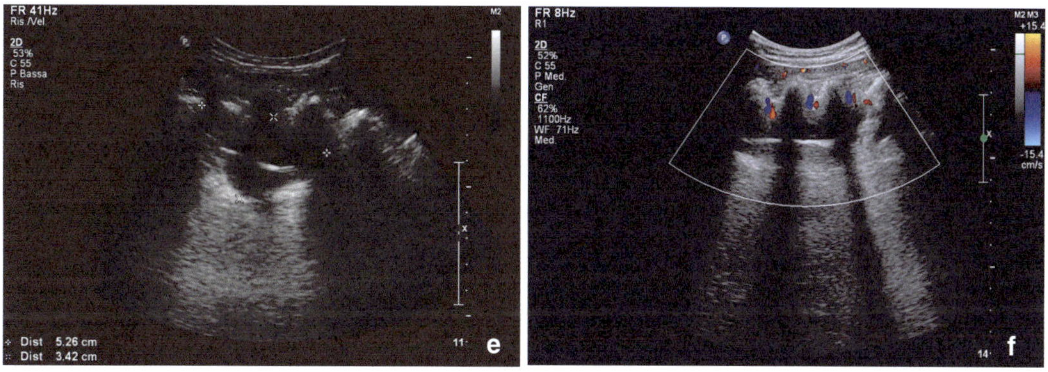

Fig. 16.14 (continued)

TUS showed an oval lesion with air-fluid level (Fig. 16.14e); the dimensions were 50 × 18 mm. After 1 week, the diameters of the lesion were increased reaching 63 × 32 mm. Color Doppler showed flow signals within the intercostal arteries (Fig. 16.14f).

Traumatic pneumatoceles occur primarily in young adults and children, with 85% of patients being younger than 30 years [17]. They generally result from non-penetrating chest trauma, often as a consequence of road accidents, or mechanical ventilation with positive airway pressure [18]. Chest X-ray has a sensitivity of 24% in diagnosing pneumatoceles, while CT gives a reported sensitivity of 96% [18–20]. Youths have a more compressible thoracic cage elastic recoil of the lungs than adults; these factors may result in increased negative intrathoracic pressure leading to laceration. The size of the cavity continues to increase until a balance is achieved between lung pressures and the surrounding tissues. Differential diagnosis should exclude congenital cysts, tuberculosis infection, post-pneumonia pneumatoceles, or cavitating pulmonary carcinoma and pulmonary abscess.

References

1. Lee RK, Griffith JF, Ng AW, Sitt JC. Sonography of the chest wall: a pictorial essay. J Clin Ultrasound. 2015;43:525–37. https://doi.org/10.1002/jcu.22286.
2. Maw AM, Hassanin A, Ho PM, McInnes MDF, Moss A, Juarez-Colunga E, Soni NJ, Miglioranza MH, Platz E, DeSanto K, Sertich AP, Salame G, Daugherty SL. Diagnostic accuracy of point-of-care lung ultrasonography and chest radiography in adults with symptoms suggestive of acute decompensated heart failure: a systematic review and meta-analysis. JAMA Netw Open. 2019;2(3):e190703. https://doi.org/10.1001/jamanetworkopen.2019.0703.
3. Ozdemir N, Ersu R, Akalin F, et al. Tracheobronchial calcification associated with Keutel syndrome. Turk J Pediatr. 2006;48(4):357–61.
4. Joshi A, Berdon WE, Ruzal-Shapiro C, Barst RJ. CT detection of tracheobronchial calcification in an 18-year-old on maintenance warfarin sodium therapy, cause and effect? AJR. 2000;175(3):921–2.
5. Mundinger GS, Weiss C, Fishman EK. Severe tracheobronchial stenosis and cervical vertebral subluxation in X-linked recessive chondrodysplasia punctata. Pediatr Radiol. 2009;39(6):625–8.
6. Simsek PO, Ozcelik U, Demirkazik F, et al. Tracheobronchopathia osteochondroplastica in a 9-year-old girl. Pediatr Pulmonol. 2006;41(1):95–7.

7. Fonseca AR, de Oliveira SK, Rodrigues MC, Aymoré IL, Domingues RC, Sztajnbok FR. Relapsing polychondritis in childhood: three case reports, comparison with adulthood disease and literature review. Rheumatol Int. 2013;33(7):1873–8.
8. Ceyhan M, Nural MS, Elmali M, Bayrak IK. Idiopathic isolated laryngotracheobronchial cartilage calcification in a child. Clin Imaging. 2008;32(1):51–3. https://doi.org/10.1016/j.clinimag.2007.04.026.
9. Lichtenstein D, Mézière G, Biderman P, et al. The comet-tail artifact an ultrasound sign of alveolar-interstitial syndrome. Am J Respir Crit Care Med. 1997;156:1640–6.
10. American Thoracic Society. Diagnosis and initial management of nonmalignant diseases related to asbestos. Am J Respir Crit Care Med. 2004;170:691–715.
11. Koh DM, Burke S, Davies N, Padley SP. Transthoracic US of the chest: clinical uses and applications. Radiographics. 2002;22(1):1.
12. Cugell DW, Kamp DW. Asbestos and the pleura. A review. Chest. 2004;125:1103–17.
13. Hosoda Y, Hiraga Y, Sasagawa S. Railways and asbestos in Japan (1928–1987)-epidemiology of pleural plaques, malignancies and pneumoconioses. J Occup Health. 2008;50(4):297–307.
14. Smargiassi A, Pasciuto G, Pedicelli I, Lo Greco E, Calvello M, Inchingolo R, Schifino G, Capoluongo P, Patriciello P, Manno M, Cirillo A, Corbo GM, Soldati G, Iavicoli I. Chest ultrasonography in health surveillance of asbestos-related lung diseases. Toxicol Ind Health. 2017;33(6):537–46. https://doi.org/10.1177/0748233716686916.
15. Feletti F, Mucci V, Aliverti A. Chest ultrasonography in modern day extreme settings: from military setting and natural disasters to space flights and extreme sports. Can Respir J. 2018;2018:8739704.
16. Feletti F, Gardelli G, Mughetti M. L'Ecografia toracica—Applicazioni ed imaging integrato. Modena: Athena; 2009. p. 140–71.
17. Yang T-C, Huang C-H, Yu J-W, Hsieh F-C, Huang Y-F. Traumatic pneumatocele. Pediatr Neonatol. 2010;51(2):135–8.
18. Matuszczak E, Oksiuta M, Hermanowicz A, Dębek W. Traumatic pneumatocele in an 11-year-old boy—report of a rare case and review of the literature. Pol J Cardiothorac Surg. 2017;1:59–62.
19. Cheung NK, James A, Kumar R. Large traumatic pneumatocele in a 2-year-old child. Case Rep Pediatr. 2013;2013:1–3.
20. Athanassiadi K, Kalavrouziotis G, Athanassiou M, Vernikos P, Skrekas G, Poultsidi A, Bellenis I. Blunt diaphragmatic rupture. Eur J Cardiothorac Surg. 1999;15(4):469–74.

MIX
Papier aus verantwortungsvollen Quellen
Paper from responsible sources
FSC® C105338

If you have any concerns about our products,
you can contact us on
ProductSafety@springernature.com

In case Publisher is established outside the EU,
the EU authorized representative is:
Springer Nature Customer Service Center GmbH
Europaplatz 3, 69115 Heidelberg, Germany

Printed by Libri Plureos GmbH
in Hamburg, Germany